WORKBOOK AND LABORATORY MANUAL for
Radiologic Science for
Technologists

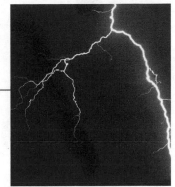

WORKBOOK AND LABORATORY MANUAL for
Radiologic Science for Technologists

NINTH EDITION

Stewart Carlyle Bushong,
ScD, FACR, FACMP
Professor of Radiologic
Science
Baylor College of
Medicine
Houston, Texas

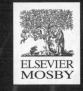

ELSEVIER
MOSBY

11830 Westline Industrial Drive
St. Louis, Missouri 63146

WORKBOOK AND LABORATORY MANUAL
FOR RADIOLOGIC SCIENCE FOR TECHNOLOGISTS   ISBN: 978-0-323-04838-5

Notice

International Standard Book Number 978-0-323-04838-5

Acquisitions Editor: Jeanne Wilke
Senior Developmental Editor: Rebecca Swisher
Book Production Manager: Linda McKinley
Project Manager: Stephen Bancroft
Designer: Julia Dummitt

Printed in the United States of America

Last digit is the print number: 9   8   7   6   5   4   3   2

Working together to grow
libraries in developing countries

www.elsevier.com | www.bookaid.org | www.sabre.org

ELSEVIER   BOOK AID International   Sabre Foundation

Contents

Preface

Readers familiar with Bushong's *Radiologic Science* will recognize the author's signature on this new edition of the *Workbook and Laboratory Manual*. Straightforward and fun, the workbook stimulates discussion while helping students review information and hone the skills necessary to become informed and competent radiologic technologists.

This edition retains the traditional way the previous editions have been divided into three parts: Worksheets, Math Tutor, and Experiments. The worksheets are organized by topic and numbered according to the textbook chapters. The worksheet numbers and descriptive titles make it easy to find worksheets to test specific topics or coordinate with the major concepts of a textbook chapter; they primarily contain multiple-choice questions that can be quickly graded and returned.

Each worksheet features "Penguins" to aid in the successful completion of the exercises. The penguin provides a concise summary of information that is relevant to the exercise questions. Lighthearted and to the point, Penguins make it easier than ever to review major textbook concepts.

The author wishes to thank the following reviewers for their valuable input: **Alberto Bello, Jr., RT, (R)(CV), MEd,** Oregon Institute of Technology; **Deb Schroth,** St. Anthony Hospitals; **Edmund Arozoo, EPA,** South Australia; **Mahadevappa Mahesh, PhD,** Johns Hopkins University; **Nancy Wardlow, MS,** Tyler Junior College; **Pamela Lee, MEd,** Tacoma Community College; **Richard Bayless, MEd,** University of Montana; **Rob Morrison,** Frank Barker Associates; **Steve Strickland, PhD,** Aiken Technical College; **Tim Gienapp, BS,** Apollo College.

As always, Mosby welcomes your comments about this book or any of our other imaging sciences publications.

The author especially appreciates your comments regarding any of the material in this volume, including specific questions, Penguins, Math Tutor, and Laboratory Experiments. Please email me at sbushong@bcm.tmc.edu so that together we can make this material even more instructive and "Physics even more Phun."

Stewart Carlyle Bushong

WORKSHEETS

Some representative radiation levels are as follows:

IN OUR DAILY LIVES

Living next to a nuclear power station	0.5 mrem/yr (5 μGy_t /yr)
Cross-country jet flight	2 mrem (20 μGy_t)
Fallout at the height of atomic weapons testing	5 mrem (50 μGyt)
Consumer products (e.g., smoke detectors, watch dials)	3 mrem/yr (30 μGy_t/yr)

NATURAL BACKGROUND

Sea level	100 mrem/yr (1 mGy_t/yr)
Mountains	500 mrem/yr (5 mGy_t/yr)

THE HEALING ARTS

^{99m}Tc thyroid image	10 mrad (100 μGy_t)
Genetically significant dose (GSD)	20 mrad (200 μGy_t)
Mean marrow dose Entrance skin exposure (ESE)	100 mrad (1 mGy_t)
Posterior-anterior (PA) chest examination	10 mR (100 μGy_a)
Panoramic dental x-ray	200 mR (2 mGy_a)
Lumbar spine examination	1000 mR (10 mGy_a/min)
Fluoroscopic examination	4000 mR/min (40 mGy_a/min)

COMPUTED TOMOGRAPHY

Head examination	4000 mrad (40 mGyt)
Body examination	2000 mrad (20 mGyt)

OCCUPATIONAL DOSE LIMIT

Radiographer	5000 mrem/yr (50 mSv/yr)
Public	100 mrem/yr (1 mSv/yr)

EXERCISES

1. Which of the following items is considered to be matter?
   a. Airport surveillance x-rays
   b. Anode heat
   c. Cell phone signals
   d. Light from a movie projector
   e. Wet snow

2. Which of the following is the principal difference between mass and weight?
   a. Mass is measured in pounds (lb); weight is measured in kilograms (kg).
   b. Mass is the equivalence of energy; weight is the force exerted by gravity.
   c. There is no difference; mass and weight are equal.
   d. Weight does not change with position; mass does.
   e. Weight is energy; mass requires gravity.

3. *Energy* is defined as:
   a. A force exerted by a body
   b. Anything that occupies space and has shape
   c. The ability to do work
   d. The degree of gravity
   e. The quantity of matter

4. Which of the following examples *best* represents energy?
   a. A snowman
   b. A thrown snowball
   c. Anode mass

d. The metal plates in a battery
e. The terminals of a battery

5. Which of the following is an example of potential energy?
   a. A heated anode
   b. A mobile x-ray imaging system in motion
   c. An x-ray beam
   d. An x-ray imaging system
   e. Visible light

6. In Einstein's famous $E = mc^2$ equation, c stands for which of the following?
   a. Acceleration of mass
   b. Force
   c. Mass-energy equivalence
   d. The speed of light
   e. The theory of relativity

7. Radiation is:
   a. Energy transferred
   b. Isotropic emission
   c. Kinetic particles
   d. Mass with a charge
   e. Measured in joules

8. The roentgen relates to which of the following?
   a. A dose equivalent
   b. A radiation-absorbed dose
   c. Ions produced in the air
   d. Isotropic emission
   e. Non-ionizing radiation

9. Which of the following is an example of electromagnetic radiation?
   a. Alpha radiation
   b. Beta rays
   c. Sound
   d. Ultrasound
   e. Visible light

10. When ionization occurs, which of the following is *true?*
    a. The negative ion is electromagnetic radiation.
    b. The negative ion is the ion pair.
    c. The negative ion is the target atom.
    d. The positive ion is electromagnetic.
    e. The positive ion is the resulting atom.

11. X-rays are *most* like:
    a. Alpha rays
    b. Beta rays
    c. Diagnostic ultrasound
    d. Gamma rays

e. Radio waves

12. Which of the following is the largest source of human exposure to man-made radiation?
    a. Cosmic rays
    b. Medical diagnostic x-rays
    c. Nuclear power–generating stations
    d. Radioactive fallout
    e. Radioactive materials in consumer products

13. What is the approximate annual effective dose from natural environmental radiation at sea level?
    a. 5 mrem/yr (50 μSv/yr)
    b. 10 mrem/yr (100 μSv/yr)
    c. 50 mrem/yr (500 μSv/yr)
    d. 100 mrem/yr (1 mSv/yr)
    e. 500 mrem/yr (5 mSv/yr)

14. Which of the following results in the highest annual radiation dose?
    a. Cosmic rays
    b. Diagnostic x-rays
    c. Nuclear power
    d. Radiation from inside the earth

15. Which of the following contributes more than 50 mrad per year to each of us?
    a. Consumer Products
    b. Medical Imaging
    c. Microwave oven radiation
    d. Radioactive fallout
    e. Radioisotopes in nuclear medicine

16. The rad is related *most* closely to which of the following?
    a. Dose equivalent
    b. Radiation exposure
    c. The gray
    d. The joule
    e. The sievert

17. Which of the following is ionizing electromagnetic radiation?
    a. Beta rays
    b. Gamma rays
    c. Microwaves
    d. Radio waves
    e. Ultrasound

18. Which of the following is a unit of mass?
    a. Joule
    b. Kilogram
    c. mrad
    d. Pound
    e. Volt

WORKSHEET 1-2

Discovery of X-Rays
Development of Modern Radiology

 • X-rays were discovered in 1895 by Roentgen.
- The cadmium tungstate ($CdWO_4$) radiographic intensifying screen was developed by Edison and was first used in 1898.
- Clarence Dally, who was an assistant to Edison, died of radiation injuries in 1904.
- In 1913, Coolidge developed the modern heated filament x-ray tube.
- The National Council on Radiation Protection (NCRP) reduced the occupational dose limit to 5000 mrem/yr in 1957.
- The image-intensifier tube became available in the early 1960s.
- Diagnostic ultrasonography was introduced in the early 1960s.
- Computed tomography appeared in 1972.
- Magnetic resonance imaging was introduced for clinical use in 1980.
- The first federal imaging regulation—the Mammography Quality Standards Act (MQSA)—was passed in 1992.
- The first all-digital department of radiology (Baltimore Veterans Affairs Medical Center [VAMC]) opened in 1993.
- Solid-state digital image receptors were introduced in 1996.
- The Radiological Society of North America (RSNA) presented the first annual showing of Integrating the Healthcare Environment (IHE) in 1997.
- Multislice spiral computed tomography appeared in 1998.
- Digital mammography was approved by the U.S. Food and Drug Administration (FDA) in 2000.

- Positron emission tomography (PET) assumed a role in clinical practice in 2002.
- Sixteen-slice computed tomography was offered in 2003.

EXERCISES

1. What was the device with which Roentgen discovered x-rays?
   a. Anode tube
   b. Coolidge tube
   c. Crookes tube
   d. Geissler tube
   e. Snook interrupterless transformer

2. The phosphor that Roentgen used in early experiments with x-rays was which of the following?
   a. Barium platinocyanide
   b. Cadmium tungstate
   c. Calcium tungstate
   d. Rare Earth
   e. Zinc cadmium sulfide

3. How are x-ray tube voltages measured?
   a. Kilovolt
   b. Megavolt
   c. Microvolt
   d. Millivolt
   e. Volt

4. Which of the following early pioneers developed the fluoroscope?
   a. Alexander G. Bell
   b. J.J. Thomson
   c. Thomas Edison

d. Wilhelm Roentgen
e. William Crookes

5. Who first applied x-ray beam collimation and filtration in medical imaging?
   a. Wilhelm Roentgen
   b. William Coolidge
   c. William Crookes
   d. William Longfellow
   e. William Rollins

6. Which of the following is the type of x-ray tube that is used today?
   a. Coolidge tube
   b. Crookes tube
   c. Geissler tube
   d. Leonard tube
   e. Snook tube

7. The Bucky grid, which was introduced in 1921, does what?
   a. Improves image contrast
   b. Improves spatial resolution
   c. Provides x-ray collimation
   d. Reduces examination time
   e. Reduces patient exposure

8. Which of the following regarding x-ray–induced death is *true?*
   a. Clarence Dally was the first American to die because of x-ray exposure.
   b. No medical radiation deaths have occurred.
   c. Radiology has always been considered a completely safe occupation.
   d. The first x-ray–induced death did not occur until approximately 1920.
   e. The first x-ray–induced death occurred within a year of Roentgen's discovery.

9. Which of the following describes the Coolidge x-ray tube?
   a. It has a heated cathode.
   b. It has a rotating anode.
   c. It is not as good as the Crookes tube.
   d. It is not in use today.
   e. It was used by Roentgen shortly after he discovered x-rays.

10. Roentgen originally identified x-rays as which of the following?
    a. Alpha rays
    b. Cathode rays
    c. Electrons

d. X-heat
e. X-light

11. What are the two simple, general types of x-ray imaging procedures?
    a. Digital and analog
    b. Electromagnetic and ultrasonic
    c. Radiographic and fluoroscopic
    d. Radiographic and tomographic
    e. Roentgenographic and ultrasonic

12. Which of the following provides dynamic x-ray images?
    a. Digital radiography
    b. Doppler ultrasonography
    c. Fluoroscopy
    d. Mammography
    e. Tomography

13. The film base for a radiograph made in 1920 would have been made of which of the following?
    a. Calcium tungstate
    b. Cellulose acetate
    c. Cellulose nitrate
    d. Glass
    e. Tungstate cadmium

14. Collimation and filtration do which of the following?
    a. Compromise image quality
    b. Improve spatial resolution
    c. Reduce exposure time
    d. Reduce patient dose
    e. Result in patient discomfort

15. Which of the following imaging modalities was developed *most* recently?
    a. Computed tomography
    b. Diagnostic ultrasound
    c. Direct digital radiography
    d. Magnetic resonance
    e. Multislice spiral CT

16. Which of the following radiation responses was *not* reported before 1910?
    a. Aplastic anemia
    b. Death
    c. Epilation
    d. Leukemia
    e. Skin erythema

Reports of Radiation Injury
Basic Radiation Protection
The Diagnostic Imaging Team

- Radiology is a safe occupation.
- The principal concerns of medical x-ray exposure are cancer and leukemia.
- The occupational dose limit for radiologic technologists is 5000 mrem/yr (50 mSv/yr).
- Remember the principle of *ALARA:* Maintain radiation exposure *as low as reasonably achievable.*
- The three cardinal principles of radiation protection are as follows: (1) reduce time, (2) increase distance, and (3) use shielding where appropriate.
- Radiologic technologists must be American Registry of Radiologic Technologists (ARRT) certified; medical physicists must be American Board of Medical Physics (ABMP) or American Board of Radiology (ABR) certified; interpreting physicians should be ABR certified.

EXERCISES

1. One of the cardinal principles of radiation protection states that the radiologic technologist should minimize which of the following?
   a. Distance
   b. kVp
   c. mAs
   d. Shielding
   e. Time

2. Which of the following is *not* included in the 10 basic radiation control principles of diagnostic radiology?
   a. Always wear a radiation monitor while at work.
   b. Collimate the x-ray beam to the smallest approximate field size.

c. Use high-kVp technique.
d. Use high-mA technique.
e. Wear protective apparel during fluoroscopy.

3. If it is necessary to immobilize a patient during a radiographic examination, the *most* acceptable person to do this is a/an:
   a. 18-year-old brother of the patient
   b. 20-year-old female technologist
   c. 40-year-old male technologist
   d. 50-year-old female friend of the patient
   e. Hospital orderly

4. Which of the following is correctly stated for diagnostic radiology?
   a. Collimation is important only for chest examination.
   b. Copper is used most often as an x-ray filter.
   c. Gonad shields are as important for a 50-year-old woman as for a 20-year-old woman.
   d. The radiologic technologist may hold patients for routine examinations.
   e. Radiographic intensifying screens reduce patient dose.

5. Which of the following will reduce personnel exposure the *most?*
   a. Collimation of the x-ray beam
   b. Filtration of the x-ray beam
   c. Recording of fluoroscopy time
   d. A high-kVp technique
   e. Use of protective barriers for radiologic technologists

6. When abdominal radiography is conducted on a child, which of the following is *true*?
   a. Gonad shielding is not necessary.
   b. Increasing kVp will increase contrast.
   c. The parent should hold the child if necessary, and protective apparel should be provided.
   d. The parent should hold the child if necessary, and protective apparel is not necessary.
   e. The technologist should hold the child if necessary.

7. All *except* which of the following help to reduce patient dose?
   a. Cones
   b. Filtration
   c. Gonad shields
   d. Grids
   e. Intensifying screens

8. After termination of an x-ray exposure:
   a. No more x-rays are emitted.
   b. The patient continues to emit scatter radiation for a few seconds.
   c. The patient continues to emit scatter radiation for less than 1 s.
   d. The patient is momentarily radioactive.
   e. X-rays continue to be emitted for a few seconds.

9. During fluoroscopy, what should the radiologic technologist always do?
   a. Leave the radiation monitor behind the fixed protective barrier.
   b. Position the radiation monitor under the protective apron.
   c. Remain as close to the patient as possible.
   d. Wear a radiation monitor when examined as a patient.
   e. Wear protective apparel.

10. The main reason for filtering the x-ray beam is to:
    a. Absorb heat.
    b. Absorb penetrating radiation.
    c. Focus the beam.
    d. Reduce patient dose.
    e. Sharpen the image.

11. Which of the following represents implementation of a radiation protection procedure?
    a. Avoid repeat examination.
    b. Collimate to the film size.
    c. Monitor processor performance.
    d. Remove filtration.
    e. Wear protective apparel at the control console.

12. Which of the following is an example of an x-ray beam collimator?
    a. Dead-man switch
    b. Elapsed timer
    c. Filter
    d. Grid
    e. Positive-beam limitation (PBL)

13. X-ray examination of the pelvis of a woman of reproductive capacity should be limited to which of the following times?
    a. The 10-day interval after onset of menses
    b. The 10-day interval before onset of menses
    c. The first 10 days of every month
    d. The last 10 days of every month
    e. There are no restrictions; any time is fine.

14. Which of the following is *true* regarding the discovery of ionizing radiation?
    a. It was predicted by Mendeleev's Field Theory.
    b. Radioactivity was discovered within a year of Roentgen's discovery.
    c. Roentgen's discovery occurred in 1906.
    d. The apparatus that Roentgen used was called a *Coolidge tube*.
    e. The first radiation fatality occurred in 1920.

15. Generally, x-ray examinations are reserved for which of the following?
    a. Asymptomatic patients
    b. Older patients
    c. Patients who are not pregnant
    d. Symptomatic patients
    e. X-ray personnel

16. Gonad shields should be used:
    a. For all examinations of all patients
    b. On all female patients
    c. On all male patients
    d. When the gonads are in or near the useful beam
    e. When the gonads are in the useful beam

17. Which of the following is the principal reason to avoid repeat examination?
    a. The cost of the procedure is doubled.
    b. The images may be confused.
    c. The patient is inconvenienced.
    d. The patient receives twice the radiation dose.
    e. The technologist's workload is doubled.

WORKSHEET

2-1 Mathematics for Radiologic Science

- A **ratio** is the comparison of one number to another and is expressed as a **quotient** or **fraction.**
- A **proportion** relates the quantity of two or more ratios.
- **Rounding off to significance** is the procedure of reducing a complex number to a simpler number. To do this, drop the last digit of a number and raise the next-to-last digit by 1 if the last digit is 5 or greater.
- Power-of-10 notation is a scientific method used for writing very large or very small numbers. The method makes these types of numbers easy to manipulate. Numbers in power-of-ten notation can be multiplied, divided, or raised by powers of 10 according to the following rules:

$$10^x \times 10^y = 10^{x+y}$$

Numbers in power-of-10 notation are added or subtracted rarely, but when they are, the value of all the exponents must be the same.

EXERCISES

Perform the indicated operations.

ARITHMETIC

1. 649 + 88 = 737
2. 38,246 + 721 + 193,405 + 5,227 + 81,491 = 319,090
3. 69,525 − 2,820 = 66,705
4. 9413 × 4 = 37,652
5. 432.71 + 19,878 + 1,000.092 = 21,310.802
6. 419,307 − 67,227 = 352080
7. 62.58 × 0.043 = 2.69094
8. 200 × 0.05 = 10
9. 421.25 ÷ 0.31 = 1358.9
10. 360 ÷ 3.1416 = 114.5913

FRACTIONS

11. $\frac{1}{2} + \frac{2}{8} =$ 6/8 = 3/4
12. $\frac{3}{8} + \frac{5}{16} =$ 11/16
13. $\frac{1}{2} + \frac{1}{4} =$ 3/4
14. $\frac{3}{8} - \frac{3}{16} =$ 3/16
15. $\frac{3}{5} - \frac{9}{4} =$ −3 3/20
16. $\frac{3}{8} + \frac{19}{16} + \frac{7}{32} =$ 57/32 = 1 25/32
17. $\frac{15}{32} \times 1\frac{1}{3} =$ 60/96 = 5/8
18. $6\frac{7}{8} \times 2\frac{11}{16} =$ 2365/128
19. $\frac{1}{2} \div \frac{1}{3} =$ 1/2 × 3/1 = 3/2 or 1 1/2
20. $\frac{12}{9} \div \frac{2}{3} =$ 12/9 × 3/2 = 36/18 = 2

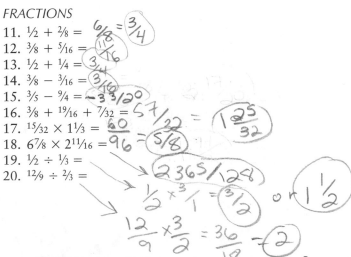

SIGNIFICANT FIGURES

21. 70.05
    6.85
    100.003
    +12.1
    189.0

22. 6.254
    −1.04
    5.21

23. 3.1416
    ×30
    94.25

24. 8.05
    ×0.693
    5.58

25. $6.02 \div 2.567 =$ *2.35*

ALGEBRA

26. $13a = 126$; $a =$ *$\frac{126}{13} = 9.7$*
27. $168 + b = 42$; $b =$ *$42 - 168 = -126$*
28. $\%_5 = \frac{3}{8}$; $c =$ *$5(\frac{3}{8}) = 1\frac{5}{8}$*
29. $3 - \frac{3}{8} + \frac{3}{4} = 16$; $x =$
30. $1\frac{3}{8} + 3x = (\frac{1}{4})2$; $x =$
31. What is the ratio of 100 mAs to 400 mAs?

32. $\dfrac{x}{8 \text{ mR}} = \dfrac{300 \text{ mAs;}}{400 \text{ mAs}}$ $x =$

33. $\dfrac{75 \text{ kVp}}{80 \text{ kVp}} = \dfrac{210 \text{ mAs;}}{x}$ $x =$

34. $\frac{3}{4} \times 500$ mAs =

35. $\dfrac{150 \text{ mR}}{50 \text{ mR}} = \dfrac{600 \text{ mAs;}}{x}$ $x =$

36. If $12x = 420$ mAs, then $x =$
37. Given $a = bc$, if $a = 189$, $b = 27$, then $c =$
38. A radiographic unit emits 3.7 mR/mAs at 80 kVp. If a given technique requires 120 mAs, what will be the entrance skin exposure (ESE)?
    a. 267 mR
    b. 444 mR
    c. 610 mR
    d. 756 mR
    e. 891 mR

39. The radiographic output intensity is 4.3 mR/mAs. If a given technique is 200 mA, 1/60 s, what will be the exposure?
    a. 3.3 mR
    b. 14.3 mR

    c. 17.6 mR
    d. 26.8 mR
    e. 41.1 mR

Convert each to power-of-10 notation.
40. 2741.92
41. 9,174,843
42. 7713

Convert each to power-of-10 notation and perform the indicated operations.

43. 176
    +382

44. 931.45
    −36.63

45. 37,000
    +617

46. $3.2 \times 48.6 \times 10^{-5} =$

47. $(80{,}071)(157) =$

48. $\dfrac{921}{3705}$

49. $(10^5)^4 =$

50. $\dfrac{10 \times 10^3 \times 10^{-2} \times 10^5}{10^2 \times 10^{-4}} =$

51. $\dfrac{(10^{-18})^2 \times (10^7)^3}{10} =$

52. $(2.5 \times 10^{-10}) \times (1.2 \times 10^{18}) =$

Compute the following.
53. An iodine atom has a diameter of 4×10^{-10} m. A 60 keV x-ray has a wavelength of 2×10^{-11} m. What is the ratio of the atomic diameter to the x-ray wavelength?

54. There are 6.02×10^{23} atoms in 131 g of ^{131}I. What is the mass of one atom of ^{131}I?

55. The nucleus of a barium atom is approximately 10^{-15} m in diameter. The atom itself is approximately 10^{-10} m in diameter. What is the ratio of the diameter of the atom to the diameter of the nucleus?

WORKSHEET

2-2

Milliampere-Second Conversions

When a radiographic technique is selected, the milliamperage (mA) and the exposure time(s) are multiplied together to produce the total **milliampere-seconds (mAs)**. The total mAs value is very important because it directly relates to how light or how dark the radiographic image will be; this is also called **optical density (OD)**. Neither the exposure time nor the mA can be considered alone in controlling the OD of the resulting image:

$$mA \times s = mAs$$

Further, mAs is actually nothing more than the total number of cathode-to-anode electrons during the exposure:

$$mAs = mA \times s = mC/s \times s = mC$$

where mC = millicoulomb

$$1 \text{ mC} = 1.6 \times 10^{18} \text{ electrons}$$

EXERCISES

Compute the following total mAs values. To benefit from this exercise, do not figure your calculations on paper; do them mentally, then write your answers. For additional help with math technique, turn to the "Math Tutor" section of this workbook, page ???.

PART I: DECIMAL/FRACTION CONVERSIONS

FRACTION	=	DECIMAL
1. $\frac{1}{5}$	=	_____
2. $\frac{1}{20}$	=	_____
3. $\frac{1}{8}$	=	_____
4. $\frac{1}{60}$	=	_____
5. $\frac{1}{15}$	=	_____

6. $\frac{1}{40}$	=	_____
7. $\frac{1}{120}$	=	_____
8. $\frac{2}{3}$	=	_____
9. $\frac{1}{30}$	=	_____
10. $\frac{2}{5}$	=	_____
11. $\frac{3}{20}$	=	_____
12. $\frac{2}{15}$	=	_____
13. $\frac{7}{10}$	=	_____
14. $\frac{3}{5}$	=	_____
15. $\frac{7}{20}$	=	_____

DECIMAL	=	FRACTION
16. 0.05	=	_____
17. 0.333	=	_____
18. 0.0125	=	_____
19. 0.02	=	_____
20. 0.4	=	_____
21. 0.0167	=	_____
22. 0.025	=	_____
23. 0.143	=	_____
24. 0.75	=	_____
25. 0.0833	=	_____
26. 0.0667	=	_____
27. 0.8	=	_____

PART II: DECIMAL TIMES

$$mA \times TIME(S) = mAs$$

28. 100 @ 0.07	=	_____
29. 100 @ 0.013	=	_____
30. 100 @ 0.033	=	_____
31. 100 @ 0.25	=	_____
32. 100 @ 0.009	=	_____
33. 200 @ 0.04	=	_____
34. 200 @ 0.07	=	_____

35. 200 @ 0.025 = _____
36. 200 @ 0.035 = _____
37. 200 @ 0.35 = _____
38. 200 @ 0.12 = _____
39. 200 @ 0.2 = _____
40. 200 @ 0.6 = _____
41. 200 @ 0.005 = _____
42. 300 @ 0.01 = _____
43. 300 @ 0.08 = _____
44. 300 @ 0.05 = _____
45. 300 @ 0.5 = _____
46. 300 @ 0.2 = _____
47. 300 @ 0.16 = _____
48. 300 @ 0.33 = _____
49. 300 @ 0.033 = _____
50. 300 @ 0.015 = _____
51. 300 @ 0.002 = _____
52. 400 @ 0.08 = _____
53. 400 @ 0.03 = _____
54. 400 @ 0.035 = _____
55. 400 @ 0.2 = _____
56. 400 @ 0.35 = _____
57. 400 @ 0.002 = _____
58. 500 @ 0.07 = _____
59. 500 @ 0.04 = _____
60. 500 @ 0.4 = _____
61. 500 @ 0.004 = _____
62. 500 @ 0.005 = _____
63. 600 @ 0.5 = _____
64. 600 @ 0.02 = _____
65. 600 @ 0.15 = _____
66. 600 @ 0.003 = _____
67. 600 @ 0.125 = _____

PART III: FRACTIONAL TIMES

$$mA \times TIME(S) = mAs$$

68. 100 @ 1/8 = _____
69. 100 @ 1/120 = _____
70. 100 @ 1/15 = _____
71. 100 @ 1/40 = _____

72. 100 @ 1/6 = _____
73. 50 @ 1/20 = _____
74. 50 @ 1/120 = _____
75. 50 @ 1/80 = _____
76. 200 @ 1/80 = _____
77. 200 @ 1/12 = _____
78. 200 @ 1/15 = _____
79. 200 @ 1/40 = _____
80. 200 @ 1/30 = _____
81. 200 @ 1/6 = _____
82. 300 @ 1/5 = _____
83. 300 @ 1/60 = _____
84. 300 @ 1/15 = _____
85. 300 @ 1/120 = _____
86. 400 @ 1/20 = _____
87. 400 @ 1/80 = _____
88. 400 @ 1/60 = _____
89. 500 @ 1/12 = _____
90. 500 @ 1/15 = _____
91. 500 @ 1/20 = _____
92. 600 @ 1/40 = _____
93. 600 @ 1/30 = _____
94. 600 @ 1/120 = _____
95. 600 @ 1/25 = _____
96. 600 @ 1/5 = _____
97. 100 @ 2/15 = _____
98. 100 @ 7/20 = _____
99. 200 @ 4/5 = _____
100. 200 @ 3/10 = _____
101. 300 @ 4/5 = _____
102. 300 @ 2/15 = _____
103. 300 @ 3/10 = _____
104. 400 @ 3/5 = _____
105. 400 @ 3/20 = _____
106. 500 @ 3/20 = _____
107. 600 @ 3/20 = _____

- A linear scale has equal value for equal length.
- A logarithmic (log) scale is used when the range of numbers is wide.

- Equal lengths on a log scale have equal ratio, which is determined by the logarithmic increment.
- An order of magnitude is 1 to 10, 10 to 100, 100 to 1000, and so on.

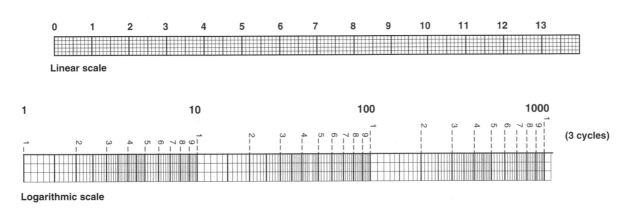

Linear scale

Logarithmic scale

(3 cycles)

EXERCISES

Locate the number indicated at the left on each side of the adjacent scales.

1. 0.493

2. −0.8

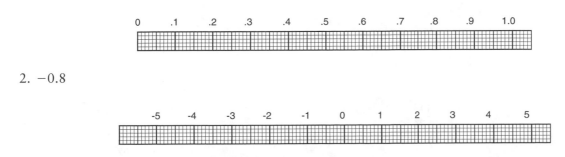

3. 3.6

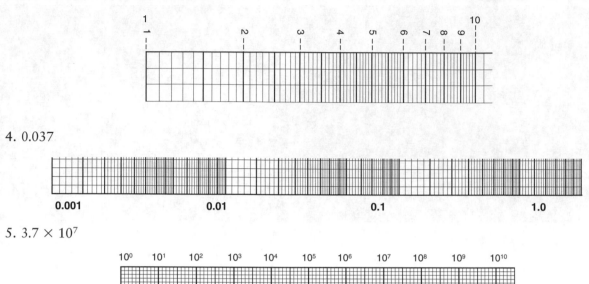

4. 0.037

5. 3.7×10^7

Plot each of the following sets of data on the linear-linear grid and on the linear-log (semilog) graph paper provided on pages 16 through 19 in this workbook.

6. A very small change in filament current results in a very large change in x-ray tube current. A special high-intensity x-ray tube design is being tested, and the following data are obtained:

X-RAY TUBE

FILAMENT CURRENT, A	CURRENT, mA
5.2	25
5.7	50
6.2	100
6.7	200
7.1	300
7.6	500
7.9	700
8.1	900
8.4	1200

7. An x-ray beam is measured to determine the necessary shielding for the walls of a radiographic room. The following data are obtained:

SHIELDING THICKNESS, mm LEAD	RADIATION INTENSITY, mR
0.0	1650
0.1	1236
0.2	995
0.4	661
0.8	343
1.2	174
1.5	129

8. Radioactive ^{131}I has a half-life of 8 days. An unknown quantity is analyzed today (t 0 days) and results in 9860 counts per minute (c/min). If analysis of this sample continues at 10-day intervals, the data might appear as follows:

TIME, DAYS	ACTIVITY, c/min
0	9860
10	4146
20	1744
30	733
40	308
50	130
60	55
70	23
80	10

9. This graph shows the relative intensity and color of light emitted by different types of radiographic intensifying screens when they are exposed to x-rays. Most of the light emitted by the fluorescent screen is of what color?
   a. Blue
   b. Green
   c. Red
   d. Ultraviolet
   e. Yellow

10. This graph shows how increasing exposure to radiation results in shorter periods of time before death. Which type of death occurs at a fixed time after a large radiation dose range?
   a. Central nervous system
   b. Gastrointestinal
   c. Hematologic
   d. Nonlethal
   e. Prodromal

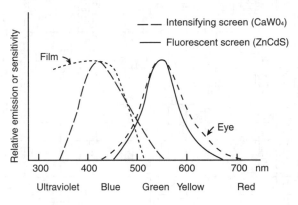

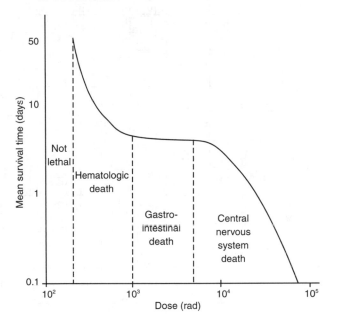

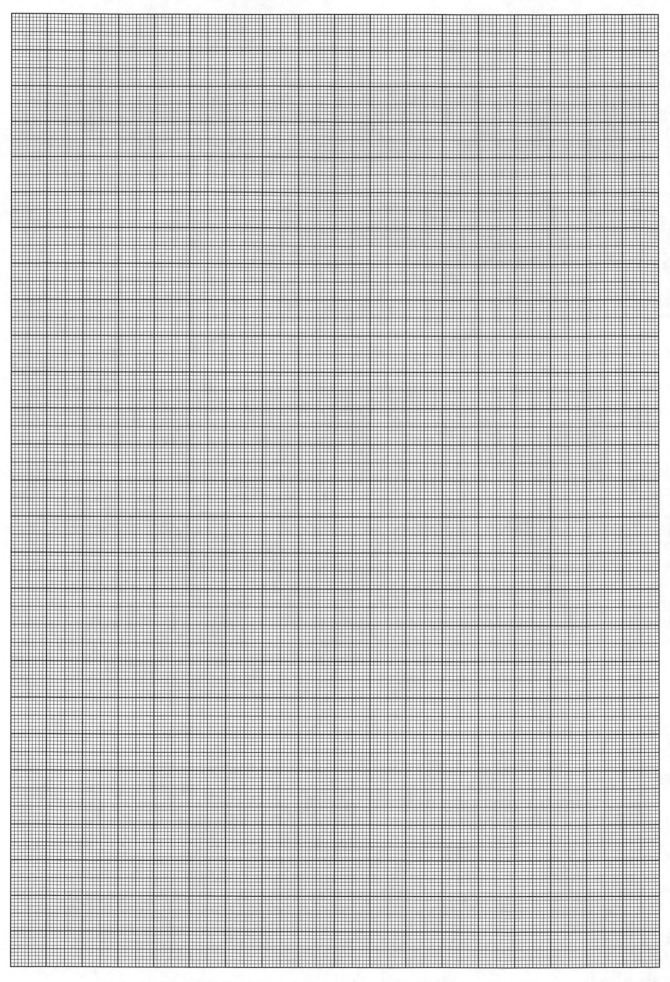

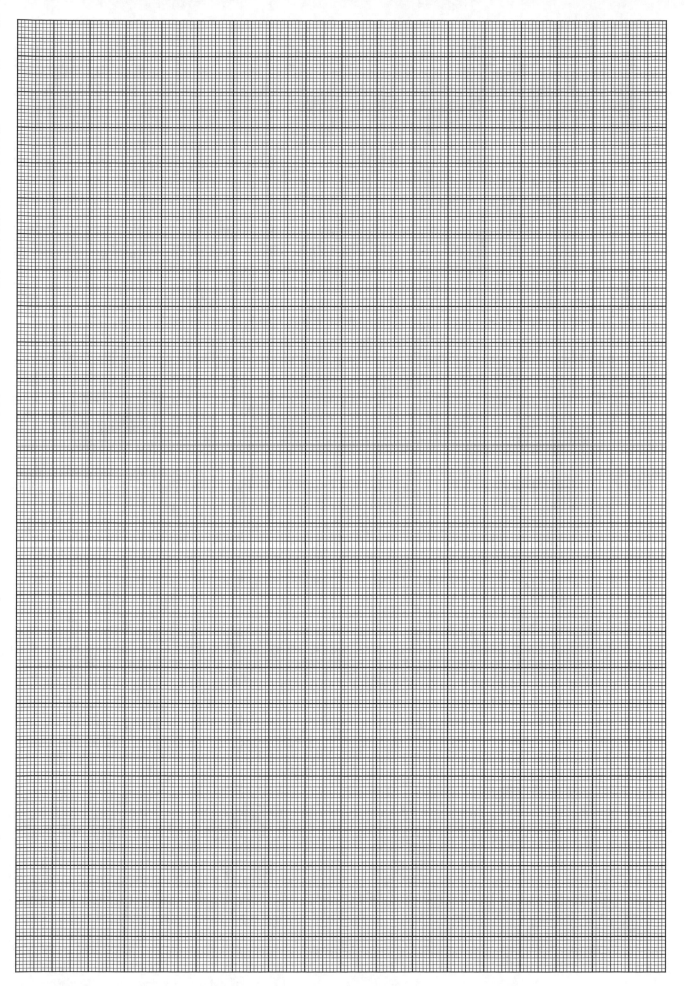

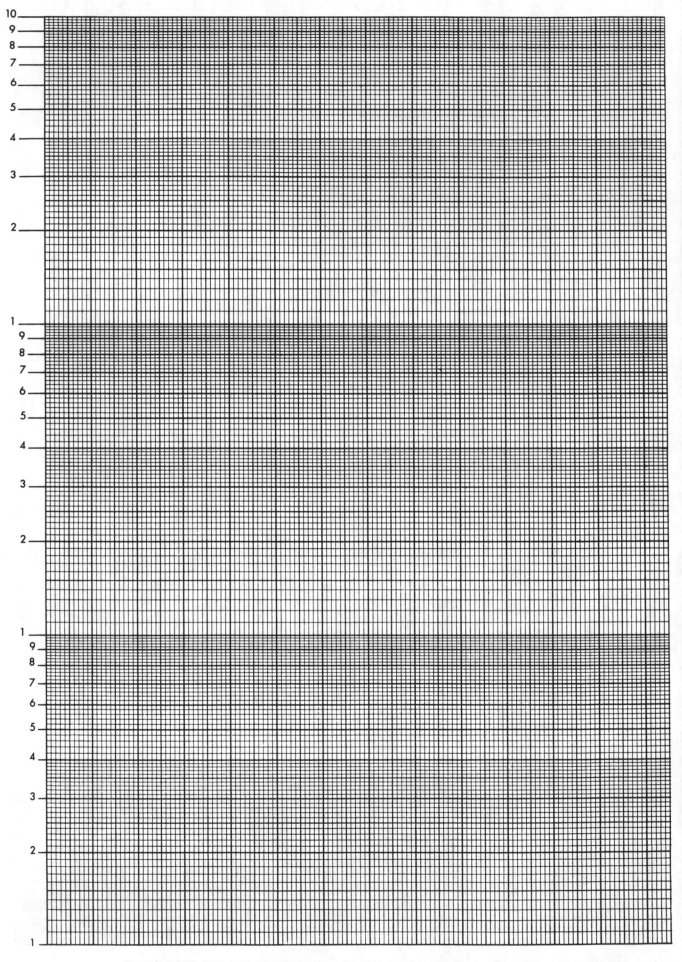

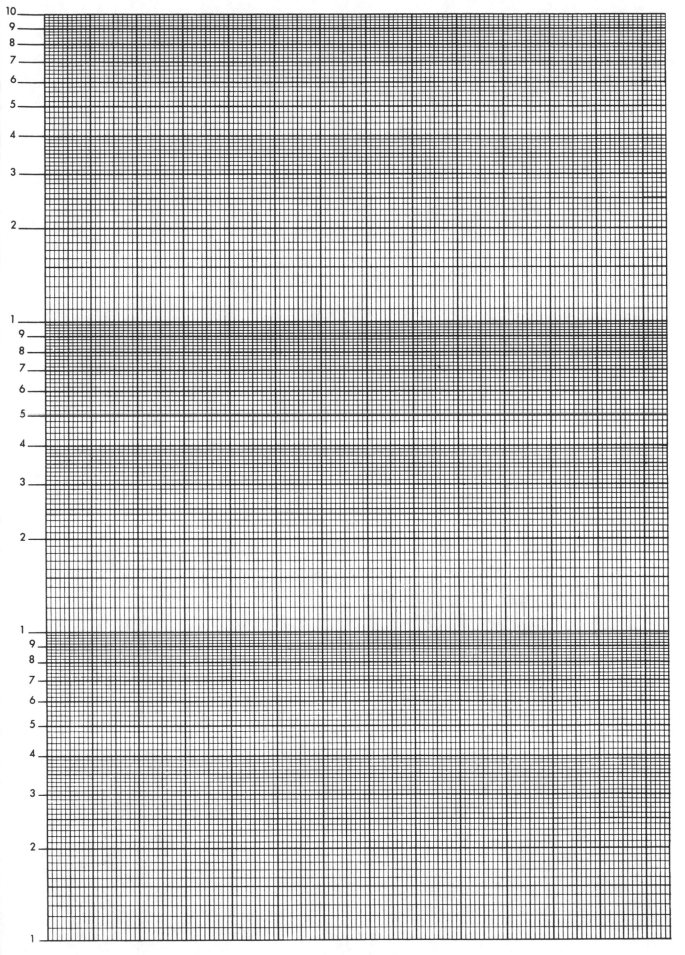

11. This graph shows the relationship between the amount of exposure received by two films and resultant optical densities. At log relative exposure (LRE) less than 1.5, what can be concluded about optical density (OD)?
   a. Film A will have higher OD (darker).
   b. Film B will have higher OD (darker).
   c. The OD is constant for both.
   d. The graph does not give enough information.
   e. The films have equal OD.

13. This graph shows how frequently two types of x-ray interactions (Compton and photoelectric) occur in bone and in soft tissue at different x-ray energies. In soft tissue, at approximately what x-ray energy is the probability the same for Compton interaction and photoelectric interaction?
   a. 10 keV
   b. 20 keV
   c. 40 keV
   d. 60 keV
   e. 90 keV

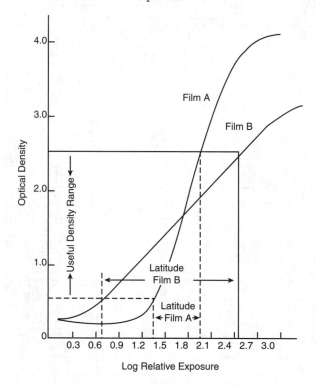

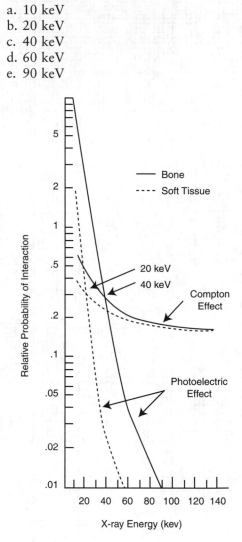

12. Review this graph again. In the "straight line" portion of the two curves, which film is getting dark (higher OD) faster?
   a. Film A
   b. Film B
   c. The OD is constant for both.
   d. The graph does not give enough information.
   e. The films are getting dark equally as quickly.

14. At 70 keV in soft tissue:
    a. Compton interaction occurs more often than photoelectric.
    b. Compton interactions no longer occur.
    c. Photoelectric interaction is equal to Compton.
    d. Photoelectric interaction is more frequent than it is at 50 keV.
    e. Photoelectric interaction occurs more often than Compton.

15. The graph below shows how many x-rays are produced at each energy when two different kVp values are used. At 70 keV, x-rays are:
    a. Absent from both beams
    b. More intense in the A beam
    c. More intense in the B beam
    d. About equal in the two beams
    e. The graph does not give enough information

16. On review of the same graph, the average x-ray energy (keV):
    a. Changes with energy range
    b. Is about equal for both beams
    c. Is higher for the A beam than for the B beam
    d. Is higher for the B beam than for the A beam
    e. The graph does not give enough information

17. Review the same graph. Which of the following statements is *true*?
    a. The two beams are equally collimated.
    b. The two beams are produced with the same mAs.
    c. The A beam was produced at a higher kVp.
    d. The B beam was produced at a higher kVp.
    e. There is more filtration with the same mAs.

18. Review the same graph. At approximately what energy is x-ray emission the greatest?
    a. 25 keV, beam A
    b. 35 keV, beam B
    c. 70 keV, both beams
    d. 72 keV, beam A
    e. 80 keV, beam B

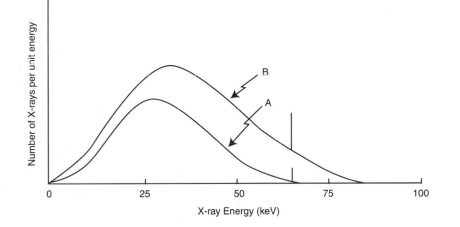

WORKSHEET
2-4

Numeric Prefixes

 The numeric prefixes most often encountered in radiology are as follows:

MULTIPLE	PREFIX	SYMBOL
10^{-12}	pico-	p
10^{-9}	nano-	n
10^{-6}	micro-	μ
10^{-3}	milli-	m
10^{-2}	centi-	c
10^{3}	kilo-	k
10^{6}	mega-	M
10^{9}	giga-	G
10^{12}	tera-	T

EXERCISES

1. 10 kilometers (km) is equivalent to:
   a. 100 m
   b. 1000 m
   c. 10,000 m
   d. 100,000 m
   e. 1,000,000 m

2. A radiographic exposure that lasts $\frac{1}{10}$ s is equivalent to:
   a. 100 μs
   b. 1 ms
   c. 10 ms
   d. 100 ms
   e. 1000 ms

3. A PA chest examination is conducted at 120 kVp. The peak x-ray tube voltage is:
   a. 120 V
   b. 1200 V
   c. 12,000 V
   d. 120,000 V
   e. 1,200,000 V

4. A radiographic exposure made on the 200 mA station is equivalent to:
   a. 2000 μA
   b. 20,000 μA
   c. 200,000 μA
   d. 2,000,000 μA
   e. 20,000,000 μA

5. If you are 160 cm tall, your height is also:
   a. 0.16 m
   b. 16 mm
   c. 16,000 mm
   d. 1.6×10^{6} μm
   e. 1.6×10^{6} nm

6. Which of the following is *correct?*
   a. 1,000,000 eV = 1 keV
   b. 0.001 A = 1 pA
   c. 10^{-7} m = 1 nm
   d. 10 μA = 0.1 mA
   e. $\frac{1}{60}$ s = 17 ms

7. If your mass is 70 kg, it is also:
   a. 0.07 mg
   b. 7000 g
   c. 70,000 g
   d. 7,000,000 mg
   e. 70,000,000 μg

8. Which of the following scientific prefixes is *correct?*
   a. A $\frac{1}{120}$ s exposure is 8 ms.
   b. A 35-keV x-ray has 35×10^{6} eV of energy.

c. 1 nm is 10^{-12} m.
d. 1 μCi is 10^{-3} Ci.
e. 10 kVp is 1000 Vp.

9. A KUB radiograph (radiography of the kidneys, ureters, and bladder) is made at 82 kVp/200 mA/0.25 s. This is equivalent to:
a. 0.82×10^3 kVp/2 $\times 10^{-5}$ μA/2.5 $\times 10^4$ ms
b. 0.82×10^4 kVp $\times$ 0.2 A $\times$ 25 ms
c. 8.2×10^6 mVp/2 $\times 10^2$ mA/2.5 $\times 10^2$ ms
d. 8.2×10^7 μVp/2 $\times 10^5$ μA/2.5 $\times 10^6$ μs
e. 82×10^3 Vp/2 $\times 10^{-1}$ A/250 ms

10. The normal source-to-image receptor distance (SID) for an upright chest radiograph is 180 cm. This is equivalent to:
a. 1.8 m
b. 18 mm
c. 180 mm
d. 1800 μm
e. 18,000 μm

11. When the radiographic exposure time is ½ s, it is also:
a. 50 ms
b. 200 ms
c. 500 ms
d. 2000 ms
e. 5000 ms

12. A fluoroscopic examination is conducted at 1.5 A. This is equivalent to:
a. 15 mA
b. 150 mA
c. 1500 mA
d. 15,000 mA
e. 1500 μA

13. The normal x-ray tube potential for a mammogram is 26 kVp. This is equivalent to:
a. 2.6×10^{-2} Vp
b. 2.6×10^{-1} Vp
c. 2.6×10^2 Vp
d. 2.6×10^3 Vp
e. 2.6×10^4 Vp

14. The SID for a mobile radiograph is often 90 cm. This is equivalent to:
a. 9×10^{-2} m
b. 9×10^{-1} m
c. 9×10^0 m
d. 9×10^2 m
e. 9×10^3 m

15. A radiographic exposure requires 400 ms. This is also:
a. 0.0004 s
b. 0.004 s
c. 0.04 s
d. 0.4 s
e. 4 s

16. A radiographic exposure is made at 600 mA, 200 ms. This is equivalent to:
a. 1.2 mAs
b. 1.2×10^1 mAs
c. 1.2×10^2 mAs
d. 1.2×10^3 mAs
e. 1.2×10^4 mAs

17. A high kVp chest radiograph is conducted at 125 kVp. This is equivalent to:
a. 1.25×10^2 Vp
b. 1.25×10^3 Vp
c. 1.25×10^4 Vp
d. 1.25×10^5 Vp
e. 1.25×10^6 Vp

18. An average monthly exposure for a radiologic technologist is approximately 5 mrem. This is equivalent to:
a. 5×10^{-3} rem
b. 5×10^{-2} rem
c. 5×10^{-1} rem
d. 5×10^0 rem
e. 5×10^2 rem

19. A lateral chest radiograph will expose a patient to approximately 20 mR. This is equivalent to:
a. 2×10^1 μR
b. 2×10^2 μR
c. 2×10^3 μR
d. 2×10^4 μR
e. 2×10^5 μR

Express each of the following as a whole number and in power-of-10 notation (without a prefix):

WHOLE NUMBER		POWER OF 10
20. 1 μL	= _____	_____
21. 10 cm	= _____	_____
22. 10,000 g	= _____	_____
23. 1200 mA	= _____	_____
24. 7 mR	= _____	_____

Convert the following:
25. 1.0 g/cm²/s/s = _____ kg/m²/s/s

WORKSHEET

2-5

Units of Measurement

The International System of Units (SI) has been adopted by nearly all countries. It incorporates seven **base units** as its foundation. The base units then are used to develop **derived units,** some of which are identified by **special names.** The radiologic units are examples of derived units with special names.

SEVEN SI BASE UNITS

QUANTITY	NAME	SYMBOL
Amount of substance	Mole	mol
Electric current	Ampere	A
Length	Meter	m
Luminous intensity	Candela	cd
Mass	Kilogram	kg
Temperature	Kelvin	K
Time	Second	s

SI-DERIVED UNITS WITH SPECIAL NAMES

QUANTITY	NAME	SYMBOL	EXPRESSION IN TERMS OF BASE UNITS
Electric charge	Coulomb	C	As
Electric potential	Volt	V	mkg/sA
Energy, work	Joule	J	mkg/s
Force	Newton	N	mkg/s
Frequency	Hertz	Hz	1/s
Power	Watt	W	mkg/s

EXERCISES

1. Which of the following is *not* a base quantity in the SI?
   a. Electric current
   b. Exposure
   c. Mass
   d. Temperature
   e. Time

2. Which of the following is an SI base unit?
   a. Becquerel
   b. Coulomb
   c. Coulomb/kilogram
   d. Gray
   e. Kilogram

3. Which of the following standards of SI measure is *correct?*
   a. The foot was measured by King Henry VIII.
   b. The meter is related to the visible emission from the sun.
   c. The meter is the length of an engraved platinum-iridium bar.
   d. The second is based on the rotation of the earth around the sun.
   e. The second is based on the vibrations of cesium atoms.

4. Water has a mass density of 1 g/cm^3. Its density is also:
   a. 10^{-3} kg/m^3
   b. 1 kg/m^3
   c. 10 kg/m^3
   d. 10^3 kg/m^3
   e. 10^5 kg/m^3

5. SI stands for which of the following?
   a. Inconsistent system
   b. Incorrect system
   c. Le Système Institutional
   d. Le Système International d'Unités
   e. System International

6. Which of the following is *not* a system of units?
   a. British
   b. CGS
   c. French
   d. MKS
   e. SI

7. Which of the following is an SI name for a base unit?
   a. Celsius
   b. Kilovolt
   c. Milliampere
   d. Newton
   e. Second

8. Which of the following is a unit of energy?
   a. Gray
   b. Joule
   c. Newton
   d. Rad
   e. Sievert

9. Which of the following is expressed in the proper units?
   a. Absorbed dose: Sv
   b. Activity: rem
   c. Dose equivalent: rad
   d. Exposure: Bq
   e. Exposure: mGy_a

10. Which of the following is an SI-derived unit?
    a. Dyne
    b. Horsepower
    c. Joule
    d. Kelvin
    e. Roentgen

11. Which of the following has units of s^{-1}?
    a. Dose
    b. Exposure
    c. Frequency
    d. Time
    e. Velocity

12. The unit of measure that is the same for all systems of measure is the:
    a. Calorie
    b. Kilogram
    c. Meter
    d. Pound
    e. Second

13. A kilogram is the:
    a. Energy required to raise 1 lb of water 1°C
    b. Mass of a standard gold bar
    c. Mass of 1 lb of water
    d. Mass of $1000 \ cm^3$ of water
    e. Temperature rise of 1 lb of water

14. What unit results when a coulomb is divided by a second?
    a. Ampere
    b. Hertz
    c. Ohm
    d. Rad
    e. Volt

15. What common radiologic unit results from the following? $\underline{millicoulomb} \times second = second$
    a. ESE
    b. kVp
    c. mAs
    d. PBL
    e. SID

16. The radiologic unit milliampere-second (mAs) is actually a measure of:
    a. Charge
    b. Electric potential
    c. Number of electrons
    d. Potential difference
    e. X-ray intensity

2-6

Radiologic Units

 Exposure:
1 roentgen (R) = 2.58 = 10^{-4} coulombs per kilogram (C/kg) of air 1 gray in air (Gy_a)

Absorbed dose:
1 radiation absorbed dose (rad) — 10^2 ergs per gram
(erg/g) = 10^{-2} gray in tissue (Gyt) 1 Gyt = 1 J/kg 10^2 rad

Dose equivalent:
1 roentgen equivalent man (rem) 10^2 ergs per gram (erg/g) 10^{-2} sieverts (Sv)
1 Sv = 1 J/kg = 10^2 rem

Radioactivity:
1 curie (Ci) = 3.7×10^{10} atoms disintegrating per second (s^{-1})
3.7×10^{10} becquerel (Bq)
1 Bq = 1 s^{-1}

EXERCISES

1. A radiation monitoring report would express a radiologic technologist's dose equivalent in which of the following?
   a. Curie
   b. Gray
   c. Rad
   d. Rem
   e. Roentgen

2. A PA chest radiograph delivers approximately what dose to the patient?
   a. 10 eV
   b. 10 J
   c. 10 mR
   d. 10 mrad
   e. 10 rem

3. To produce death, mice must be irradiated to a total dose of approximately:
   a. 600 eV
   b. 600 J
   c. 600 rad
   d. 600 rem
   e. 600 Sv

4. The approximate output intensity of a radiographic x-ray tube is:
   a. 5 mCi/mAs
   b. 5 mJ/mAs
   c. 5 mR/mAs
   d. 5 mrad/mAs
   e. 5 mrem/mAs

5. 99^mTc is the *most* often used radionuclide in diagnostic nuclear medicine. It is used in quantities of:
   a. mBq
   b. mCi
   c. mJ
   d. mrad
   e. mrem

6. The roentgen is a unit of measure that specifies which of the following?
   a. Absorption of x-rays
   b. Attenuation of x-rays
   c. Character of x-rays
   d. Intensity of x-rays
   e. Quality of x-rays

7. Which of the following adequately describes the use of the rad?
   a. To measure energy absorbed by tissue
   b. To measure radiation exposure in air
   c. To measure the amount of radioactive material
   d. To measure the occupational exposure received by a radiologic technologist
   e. To measure the output intensity of an x-ray machine

8. Which of the following is a classic radiologic unit?
   a. Ampere
   b. Coulomb/kilogram
   c. Joule
   d. Rem
   e. Sievert

9. If 2 rad is delivered to 2 g of soft tissue, 1 g of this tissue receives:
   a. 0.5 rad
   b. 1 g-rad
   c. 1 rad
   d. 2 g-rad
   e. 2 rad

10. Absorbed dose can be measured in:
    a. ergs
    b. Gy
    c. J
    d. keV
    e. kg-Gy

11. Which of the following is *not* a unit of energy?
    a. Calorie
    b. Electron volt
    c. Erg
    d. Joule
    e. Rad

12. Which of the following statements is equivalent?
    a. $1 \text{ Gy}_t = 1 \text{ J/kg}$
    b. $1 \text{ mCi} = 37 \text{ }\mu\text{C/kg}$
    c. $1 \text{ Sv} = 100 \text{ erg/g}$
    d. $200 \text{ mrad} = 2 \text{ cGy}$
    e. $500 \text{ mR} = 5 \text{ mGy}_a$

13. Which of the following is a unit of radioactivity?
    a. Ci
    b. Gy
    c. J

d. R
e. Rad

14. Absorbed dose can be expressed in:
    a. Bq
    b. Ci
    c. Ergs
    d. eV
    e. J/kg

15. Which of the following demonstrates the proper use of the unit *roentgen*?
    a. An angiographer receives an occupational exposure of 10 mR.
    b. 100 mR of ^{131}I is administered to image the thyroid.
    c. Patient treatment dose with a linear accelerator unit is 6000 R.
    d. The dose limit (DL) for radiologic technologists is 5000 mR/yr.
    e. X-ray intensity from a linear accelerator unit is 200 R/min.

16. In diagnostic radiology, it is acceptable to assume that 1 R is equal to:
    a. 1 Ci
    b. 1 erg
    c. 1 J
    d. 1 keV
    e. 1 rem

17. In the SI system:
    a. Dose equivalent is expressed in Gy.
    b. kVp is equal to keV.
    c. 1 J is approximately equal to 1 MeV.
    d. 1000 rad is equivalent to 10 Gy.
    e. 1000 rad is equivalent to 100 Sv.

18. Dose rate could be expressed in units of:
    a. Ergs/g
    b. J/kg/min
    c. keV/min
    d. kVp/s
    e. R/min

19. When SI is used, radiation exposure is defined in units of coulombs/kilogram. With regard to this unit of measure, which of the following is *true*?
    a. *Coulomb* refers to electrons released in ionization.
    b. *Coulomb* refers to energy absorbed.
    c. *Kilogram* refers to mass of radiation.
    d. *Kilogram* refers to the patient's mass.

• **Newton's first law**—*Inertia:* When no force is acting on an object, it will continue in its present state of motion or rest.
• **Newton's second law**—*Force:* The force required to change the state of motion of an object is directly proportional to the product of the mass of the object and the acceleration.
• **Newton's third law**—*Reaction:* For every force, there is an equal but opposite force.
  • **Mass** is the property of matter that tends to keep a stationary object at rest or that resists a change in the motion of an object that is already moving (Newton's first law).
  • **Force** is a push or a pull. Newton's second law, which expresses the concept of force, is his greatest and is represented by the equation:

$$F = ma \text{ where}$$
Force (newtons [N]) = Mass (kg) × Acceleration
$$(m/s^2)$$

  • The weight of an object is actually the force of gravitational attraction on its mass. In mathematical terms:

$$W = mg$$

Weight (N) = Mass (kg) × Acceleration (m/s²)

EXERCISES

1. Which of the following is *not* a correct statement of Newton's laws?
   a. Acceleration is equal to initial velocity plus final velocity, divided by 2.
   b. Force is equal to mass times acceleration.
   c. Momentum is equal to mass times velocity.
   d. Velocity is equal to distance divided by time.
   e. Weight is equal to mass times acceleration.

2. Which of the following correctly states Newton's first law of motion?
   a. An object at rest will remain at rest unless acted on by an external force.
   b. An object with mass (m) and acceleration (a) is acted on by a force, given by the equation F = ma.
   c. For every action, there is an opposite and equal reaction.
   d. Matter and energy are related.
   e. The total momentum before any interaction is equal to the total momentum after the interaction.

3. Another name for velocity is:
   a. Energy
   b. Mass
   c. Speed
   d. Time
   e. Work

4. When you travel 50 mph, you are also going approximately:
   a. 80 km/hr
   b. 100 km/hr
   c. 1100 ft/min
   d. 2200 ft/min
   e. 3300 ft/min

5. Acceleration is also:
   a. The product of time and distance
   b. The rate of change of time with velocity
   c. The rate of change of velocity with distance

d. The rate of change of velocity with time
e. Time squared

6. An automobile travels 30 miles in 30 min. Its average velocity is approximately:
   a. 1 mi/min
   b. 33 mi/min
   c. 60 mi/min
   d. 88 mi/min
   e. 99 mi/min

7. The final speed of a dragster in a quarter mile is 80 mph. The average velocity is:
   a. 4 mi/hr
   b. 8 mi/hr
   c. 16 mi/hr
   d. 32 mi/hr
   e. 40 mi/hr

8. A dragster requires 8 s to reach a speed of 80 mph. What is its acceleration?
   a. 1.1 m/s^2
   b. 2.2 m/s^2
   c. 3.3 m/s^2
   d. 4.5 m/s^2
   e. 5.5 m/s^2

9. Inertia is:
   a. Mass times acceleration
   b. Newton's second law of motion
   c. Resistance to a change in motion
   d. Velocity divided by time
   e. Velocity times time

10. Which of the following statements refers to a vector quantity?
    a. The car was speeding north at 80 mph.
    b. The speed of light is 3×10^8 m/s.
    c. The standard man has a mass of 70 kg.
    d. The standard man weighs 70 kg.
    e. The units of Planck's constant are J-s.

11. A Roger Clemens fast ball was clocked at 90 mph. How long did that ball take to travel the 90 feet to the plate?
    a. Less than 1 s
    b. 1.0 s
    c. Longer than 2 s
    d. 1.5 s
    e. 2 s

12. How many fundamental laws of motion did Newton formulate?
    a. 1
    b. 2

c. 3
d. 4
e. 5

13. If someone were to fall off the edge of the south rim of the Grand Canyon, the force exerted would be measured in:
    a. kg
    b. J
    c. m/s
    d. N
    e. lb

14. If the acceleration caused by gravity is 9.8 m/s^2, what is the gravitational force acting on a 50-kg sack pushed off the roof of a 50-story building?
    a. 0.2 N
    b. 5.1 N
    c. 40.2 N
    d. 80 N
    e. 490 N

15. How is momentum *best* described?
    a. For every action, there is an equal and opposite reaction
    b. It is the force of an object caused by the downward pull of gravity
    c. It is the product of the mass of an object and its velocity
    d. It is the relationship between matter and energy
    e. Objects falling to the earth accelerate at a constant rate

16. The total momentum before any interaction is:
    a. An equal and opposite reaction.
    b. Decreased by the property of friction, so it is less after the interaction.
    c. Equal to the total momentum after the interaction.
    d. Greater than the total momentum during the interaction.
    e. Less than the total momentum during the interaction.

17. Which of the following is a unit of work?
    a. Gray
    b. Hertz
    c. Joule
    d. Newton
    e. Rad

Newton's Laws of Motion page 31 worksheet

18. Which of the following statements about work is *true?*
    a. It can be measured in watts.
    b. It depends on time.
    c. It involves the same units as energy.
    d. It involves time.
    e. It is performed when a large weight is held motionless.

19. When a force is exerted to push a mobile radiographic imaging system, the force would be expressed in what unit?
    a. Joule
    b. Kilogram
    c. Kilovolt
    d. Newton
    e. Rad

WORK

If one exerts a **force** (a push or pull) on a box and moves it across the floor, one does **work** on the box. The following is the formula for work:

$$W = Fd$$

The unit of work is the **joule** (J) if the force is measured in newtons and the distance in meters ($1 \text{ J} = 1 \text{ N} \times 1 \text{ m}$).

ENERGY

A system that is capable of doing work is said to have energy. Energy is the ability to do work, and it can take many forms, including heat energy, electric energy, nuclear energy, and mechanical energy. Mechanical energy may be potential or kinetic:

1. **Potential energy (PE):** The energy of an object is a result of its position. For example, a brick raised over your head or a coiled spring has potential energy.
2. **Kinetic energy (KE):** The energy of an object is a result of its motion.

$$KE \ 1/2 \ mv^2$$

The basic unit of energy is the **joule.** Other units are also used:

1 electron volt (eV) = 1.6×10^{-19} J
1 erg = 10^{-7} J
1 British thermal unit (BTU) = 1.06 J
1 foot-pound (ft-lb) = 1.36 J
1 kilowatt-hour (kW-hr) = 3.6×10^6 J

POWER

Power is the rate at which work is done. The following is the formula for power:

$$P = W/t$$

The unit of power is the **watt** (1 watt = 1 J/s). A commonly used unit of power is the **kilowatt,** which is equal to 1000 watts. Another frequently used unit of power is the **horsepower** (hp):

$$1 \text{ hp} = 746 \text{ watts}$$

EXERCISES

A radiologic technologist lifts a box onto a platform. Choose one or more of the following choices, a through f, to use as you complete Exercises 1 to 5.

    a. The distance the box is lifted
    b. The force used by the man to lift the box
    c. The mass of the box
    d. The size of the box
    e. The time required to lift the box
    f. The velocity of the box

1. The **KE** of the box depends on _____.
2. The man's **power** output depends on _____.
3. The **PE** of the box depends on _____.
4. The total **energy** used depends on _____.
5. The **work** done depends on _____.
6. Which of the following statements about work is *true?*
    a. It can be measured in watts.
    b. It depends on time.
    c. It has units the same as energy.

d. It is measured in newtons.
e. It is performed when a large weight is held
    motionless.

7. A one-bedroom apartment might use 1000 kW-hr
   of electricity. The kilowatt-hour is a unit of:
   a. Energy
   b. Force
   c. Heat
   d. Potential energy
   e. Power

8. Kinetic energy (KE) is directly proportional to:
   a. A vector quantity
   b. Acceleration
   c. Force
   d. Mass
   e. Velocity

9. Which of the following units of energy is *most*
   fundamental?
   a. Calorie
   b. Electron volt
   c. Erg
   d. Joule
   e. Kilowatt-hour

10. Which of the following is the primary method
    of heat dissipation from the rotating anode of
    an x-ray tube?
    a. Conduction
    b. Convection
    c. Convention
    d. Radiation
    e. Reduction

11. Which of the following statements about energy
    is *true?*
    a. Energy is a force.
    b. Energy is form of power.
    c. Energy is the ability to do work.
    d. Energy is the rate of doing work.
    e. X-rays can be described by their potential
       energy.

12. How much work is done in lifting a 1 kg box
    of film from the floor to a shelf that is 2 m
    high? (*Hint:* 1 kg = 2.2 lb = 9.8 N)
    a. 1 J
    b. 2.2 J
    c. 4.5 J
    d. 19.6 J
    e. 9 N

13. A car with a 300 hp engine is very fast. The
    power of the engine is equivalent to how many
    kilowatts?
    a. 0.4 kW
    b. 2.5 kW
    c. 25 kW
    d. 224 kW
    e. 300 kW

14. Heat is transferred from a glass-enclosed fire-
    place primarily by:
    a. Conduction
    b. Convection
    c. Convention
    d. Radiation
    e. Temperature

15. A 1° change is equal in thermal energy for
    which two scales?
    a. Absolute and kelvin
    b. Celsius and absolute
    c. Celsius and Fahrenheit
    d. Celsius and kelvin
    e. Fahrenheit and kelvin

16. Which British unit is equivalent to the newton?
    a. Foot-pound
    b. Gram
    c. Joule
    d. Kilogram
    e. Pound

Match the following:

_____ 17. Energy   a. Push and pull
_____ 18. Force   b. The ability to do work
_____ 19. Kinetic energy c. The energy of motion
_____ 20. Power   d. The product of force
                              and distance
_____ 21. Work   e. The rate of doing work

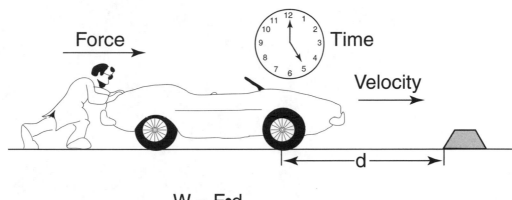

$$W = F{\bullet}d$$
$$KE = \tfrac{1}{2}mv^2$$
$$P = \frac{F{\bullet}d}{t} = \frac{W}{t}$$

3-1

Centuries of Discovery

THE PERIODIC TABLE

- The periodic table is a systematic grouping of the elements that is based on similarity of chemical properties.
- The vertical columns are called *groups*. The horizontal rows are *periods*.
- As you proceed from left to right in a period, the number of easily removable electrons, called *valence electrons*, increases by one from one group to the next.

EXERCISES

1. Which of the following statements is *true* regarding our understanding of atomic structure?
   a. Rutherford described the nuclear atom.
   b. Rutherford identified cathode rays as particles, and constituents of all are correct atoms.
   c. Rutherford is known as the "Father of Radioactivity."
   d. Rutherford is responsible for the periodic table.
   e. Rutherford was an epicurean and envisioned the atom as something familiar to him—plum pudding.

2. In the rendering of the atom by J. J. Thomson:
   a. Electrons were in orbits.
   b. Electrons were distributed throughout the nucleus as plums in a pudding.
   c. Eyes and hooks represented electrons.
   d. He called it the "cathode ray atom."
   e. Uniform positive electrification was theorized.

3. The periodic table presents the elements in the order of:
   a. Atomic charge
   b. Atomic mass
   c. Atomic number
   d. Natural occurrences
   e. Number of isotopes

4. Approximately how many known elements are there?
   a. 50
   b. 100
   c. 150
   d. 200
   e. 300

5. The only element that is *not* placed in any group of the periodic table is:
   a. Helium
   b. Hydrogen
   c. Plutonium
   d. Tungsten
   e. Uranium

6. The horizontal rows in the periodic table are called:
   a. Articles
   b. Compounds
   c. Groups
   d. Molecules
   e. Periods

7. As you move from left to right across the periodic table, what happens to the number of outer-shell electrons from one element to the next?
   a. It decreases by 1.
   b. It decreases by 2.
   c. It increases by 1.
   d. It increases by 2.
   e. It remains constant.

8. Which group in the periodic table contains elements that have only one electron in the outer shell?
   a. Actinide metals
   b. Alkali metals
   c. Halogens
   d. Rare Earths
   e. Vapors

9. Which of the following is a transitional element?
   a. Barium
   b. Carbon dioxide
   c. Iodine
   d. Tungsten
   e. Xenon

10. Atoms with all electron shells filled are:
    a. Chemically stable
    b. Chemically very reactive
    c. Found in group 1 of the periodic table
    d. Gases
    e. Radioactive

11. Atoms with three electrons in the outer shell:
    a. Are compounds
    b. Are molecules
    c. Are probably inert gases
    d. Are probably radioactive
    e. Have three valence electrons

12. In the periodic table of the elements, the group number identifies the:
    a. Electron spin state
    b. Number of electrons allowed in the outer shell
    c. Principal quantum number of the outermost shell
    d. Total number of electrons in the atom
    e. Valence state of the atom

13. All of the following are elements *except*:
    a. Carbon
    b. Molybdenum
    c. Oxygen
    d. Steel
    e. Tungsten

14. How many atoms are there in one molecule of sodium bicarbonate ($NaHCO_3$)?
    a. 1
    d. 6
    b. 3
    c. 4
    e. 8

15. Which of the following physicists had a major part in describing the atom as we know it today?
    a. Becquerel
    b. Bohr
    c. Curie
    d. Einstein
    e. Roentgen

16. Which of the following statements is *true*?
    a. A 6000 yd golf course is approximately 10^4 m long.
    b. A football field is approximately 10^3 m long.
    c. An atomic nucleus has a diameter of approximately 10^{-10} m.
    d. In 1 yr, light can travel approximately 10^{16} m.
    e. The wavelength of a 100 keV x-ray is approximately 10^{-8} m.

17. The periodic chart of elements is attributed to:
    a. Dimitri Mendeleev
    b. Ernest Rutherford
    c. J. J. Thomson
    d. John Dalton
    e. Niels Bohr

18. Rutherford made what significant contribution to science?
    a. Description of the electron shells
    b. Description of the nuclear atom
    c. Discovery of artificial radioactivity
    d. Discovery of negatively charged electrons
    e. Periodic table of the elements

19. Which of the following statements about atoms is *true?*
    a. Atomic mass is divided equally between the nucleus and the electrons.
    b. Most of the atom is made up of empty space.
    c. The nucleus is held together by the electrostatic proton–proton attraction.
    d. The number of electrons surrounding the nucleus equals the number of neutrons.
    e. The number of electrons surrounding the nucleus equals the number of protons plus the number of neutrons.

20. Which of the following statements about atoms is *true?*
    a. Atoms that have the same atomic mass interact the same way chemically.
    b. Atoms that have the same atomic number are atoms of the same element.
    c. Electrons are more tightly bound in little atoms than in big atoms.
    d. M-shell electrons are more tightly bound than L-shell electrons.
    e. Neutron number determines chemical properties.

Matter is composed of atoms. Atoms are composed of fundamental particles called **protons, neutrons,** and **electrons.** The positively charged protons and uncharged neutrons make up the **nucleus** of the atom. The negatively charged electrons revolve around the nucleus in definite orbits, just as the planets orbit the sun.

The electron is the lightest of the fundamental particles. The mass of the proton is 1836 times larger than the mass of the electron. The neutron mass is 1839 times larger than that of the electron.

The closer electrons are to the nucleus, the more tightly bound they are. The number of electrons in any shell increases to a maximum of $2n^2$, where n is the shell number. No matter how large the atom becomes, however, it normally has the same number of electrons as protons. If this is not the case, the atom is an **ion.**

EXERCISES

1. If $^{129}_{53}$I is a stable, electrically neutral atom, then how many neutrons are there in such an atom?
   a. 53
   b. 76
   c. 129
   d. 182
   e. The question does not give enough information.

2. When oxygen ($^{16}_{8}$O) combines with two atoms of hydrogen ($^{1}_{1}$H) to form water, the resultant molecule has a total of:
   a. 8 electrons
   b. 10 protons
   c. 16 electrons
   d. 18 protons
   e. 20 nucleons

3. The atomic mass number of an atom is given by the number of:
   a. Electrons
   b. Neutrons
   c. Protons
   d. Protons plus neutrons
   e. Protons plus neutrons plus electrons

4. The atomic number:
   a. Has the symbol "A"
   b. Has the symbol "N"
   c. Is the number of neutrons
   d. Is the number of protons
   e. Is the number of protons plus neutrons

5. Isotopes are atoms:
   a. In the same molecule
   b. Of the same element
   c. That are ions
   d. That contain the same number of neutrons plus protons
   e. With the same number of nucleons

6. Electrons in the M-shell:
   a. Have lower binding energy than those in the N-shell
   b. Never exceed 8 in number
   c. Do not exceed 18 in number
   d. Do not exist in an atom of carbon ($^{12}_{6}$C)
   e. Probably are closer to the nucleus than those in the L-shell

7. $_{6}^{12}$C and $_{6}^{14}$C have the same:
   a. A number
   b. N number
   c. Number of neutrons
   d. Number of nucleons
   e. Number of protons

8. The binding energy of an electron to a nucleus:
   a. Increases with increasing distance from the nucleus
   b. Is higher for an L-shell electron than for an M-shell electron
   c. Is higher for a low-Z atom than for a high-Z atom
   d. Is higher for an N-shell than for an M-shell
   e. Depends on the size of an electron

9. How many nucleons does $_{53}^{131}$I have?
   a. 53
   b. 78
   c. 131
   d. 184
   e. 237

10. The number of protons in the nucleus is called the:
    a. Atomic number
    b. Elemental charge
    c. Ionization state
    d. Mass
    e. Valence

11. A neutron has approximately:
    a. 1/2000 atomic mass unit (amu) and no charge
    b. 1 amu and no charge
    c. 1 amu and a charge of +1
    d. 4 amu and a charge of +2
    e. 4 amu and no charge

12. How many different types of nucleons are there?
    a. 1
    b. 2
    c. 3
    d. 4
    e. 6

13. Which of the following is a fundamental particle?
    a. Alpha
    b. Beta
    c. Electron
    d. Gamma
    e. Hydrogen

14. What is the maximum number of electrons allowed in the outermost shell of an atom in the third period, n = 3?
    a. 2
    b. 8
    c. 18
    d. 32
    e. 50

15. Tungsten $_{74}^{184}$W has how many neutrons?
    a. 74
    b. 110
    c. 184
    d. 258
    e. 332

16. What is the maximum number of electrons permitted in the N-shell?
    a. 8
    b. 18
    c. 24
    d. 32
    e. 50

17. Regarding atomic nomenclature:
    a. Atomic mass is the number of neutrons.
    b. Atomic mass is the number of protons.
    c. Atomic mass is the number of protons minus neutrons.
    d. Atomic mass number determines chemical properties.
    e. Atomic mass number is a whole number.

18. The following atoms are all stable; which has the highest K-shell electron binding energy?
    a. Al (aluminum)
    b. Hg (mercury)
    c. S (sulfur)
    d. Sr (strontium)
    e. Tc (technetium)

Certain naturally occurring and artificially produced atoms can emit radiation spontaneously. Such atoms are said to be **radioactive.** Radioactivity is the result of instability in the nucleus. Three types of radiation come from the nucleus of a radioactive atom: **alpha (α) particles, beta (β) particles, and gamma (γ) rays.**

- Alpha particles consist of two protons and two neutrons.
- Beta particles are actually electrons that are emitted from the nucleus.
- Gamma rays are the product of electromagnetic radiation of high energy and high penetrability (much like x-rays).

EXERCISES

Match the following.

_____ 1. Alpha particle
_____ 2. Beta particle
_____ 3. Cyclotron
_____ 4. Gamma ray
_____ 5. Gold
_____ 6. Isotope
_____ 7. Radioactive
_____ 8. Radioactivity
_____ 9. Radioisotope
_____ 10. Uranium

a. A particle accelerator used to produce radioisotopes
b. A particle with a charge of -1.602×10^{-19} C
c. A stable atom that can be made radioactive
d. A substance composed of atoms with unstable nuclei
e. An atom that is naturally radioactive
f. Atoms with the same number of protons but different numbers of neutrons
g. Radiation that cannot penetrate a sheet of paper material
h. Spontaneous emission of energy or particles from unstable nuclei
i. Uncharged radiation; highly penetrating
j. Usually produced by particle accelerators from common elements

11. When a radioisotope emits a beta particle:
    a. A gamma ray is always emitted.
    b. A neutron is converted to a proton.
    c. A proton is converted to a neutron.
    d. An electron is converted to a beta particle.
    e. An x-ray is always emitted.

12. Which of the following pairs of atoms are isobars?
    a. ^{129}I and ^{131}I
    b. ^{131}I and ^{198}Hg
    c. ^{2}H and ^{3}H

    d. ^{3}He and ^{3}H
    e. ^{131}I and ^{137}Cs

13. Potassium ($^{40}_{19}$K) is a naturally occurring radioisotope that decays by beta emission. Therefore, the daughter atom:
    a. Has a mass of approximately 19 amu
    b. Will also be radioactive
    c. Will have 19 neutrons
    d. Will have 40 nucleons
    e. Will have 90 protons

14. Isotopes are:
    a. Atoms that have identical mass and atomic number
    b. Atoms that have the same atomic mass number but different atomic numbers
    c. Atoms that have the same atomic number but different atomic mass numbers
    d. Molecules that consist of identical atoms
    e. Molecules that have the same number of atoms

15. The number of disintegrations per second in 2 mCi of ^{99m}Tc is:
    a. 3.7×10^7
    b. 3.7×10^{10}
    c. 3.7×10^{12}
    d. 7.4×10^7
    e. 7.4×10^{10}

16. With regard to $^{90}_{38}\text{Sr}^{+2}_3$:
    a. The atomic number is 90.
    b. The symbolism indicates that this is a radioactive nuclide.
    c. The valence is 3.
    d. There are 90 neutrons in the nucleus of this atom.
    e. There are a total of 36 electrons in one such atom.

17. Beta emission:
    a. Occurs only with heavy elements
    b. Occurs only with light elements
    c. Occurs only with radioisotopes with long half-lives
    d. Results in the gain of a proton
    e. Results in the loss of 1 amu

18. Alpha emission:
    a. Occurs only with light elements
    b. Occurs only with radioisotopes with long half-lives
    c. Results in the gain of a proton
    d. Results in the loss of 2 amu
    e. Results in the loss of 4 amu

19. After beta emission, the nucleus has:
    a. Decreased in A number by 1
    b. Decreased in Z and A numbers by 1
    c. Decreased in Z number by 1
    d. Increased in A number by 1
    e. Increased in Z number by 1

20. 1 Ci is equivalent to disintegration of how many atoms every second?
    a. 3×10^8
    b. 3×10^{10}
    c. 3.7×10^8
    d. 3.7×10^{10}
    e. 2.2×10^{12}

21. 10 mCi is equivalent to:
    a. $3.7 \ 10^8$ Bq
    b. 10^{-6} Ci
    c. 3.7×10^{10} d/s
    d. 10^{-2} nCi
    e. 2.2×10^{12} d/min

22. Which of the following statements about atoms is *true?*
    a. $A = Z + N$.
    b. $A = Z - N$.
    c. An alpha emission contains four units of mass and four units of charge.
    d. In a radioactive atom, the number of protons does not equal the number of electrons.
    e. Nucleons are electrons, protons, and neutrons.

23. Which of the following pairs of atoms consists of isotones?

    a. $^1_1$H and $^2_1$H

    b. $^{130}_{56}$Ba and $^{132}_{56}$Ba

    c. $^{130}_{53}$I and $^{131}_{54}$Xe

    d. ^{99}Tc and ^{99m}Tc

    e. $^{133}_{54}$Xe and $^{133}_{55}$Cs

24. Isomers are atoms that have different:
    a. Energy states
    b. Filled electron shells
    c. Numbers of neutrons
    d. Numbers of protons
    e. States of ionization

25. Radioisotopes:
    a. Are ionized
    b. Are made with x-rays
    c. Are stable atoms

d. Have closed electron shells
e. Have unstable nuclei

26. Which of the following statements about $^{40}_{19}$K, a naturally occurring radionuclide deposited in body tissues, is *true?*
    a. It can be detected by x-rays.
    b. It can be produced by x-rays.
    c. It contributes to our total radiation exposure.
    d. It has 40 electrons.
    e. It has 40 protons.

27. Electrons are:
    a. Arranged in orbits around the nucleus
    b. Composed of neutrons and protons
    c. Organized inside the nucleus
    d. Positively charged
    e. Usually bundled together

3-4

Radioactivity

Radioactivity is due to natural or artificially induced instability in the nucleus of an atom. To become stable, the nucleus decays by emitting alpha, beta, or gamma radiation. Radioactivity is measured in curies or becquerels:

$$1 \text{ curie (Ci)} = 3.70 \times 10^{10} \text{ disintegrations/s}$$
$$1 \text{ becquerel (Bq)} = 1 \text{ disintegration/s}$$

Radioactivity decreases with time. The time required for the activity of a sample to decay to half of its original value is called the radioactive half-life ($t_{1/2}$).

EXERCISES

1. Radioactive half-life is the time:
   a. It takes for half of the dose to be delivered
   b. It takes for half of the mass to disappear
   c. It takes for one atom to disintegrate
   d. Required for radioactivity to reach one half of its original value
   e. When half of the quantity now present remains

2. How many half-lives must elapse before the remaining activity is less than 0.1% of the original activity?
   a. 4 half-lives
   b. 6 half-lives
   c. 8 half-lives
   d. 10 half-lives
   e. 12 half-lives

3. Given a 50 μCi (0.19 MBq) sample of ^{131}I ($t_{1/2}$ = 8 days), the radioactivity will be 3 μCi after approximately how many days?
   a. 24 days
   b. 32 days
   c. 36 days
   d. 40 days
   e. 44 days

4. A 10 mCi quantity of technetium ^{99m}Tc ($t_{1/2}$ = 6 hr) is available at 8:00 AM. At 12:00 noon on that same day, the radioactivity will be closer to:
   a. 1 mCi than to 3 mCi
   b. 3 mCi than to 5 mCi
   c. 5 mCi than to 8 mCi
   d. 10 mCi than to 8 mCi
   e. 15 mCi than to 10 mCi

5. ^{14}C ($t_{1/2}$ = 5730 yr) is used for archeologic dating. Approximately how old is a tree specimen that contains 3 nCi/g (110 Bq/g) if the original concentration of radioactivity is known to be 12 nCi/g (444 Bq/g)?
   a. 5730 years
   b. Approximately 11,000 years
   c. Approximately 17,000 years
   d. Younger than 5730 years
   e. Older than 17,000 years

6. One hundred mCi (3.7 GBq) of an unknown radionuclide has a half-life of 15 days. Therefore:
   a. 400 mCi should have been available 15 days earlier.
   b. In 15 days, only 25 mCi will remain.

c. In 1 mo, 25 mCi will have decayed.
d. In 1 mo, only 75 mCi will remain.
e. In 3½ mo, the activity will be less than 1 mCi.

7. How much ^{99m}Tc (t½ = 6 hr) decays in 24 hr?
   a. 3%
   b. 6%
   c. 14%
   d. 86%
   e. 94%

8. In approximately how many half-lives will the activity of 10 mCi (0.37 GBq) of $^{131}_{53}$I (t½ = 8 days) be reduced to 0.1 mCi (3.7 MBq)?
   a. 3.3 half-lives
   b. 10 half-lives
   c. 12.5 half-lives
   d. 50 half-lives
   e. 100 half-lives

9. Which of the following statements about a given radioisotope is *true?*
   a. As the number of atoms decreases, the half-life decreases.
   b. The half-life increases as the decay constant increases.
   c. The number of radioactive atoms decreases linearly with time.
   d. The percentage of atoms decaying per unit of time decreases.
   e. The percentage of atoms decaying per unit of time is constant.

10. If the half-life of $^{131}_{53}$I is 8 days, approximately how much $^{131}_{53}$I remains of an original shipment of 50 μCi (1.9 MBq) after 24 days?
    a. 25 nCi
    b. 25 nCi
    c. 3 μCi
    d. 6 μCi
    e. 12 μCi

11. 10 mCi of ^{99m}Tc is a normal patient dose for imaging. How many becquerels is this?
    a. 2.2×10^8 Bq
    b. 3.7×10^8 Bq
    c. 2.2×10^{11} Bq
    d. 3.7×10^{11} Bq
    e. 3.7×10^{12} Bq

12. $^{131}_{53}$I has a half-life of 13 hr. If 150 μCi (5.7 MBq) is available at 12:00 noon on Wednesday, approximately how much will remain at 5:00 PM on Friday?
    a. 10 μCi
    b. 20 μCi
    c. 30 μCi
    d. 40 μCi
    e. 50 μCi

13. An unknown radioisotope is assayed to be 40 μCi (15 MBq) at 9:00 AM on Monday. An assay at 9:00 PM on Tuesday yields a result in 2.5 μCi (0.1 MBq). What is the half-life of the radioisotope?
    a. 3 hr
    b. 6 hr
    c. 9 hr
    d. 12 hr
    e. 18 hr

14. Use the following graph to estimate the percentage of radioactivity that remains after 2½ half-lives.

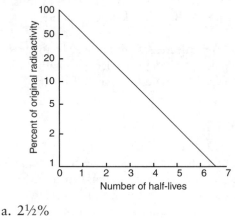

    a. 2½%
    b. 5%
    c. 16%
    d. 50%
    e. 75%

15. The shape of the radioactive decay curve is:
    a. A concave-down curve on linear paper
    b. A concave-up curve on semilog paper
    c. A straight line on linear paper
    d. A straight line on semilog paper
    e. Linear and nonthreshold

• Radiation is the transfer of energy from one position or medium to another.
- There are two types of radiation: ionizing and non-ionizing.
- There are two sources of radiation: naturally occurring radiation and that produced by humans.
- Ionizing radiation is any radiation that is capable of removing an orbital electron from an atom.
- There are two types of ionizing radiation: particulate and electromagnetic.

I. Particulate
  a. Alpha (α) particles
  b. Beta (β) particles
  c. Other nuclear particles
II. Electromagnetic
  a. Gamma (γ) rays
  b. X-rays

EXERCISES

1. The difference between electrons and beta particles is:
  a. Beta particles are ionizing.
  b. Beta particles have higher energy.
  c. Electrons have higher mass.
  d. Electrons have higher velocity.
  e. Their origin

2. In the air:
  a. A gamma ray does not normally travel farther than 10 m.
  b. Alpha particles have a range of 1 to 10 cm.
  c. Alpha particles travel farthest.
  d. An x-ray does not normally travel farther than 1 m.
  e. Beta particles have a range of 1 to 10 mm.

3. The amount of energy acquired when an electron is accelerated by a potential difference of 1 V is:
  a. 1 Ci
  b. 1 eV
  c. 1 J
  d. 1 R
  e. 1 rad

4. Alpha particles:
  a. Are similar to hydrogen nuclei
  b. Are useful in nuclear medicine
  c. Contain two electrons
  d. Have an A number of 4
  e. Have a Z number of 4

5. Of the following radiations, the *most* penetrating is a:
  a. 10 keV x-ray
  b. 100 keV gamma ray
  c. 0.01 MeV x-ray
  d. 2.1 MeV beta particle
  e. 4.8 MeV alpha particle

6. The difference between x-rays and gamma rays is:
  a. Gamma rays always have higher energy than x-rays.
  b. Gamma rays have higher mass.
  c. Gamma rays travel faster.

d. Their origin
e. X-rays produce bremsstrahlung radiation and gamma rays do not

7. X-rays have:
   a. 1 amu and are neutral
   b. A negative charge and no rest mass
   c. No mass and a charge of -1
   d. No mass and a charge of $+2$
   e. No mass and no charge

8. Given the general characteristics of ionizing radiation:
   a. All photons travel in straight lines, even in the presence of a magnetic field.
   b. As x-ray energy increases, so does linear energy transfer (LET).
   c. The neutron is a chargeless particle and is therefore non-ionizing radiation.
   d. The range of a beta particle in tissue can extend to a depth of 10 cm.
   e. The range of gamma rays in air normally does not exceed 1 m.

9. Which of the following types of radiation are emitted from outside of the nucleus?
   a. Alpha particles
   b. Beta particles
   c. Gamma rays
   d. Neutrinos
   e. X-rays

10. As compared with particulate radiation, electromagnetic radiation:
    a. Has a higher electrostatic charge
    b. Has higher LET
    c. Is heavier
    d. Is more densely ionizing
    e. Is more penetrating

11. When electromagnetic radiation is compared with particulate radiation, it is *true* that:
    a. Both interact by ionization and excitation.
    b. Particulate radiation exists only at the speed of light.
    c. They are equally penetrating.
    d. They have equal mass.
    e. They have nearly equal LET.

12. Particulate ionizing radiation:
    a. Can include any type of subatomic particle
    b. Has greater range than electromagnetic radiation
    c. Includes ultrasound
    d. Travels at the speed of light
    e. Usually has low LET

13. Electromagnetic ionizing radiation:
    a. Comes from both inside and outside of the nucleus
    b. Has a lower velocity than light
    c. Has a lower velocity than particulate radiation
    d. Includes alpha and beta particles
    e. Includes therapeutic ultrasound

14. X-rays and gamma rays are examples of electromagnetic radiation. In addition, they both have:
    a. No electrostatic charge
    b. Small mass
    c. The same origin
    d. The velocity of ultrasound
    e. Variable velocity

15. Which of the following is an example of ionizing radiation?
    a. Energetic protons
    b. Microwaves
    c. MRI
    d. Therapeutic ultrasound
    e. Ultraviolet radiation

16. How does the energy of a gamma ray compare with the energy of an x-ray?
    a. The question does not give enough information.
    b. They are equal.
    c. The energy of gamma rays is greater than the energy of x-rays.
    d. The energy of gamma rays is less than the energy of x-rays.
    e. The energy of gamma rays is much greater than the energy of x-rays.

17. What are the two principal classes of ionizing radiation?
    a. Diagnostic and particulate
    b. MRI and electromagnetic
    c. MRI and ultrasound
    d. Particulate and electromagnetic
    e. Particulate and ultrasound

18. Which of the following is *not* ionizing radiation?
    a. Auger electrons
    b. Beta particles
    c. Neutrons
    d. Therapeutic ultrasound
    e. X-rays

WORKSHEET

4-1 Photons

 The wave equation is as follows:

$$v = \lambda \times f \ \textit{or} \ \text{Velocity} = \text{Wavelength} \times \text{Frequency}$$

Electromagnetic radiation always travels at the speed of light (3×10^8 m/s), so $v = c$ and, for electromagnetic radiation, $c = f$. The unit of frequency is the hertz (1 Hz = 1 cycle per second).

EXERCISES

1. X-ray wavelength is:
   a. Directly proportional to frequency
   b. Directly proportional to velocity
   c. Inversely proportional to frequency
   d. Inversely proportional to velocity
   e. Usually designated by "c"

2. Which of the following is *true* for both a 100 keV x-ray and a 10 keV gamma ray?
   a. They have equal frequencies.
   b. They have equal negative charges.
   c. They have equal wavelengths.
   d. They have the same origin.
   e. They have zero mass.

3. A frequency of 1 MHz is:
   a. 1 cycle/s
   b. 10^2 cycles/s
   c. 10^3 cycles/s
   d. 10^6 cycles/s
   e. 10^9 cycles/s

4. When the frequency of electromagnetic radiation is increased tenfold:
   a. The velocity decreases to $\frac{1}{10}$.
   b. The velocity increases times 10.
   c. The wavelength remains constant.
   d. The wavelength decreases to $\frac{1}{10}$.
   e. The wavelength increases times 10.

5. A single unit of electromagnetic radiation is also called a/an:
   a. Ion
   b. Photon
   c. Proton
   d. Quark
   e. Strange

6. Light has a constant velocity of $c = 3 \times 10^8$ m/s. Therefore:
   a. Its energy increases with increasing wavelength.
   b. Its frequency decreases with increasing wavelength.
   c. Its mass increases with increasing frequency.
   d. Its velocity is also 3×10^{12} cm/s.
   e. Its velocity is also 3×10^{12} mm/s.

7. The frequency of electromagnetic radiation is:
   a. Measured in disintegrations per second
   b. Measured in hertz
   c. Measured in meters per second
   d. Proportional to the wavelength
   e. Proportional to velocity

8. When one uses the sine wave as a model:
   a. Amplitude and frequency are directly proportional.
   b. Amplitude and wavelength are directly proportional.
   c. The distance from one peak to the next is the wavelength.
   d. The distance from one valley to the next is the frequency.
   e. The energy is proportional to amplitude.

9. Given the sine wave model of electromagnetic radiation:
   a. Amplitude and velocity are inversely related.
   b. Frequency and velocity are inversely related.
   c. Frequency times amplitude is a constant.
   d. Frequency times velocity is a constant.
   e. Frequency times wavelength is a constant.

10. Which of the following has a constant value for all electromagnetic radiation?
    a. Frequency
    b. Mass
    c. Origin
    d. Velocity
    e. Wavelength

11. The velocity of light is:
    a. 3×10^8 cm/s
    b. 3×10^{10} cm/s
    c. 3×10^{12} cm/s
    d. 3.7×10^{10} m/s
    e. 3.7×10^8 m/s

12. The amplitude of a sine wave is its:
    a. Frequency
    b. Minimum to maximum
    c. Velocity
    d. Wavelength
    e. Zero to maximum

13. The frequency of a sine wave is:
    a. The distance from crest to crest
    b. The distance from crest to valley
    c. The minimum to maximum
    d. The number of seconds that pass per crest
    e. The number of valleys that pass per second

14. The wave equation is described as follows:
    a. The product of frequency and velocity is constant.
    b. Velocity is frequency divided by wavelength.
    c. Velocity is wavelength divided by frequency.

d. Wavelength is the product of velocity and frequency.
e. Wavelength is velocity divided by frequency.

15. The velocity of ultrasound in tissue is 1540 m/s. If a 1 MHz transducer is used, what will be the wavelength of the ultrasound?
    a. 15.4 μm
    b. 1.54 mm
    c. 1540 mm
    d. 15.4 cm
    e. 1540 m

16. A 1 tesla MRI device operates at a radiofrequency of 42 MHz. What is the wavelength of this radiation?
    a. 4.2 mm
    b. 7.1 mm
    c. 42 cm
    d. 7.1 m
    e. 42 m

If the figure below represents a wave traveling at 25 cm/s, compute the following:

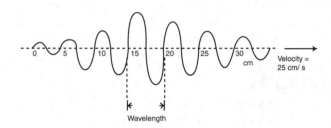

17. How many cycles occur in 1 s (frequency)?
    a. 1
    b. 2
    c. 3
    d. 4
    e. 5

18. How much time is necessary for two cycles?
    a. 0.1 s
    b. 0.2 s
    c. 0.3 s
    d. 0.4 s
    e. 0.8 s

19. What is the wavelength?
    a. 5 cm
    b. 10 cm
    c. 15 cm
    d. 20 cm
    e. 25 cm

20. What distance is traveled in 5 s?
    a. 75 cm
    b. 125 cm
    c. 175 cm
    d. 225 cm
    e. 275 cm

4-2

Electromagnetic Spectrum

The electromagnetic (EM) spectrum includes many types of electromagnetic radiation that extend over 35 orders of magnitude from low-energy radio waves to high-energy x- and y-rays. Each region of the EM spectrum can be identified by energy, wavelength, or frequency through the following equations:

$$E = hf = hc/l \text{ and } c = lf$$

Traditionally, x-rays are identified by their energy, visible light by its wavelength, and radio waves by their frequency.

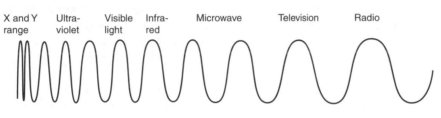

EXERCISES

1. A photon that has energy of approximately 1 eV is *most* likely:
   a. A gamma ray
   b. A radio emission
   c. An x-ray
   d. Therapeutic ultrasound
   e. Visible light

2. When the electromagnetic spectrum is considered, photons of a radio broadcast have relatively:
   a. High energy and long wavelengths
   b. High energy and short wavelengths
   c. High frequency and low energy
   d. Low energy and long wavelengths
   e. Low energy and short wavelengths

3. When white light is refracted through a prism, the following colors are emitted. Which has the longest wavelength?
   a. Blue
   b. Orange

   c. Red
   d. Ultraviolet
   e. Yellow

4. Invisible photons on the long-wavelength side of the visible-light spectrum can create a problem in the darkroom. Which of the following types of light are these photons likely to be?
   a. Green light
   b. Infrared light
   c. Laser light
   d. Maser light
   e. Ultraviolet light

5. The principal difference between x-rays and gamma rays is their:
   a. Energy
   b. Frequency
   c. Origin
   d. Velocity
   e. Wavelength

6. Radiation emitted from a standard radio broad-cast antenna:
   a. Has a higher frequency than gamma rays
   b. Has a higher frequency than microwaves
   c. Has relatively high energy
   d. Is electromagnetic radiation
   e. Is sound

7. For any electromagnetic radiation:
   a. An increase in frequency results in an increase in energy.
   b. An increase in velocity results in an increase in energy.
   c. An increase in velocity results in an increase in frequency.
   d. An increase in wavelength results in an increase in energy.
   e. An increase in wavelength results in higher frequency.

8. Electromagnetic radiation:
   a. Exists at zero velocity
   b. Exists only if its velocity is 3×10^8 m/s
   c. Has energy represented by amplitude
   d. Has mass that increases with increasing velocity
   e. Is usually shown as a square wave

9. If an x-ray imaging system is operated at 40 kVp, then:
   a. 20 keV x-rays are emitted
   b. All x-rays are emitted at 40 keV
   c. Non-ionizing x-rays are emitted
   d. X-rays up to 80 keV are emitted
   e. Zero-energy x-rays are emitted

10. A photon of red light:
   a. Comes from a nucleus
   b. Has a higher frequency than an x-ray
   c. Has a longer wavelength than a photon of green light
   d. Has more energy than blue light
   e. Has the same energy as microwaves

11. Which of the following characteristics is the same for both ultraviolet radiation and microwaves?
   a. Amplitude
   b. Energy
   c. Frequency
   d. Velocity
   e. Wavelength

12. Visible light cannot be:
   a. Absorbed
   b. Diffracted
   c. Reflected
   d. Refracted
   e. Weighed

13. X-rays can be:
   a. Attenuated
   b. Compacted
   c. Ionized
   d. Subdivided
   e. Weighed

14. The electromagnetic spectrum includes:
   a. Particulate radiation at the speed of light
   b. Radiation described by the following formula: Wavelength = Frequency × Velocity
   c. Radiation with physical properties determined by mass
   d. X-rays and radar with the speed of light in a vacuum
   e. X-rays, gamma rays, electrons, and neutrons that are used in medicine

15. Which of the following types of radiation would be classified as electromagnetic?
   a. 5 MHz therapeutic ultrasound
   b. 30 m radio broadcast
   c. 1000 Hz sound
   d. Beta radiation
   e. Heat convected from a radiator

16. Which of the following is an example of electromagnetic radiation?
   a. Alpha rays
   b. Diagnostic ultrasound
   c. Positrons
   d. Protons
   e. Ultraviolet light

17. Examples of electromagnetic radiation would *not* include:
   a. 1.5 T, 63 MHz MRI
   b. Cell phone signals
   c. Forced-air heat
   d. Light from an exit sign
   e. Phosphorescence from a watch dial

18. Which of the following is *not* an example of electromagnetic radiation?
   a. Gamma rays
   b. Grenz rays
   c. Laser radiation
   d. Star light
   e. Ultrasonic diathermy

E = hf (Quantum mechanics)

$$E = hf$$

where E = energy in joules and $h = 6.63 \times 10^{-34}$ J·s, f represents frequency, and h is Planck's constant. E – mc² (relativity).

$$E = mc^2$$

where E = energy in joules and $c = 3 \times 10^8$ m/s, the velocity of an x-ray.

To understand the true nature of photon radiation, both wave and particle concepts must be retained, because wave-like properties are exhibited in some experiments and particle-like properties are exhibited in others.

EXERCISES

1. Which of the following is *not* a characteristic of the wave model of radiation?
   a. Collision
   b. Deflection
   c. Reflection
   d. Refraction
   e. Transmission

2. Which of the following *most* closely represents the term *attenuation*?
   a. Absorption of x-rays
   b. Deflection of x-rays
   c. Light absorbed in black glass
   d. Light reflected from a mirror
   e. Light transmitted through frosted glass

3. When a radiograph is viewed, one might properly state that:
   a. Bony structures are radiolucent.
   b. Fat is radiopaque.
   c. Fat is radioreflective.
   d. Lung tissue is radiolucent.
   e. Soft tissue is radiopaque.

4. The development of modern quantum mechanics is attributed to:
   a. Albert Nobel
   b. Ernest Rutherford
   c. Max Planck
   d. Niels Bohr
   e. William Coolidge

5. According to quantum mechanics, the energy of an x-ray is:
   a. Dependent on its origin
   b. Dependent on its velocity
   c. Directly proportional to its wavelength
   d. Inversely proportional to its wavelength
   e. Proportional to its amplitude

6. The expression that relates x-ray energy and wavelength through Planck's constant is:
   a. $E = hf$
   b. $E = hc$
   c. $E = hc/\lambda$
   d. $E = h/c\lambda$
   e. $E = \lambda c/h$

7. Which of the following statements about visible light is *true*?
   a. It can travel with any velocity up to 3 × 10^8 m/s.
   b. It is deflected by a magnetic field.
   c. It sometimes behaves like a wave.
   d. Its energy is directly proportional to its wavelength.
   e. The photoelectric effect demonstrates the wave model.

8. Visible light:
   a. Consists of short-wavelength red radiation and long-wavelength blue radiation
   b. Has a higher frequency than ultraviolet light
   c. Has a shorter wavelength than microwaves
   d. Has a wavelength range of 1 to 100 mm
   e. Interacts with matter in the same way that x-rays do

9. Which of the following terms is *not* associated with visible-light interaction?
   a. Absorption
   b. Reflection
   c. Refraction
   d. Transmission
   e. Vaporization

10. Which statement about visible light is *correct*?
    a. Black glass is lucent.
    b. If matter absorbs visible light, it is transparent.
    c. If matter attenuates visible light, it is opaque.
    d. If visible light is transmitted but attenuated, the matter is transparent.
    e. If visible light is transmitted unattenuated, the matter is lucent.

11. In radiographs of bony structures embedded in soft tissue, the bone is:
    a. Radiolucent
    b. Radiopaque
    c. Radiorefracted
    d. Translucent
    e. Transopaque

12. Which of the following statements about photon interaction is *true*?
    a. Air is transparent and radiopaque.
    b. Frosted glass is transparent.
    c. Lead is radiopaque.
    d. Soft tissue is radiopaque.
    e. Window glass is opaque.

13. Which type of electromagnetic radiation is *not* used for medical imaging?
    a. Gamma rays
    b. Microwaves
    c. Radiofrequency
    d. Visible light
    e. X-rays

14. When compared with visible light, x-rays have greater:
    a. Charge
    b. Frequency
    c. Mass
    d. Velocity
    e. Wavelength

15. Which of the following types of electromagnetic radiation interacts with matter such as a particle?
    a. Gamma rays
    b. Infrared radiation
    c. Microwaves
    d. Radiofrequencies

16. At what level should visible light interact *most* readily?
    a. Atomic
    b. Molecular
    c. Nucleon
    d. Organ
    e. Tissue

17. Compared with red light, green light has greater:
    a. Charge
    b. Energy
    c. Mass
    d. Velocity
    e. Wavelength

18. The equivalent mass of an x-ray may be computed using:
    a. $m = hc/\lambda$
    b. $m = hc/f$
    c. $m = h\lambda/c^2$
    d. $m = hf/c^2$
    e. $m = hf\lambda/c^2$

19. A surface of which color reflects the *most* light?
    a. Black
    b. Blue
    c. Green
    d. Red
    e. White

WORKSHEET

4-4

Inverse Square Law

Radiation intensity decreases rapidly as the distance from the source increases. The intensity of radiation is inversely proportional to the square of the distance from the source to the object.

Inverse square law:

$$I_1/I_2 = d_2^2/d_1^2 = (d_2/d_1)^2$$

where I_1 is the intensity at distance d_1 from the source, and I_2 is the intensity at distance d_2 from the source.

EXERCISES

1. A source of ^{99m}Tc produces a radiation intensity of 150 mR/hr (1.5 μGy$_a$/hr) at 10 m. At what distance does the exposure rate equal 1000 mR/hr?
   a. 3.3 m
   b. 3.9 m
   c. 5.0 m
   d. 6.7 m
   e. 8.2 m

2. If the exposure rate 1 m from a source is 9 mR/hr (90 μGy$_a$/h), what is the exposure rate 3 m from the source?
   a. 9 mR/hr
   b. 3 mR/hr
   c. 1 mR/hr
   d. 0.9 mR/hr
   e. 0.1 mR/hr

3. The inverse square law states that:
   a. Intensity and distance are proportional.
   b. Intensity is directly proportional to the square of the distance.

   c. Intensity is inversely proportional to the square of the distance.
   d. The square of the intensity is directly proportional to the distance.
   e. The square of the intensity is inversely proportional to the distance.

4. The inverse square law is a result of:
   a. Absorption
   b. Attenuation
   c. Divergence
   d. Scatter
   e. Transmission

5. The inverse square relationship applies to which of the following sources?
   a. Gamma ray
   b. Plane
   c. Point
   d. Ultrasound
   e. X-ray

6. Which of the following emissions is likely to obey the inverse square law?
   a. Heat from an iron skillet
   b. Infrared radiation from a patient
   c. Skylight
   d. Visible light from an 8 ft fluorescent bulb
   e. X-rays from a mobile imaging system

7. To apply the inverse square law, one must know:
   a. Energy, distance, and intensity
   b. One distance and one intensity
   c. The frequency or the wavelength of radiation

   d. Two distances and one intensity
   e. Two intensities and two distances

8. If the distance from a point source is tripled, the intensity will be:
   a. Nine times
   b. One half
   c. One ninth
   d. One third
   e. Three times

9. If an instrument positioned 1 m from a point source is moved 50 cm closer to the source, the radiation intensity will:
   a. Decrease by a factor of 2
   b. Decrease by a factor of 4
   c. Increase by a factor of 2
   d. Increase by a factor of 4
   e. Remain constant

10. The distance from the earth to the sun is approximately 150 million km. If the earth were orbiting the sun at 50 million km, the solar intensity on the surface of the earth would be:
   a. 3 times more intense
   b. 9 times more intense
   c. 12 times more intense
   d. 27 times more intense
   e. The same

11. A linear source of radium is 15 mm long. Such a source of radiation obeys the inverse square law at approximately what minimum distance from the source?
   a. At contact
   b. 15 mm
   c. 25 mm
   d. 75 mm
   e. 105 mm

12. How far from a 4 ft fluorescent bulb must one be before its light approximately obeys the inverse square law?
   a. 4 ft
   b. 8 ft
   c. 12 ft
   d. 20 ft
   e. 28 ft

13. A ^{137}Cs source used for instrument calibration has an intensity of 100 mR/hr (1mGy$_a$/hr) at 20 cm. What would the intensity be 40 cm from the source?
   a. 8.25 mR/hr
   b. 12.5 mR/hr
   c. 25 mR/hr
   d. 50 mR/hr
   e. 75 mR/hr

14. The exposure rate from a ^{60}Co source used in radiation therapy is 100 R/min (1 Gy$_a$/min) at 80 cm. What would the exposure rate be 40 cm from the source?
   a. 25 R/m
   b. 50 R/m
   c. 100 R/m
   d. 200 R/m
   e. 400 R/m

15. A radiographic technique produces a patient dose of 200 mrad (2 mGy$_a$) at a source-to-skin distance (SSD) of 80 cm. What would be the patient dose at an SSD of 160 cm if the technique remains the same?
   a. 50 mrad
   b. 80 mrad
   c. 100 mrad
   d. 200 mrad
   e. 400 mrad

16. A radiographic technique produces an exposure of 200 mR (2 mGy$_a$) at a source-to-image receptor distance (SID) of 100 cm. What would the exposure be at an SID of 180 cm?
   a. 31 mR
   b. 55 mR
   c. 62 mR
   d. 111 mR
   e. 125 mR

17. A radiograph produced at an SID of 100 cm results in an exposure of 100 mR (1 mGy$_a$). What would be the exposure if the SID were reduced to 90 cm?
   a. 72 mR
   b. 81 mR
   c. 90 mR
   d. 111 mR
   e. 123 mR

X-rays also may be thought of as bundles of energy called *quanta* or *photons*. These x-ray photons travel at the speed of light, have direction, possess no mass or charge, and have electric and magnetic components that vary in a sinusoidal fashion. X rays adhere to the following mathematical relationships:

$$c = \lambda f \qquad E = mc^2$$

$$E = hf \qquad \lambda(nm) = \frac{1.24}{keV}$$

$$E = \frac{hc}{\lambda}$$

EXERCISES

1. Which of the following terms is associated with diagnostic imaging?
   a. Diffraction x-rays
   b. Grenz x-rays
   c. Megavoltage x-rays
   d. Superficial x-rays
   e. Supervoltage x-rays

2. Which of the following terms does *not* apply to an x-ray?
   a. Absorption
   b. Attenuation
   c. Diffraction
   d. Penetration
   e. Reflection

3. Given two x-rays, one of 50 keV and the other of 70 keV, the 70 keV x-ray:
   a. Is most likely radioactive
   b. Most likely came from a nucleus
   c. Has a higher velocity
   d. Has a longer wavelength
   e. Has a higher frequency

4. In the normal representation of an x-ray:
   a. Energy is amplitude.
   b. Mass is indicated by c.
   c. Velocity is the speed of light.
   d. Velocity varies from zero to the speed of light.
   e. Wavelength changes from short to long and back to short again.

5. The energy of an x-ray photon is directly proportional to its:
   a. Frequency
   b. Mass
   c. Velocity
   d. Velocity squared
   e. Wavelength

6. In a vacuum, x-rays travel with a velocity of:
   a. 186,000 km/hr
   b. 186,000 mph
   c. 3×10^{10} m/s
   d. 3×10^{10} cm/s
   e. 3.7×10^{10} cm/s

7. Which of the following is greater for a 30 keV x-ray than for a 60 keV x-ray?
   a. Charge
   b. Frequency
   c. Mass
   d. Velocity
   e. Wavelength

8. Which of the following electromagnetic radiations is in the diagnostic x-ray region?
   a. 78 eV
   b. 12,000 eV
   c. 65 keV
   d. 36 MeV
   e. 14 meV

9. The photon energy of an x-ray whose wavelength is 10 nm may be obtained *most* easily from which of the following?
   a. $E = mc^2$
   b. $E = hf$
   c. $E = hc/\lambda$
   d. $E = \lambda n$
   e. $E = \lambda/hc$

10. When x-rays are described, it can be said that:
    a. They are deflected by a very strong magnet.
    b. They can combine with other x-rays to form an atom.
    c. They can create molecules.
    d. They have a longer wavelength than radio waves.
    e. They travel in straight lines.

11. X-ray photons:
    a. Are part of the ultrasonic spectrum
    b. Are relatively long-wavelength electromagnetic radiation
    c. Have a higher frequency than visible light
    d. Have a longer wavelength than radiofrequencies
    e. Have the same velocity as ultrasound

12. The energy of an x-ray:
    a. Can be computed from its mass
    b. Depends on its charge
    c. Increases with increasing wavelength
    d. Is a function of Einstein's constant
    e. Is inversely proportional to its wavelength

13. The model used to describe an x-ray photon:
    a. Consists of an S wave
    b. Has a radiofrequency field and a visual field
    c. Has an electric field and an ultrasonic field
    d. Has an ultrasonic field and a magnetic field
    e. Is a sine wave

14. Planck's constant has units of:
    a. J
    b. J-eV
    c. J-kg
    d. J-s
    e. N-s

15. Which of the following characteristics is the same for both x-ray photons and light photons?
    a. Amplitude is the same.
    b. Energy is the same.
    c. Frequency is the same.
    d. Velocity is the same.
    e. Wavelength is the same.

16. X-rays:
    a. Have a mass of 1 amu and are neutral
    b. Have a negative charge and zero rest mass
    c. Have a positive charge and zero rest mass
    d. Have zero rest mass and a charge of plus two
    e. Have zero rest mass and are neutral

17. In the model of an x-ray:
    a. The amplitude of the sine wave is related to its energy.
    b. The frequency of the sine wave is related to its velocity.
    c. The wavelength of the sine wave is related to its velocity.
    d. Two sine waves are positioned perpendicular to each other.
    e. Two sine waves are superimposed.

18. Diagnostic x-rays are:
    a. High-energy electromagnetic radiation
    b. Long-wavelength electromagnetic radiation
    c. Observed with varying velocity
    d. Photons with intermediate mass
    e. Photons with low frequency

19. An x-ray also can be correctly called a:
    a. Mass
    b. Photon
    c. Pronon
    d. Proton
    e. Quantity

4-6

Matter and Energy

Einstein expressed the equivalence of mass and energy with the following equation:

$$E = mc^2$$

In the equation, if E is energy in joules, then c (the speed of light) must be 3×10^8 m/s, and m (the mass) must be measured in kilograms.

EXERCISES

1. Which of the following equations can be used to compute the mass equivalence of an x-ray photon?
   a. $m = Ec^2$
   b. $m = zv^2$
   c. $m = \dfrac{E}{c^2}$
   d. $m = \frac{1}{2} E^2$
   e. $m = Ev$

2. Which of the following equations can be used to compute the mass equivalence of an x-ray if its frequency is known?
   a. $m = \dfrac{E}{c^2}$
   b. $m = Ec^2$
   c. $m = \dfrac{hf}{c^2}$
   d. $m = h/\lambda f$
   e. $m = \frac{1}{2} c^2$

3. In the case of mass-energy conversions:
   a. Nuclear fission is an example.
   b. The inverse square law applies.

c. The law of conservation of energy is violated.
   d. The law of conservation of matter is violated.
   e. The wave equation is an example.

4. In Einstein's relativistic equation, $E = mc^2$:
   a. c represents the velocity of ultrasound.
   b. If the mass is measured in kg and the velocity in m/s, energy will be measured in J.
   c. If the mass is measured in g, the velocity must be measured in m/s.
   d. If the velocity is 3×10^8 m/s, mass should be in g.
   e. If the velocity is given as 186,000 mi/s, the energy will be in N.

5. When Einstein's relativistic equation is used to compute the energy equivalence of matter, it is usual to express such energy in:
   a. Calories
   b. Coulombs
   c. Ergs
   d. Joules
   e. Newtons

6. Energy can be:
   a. Created but not destroyed
   b. Destroyed but not created
   c. Expressed in newtons
   d. Measured in rad
   e. Transformed into matter

7. The energy equivalence of an electron at rest is 511 keV. It is also:
   a. 511 eV
   b. 511 MeV
   c. 0.51 eV
   d. 0.51 MeV
   e. 5.1 MeV

8. When various types of radiation are compared:
   a. The mass equivalence of a television broadcast is greater than that of red light.
   b. The mass equivalence of an FM broadcast is greater than that of ultraviolet light.
   c. The mass equivalence of blue light is greater than that of red light.
   d. The mass equivalence of microwaves is greater than that of x-rays.
   e. The mass equivalence of red light is greater than that of ultraviolet.

9. If the entire mass of an electron (m = 9.1×10^{-31} kg) could be converted into an x-ray, its energy would be approximately:
   a. 4.15×10^{-15} eV-s
   b. 4.15×10^{-15} keV-s
   c. 511,000 eV
   d. 511 eV
   e. 5.1 MeV

10. One amu equals 1.66×10^{-27} kg. Its energy equivalence is:
    a. 1.5×10^{-10} J
    b. 1.5×10^{-7} J
    c. 1.5 kJ
    d. 1.5 mJ
    e. 1.5 nJ

11. What is the mass equivalence of a 35 keV x-ray?
    a. 6.3×10^{-31} kg
    b. 6.3×10^{-32} kg
    c. 6.3×10^{-33} kg
    d. 6.3×10^{-34} kg
    e. 6.3×10^{-35} kg

12. The SI unit for energy is the:
    a. Dyne
    b. Electron volt
    c. Erg
    d. Joule
    e. Newton

13. The energy of a 70 keV x-ray can be expressed as:
    a. 1.1×10^{-16} J
    b. 1.1×10^{-14} J
    c. 1.1×10^{-12} J
    d. 1.1×10^{-10} J
    e. 1.1×10^{-9} J

14. The equivalence of mass and energy is described by:
    a. the Bohr constant
    b. Einstein's theory
    c. Joule's laws
    d. Newton's laws
    e. Planck's theory

15. The energy of diagnostic x-rays is similar to that of which of the following radiations?
    a. Diffraction x-rays
    b. Grenz x-rays
    c. Megzvoltage radiation
    d. Orthovoltage x-rays
    e. Superficial x-rays

16. In the equation E = hf, the *h*:
    a. Has units of energy
    b. Is a variable
    c. Stands for Einstein's constant
    d. Stands for the Bohr constant
    e. Relates photon energy to frequency

17. The product j of hc is equal to:
    a. 1.24 keV—nm
    b. 1.24 ev—mm
    c. 12.4 keV—nm
    d. 12.4 eV—m
    e. 1.24 eV—m

18. Longer-wavelength x-rays have:
    a. Higher energy
    b. Higher mass
    c. Higher velocity
    d. Lower energy
    e. Lower velocity

5-1

Electrostatics

 Electrostatics is the study of stationary electric charges:

- Electrified objects have excess charges.
- Objects can be electrified by contact, friction, or induction.
- Opposite charges attract; like charges repel.
- The magnitude of the attraction or repulsion is given by Coulomb's law:

$$F = k \frac{Q_a Q_b}{d^2}$$

where F is the force in newtons (attractive or repulsive), Q_a and Q_b are electrostatic charges in coulombs, d is separation distance in meters, and k is the proportionality constant ($k = 9.0 \times 10^9 \, N - m^2/C^2$).

EXERCISES

1. What is the principal reservoir for excess electric charge?
   a. Clouds
   b. Lightning rod
   c. The atmosphere
   d. The earth
   e. Water pipes

2. Regarding the movement of an electric charge from one atom to another atom:
   a. Both positive and negative charges can move.
   b. It must occur in a large atom.
   c. Only positive charges move.
   d. Usually inner-shell electrons move.
   e. Usually outer-shell electrons move.

3. Electric energy can be converted into:
   a. Chemical energy by an x-ray imaging system
   b. Electromagnetic energy by a battery
   c. Mechanical energy by a battery
   d. Nuclear energy in a nuclear reactor
   e. Thermal energy by a lamp

4. Electrostatics:
   a. Concerns resting electric charges
   b. Concerns the mass-energy conversion of electrons
   c. Governs the movement of electric charges in a conductor
   d. Is the conversion of kinetic energy
   e. Is the study of photon radiation

5. Coulomb's law states that electrostatic force is:
   a. Dependent on mAs
   b. Directly proportional to the square of the distance between charges
   c. Directly proportional to the square of the product of charges
   d. Inversely proportional to the product of charges
   e. Inversely proportional to the square of the distance between charges

6. Which of the following is a method of electrification?
   a. Diffraction
   b. Excitation
   c. Induction
   d. Resonance
   e. Transmission

7. Static electricity:
   a. Can make one's hair stand on end
   b. Can produce x-rays
   c. Can result in magnetism
   d. Is the basis for transformer operation
   e. Is the study of electric currents

8. The unit of electrostatic charge is the:
   a. Ampere
   b. Coulomb
   c. Electron volt
   d. Newton
   e. Volt

9. The principal electrostatic law states that:
   a. A neutron will repel a neutron.
   b. A proton will repel a neutron.
   c. An electron will repel a neutron.
   d. An electron will repel a proton.
   e. An electron will repel an electron.

10. Objects become electrified because of:
    a. An excess of neutrons
    b. An excess of protons
    c. The transfer of electrons
    d. The transfer of neutrons
    e. The transfer of protons

11. The phenomenon of lightning occurs when:
    a. Adjacent clouds are electrically neutral.
    b. Adjacent clouds have negative electrification.
    c. Adjacent clouds have positive electrification.
    d. One cloud is positively electrified and an adjacent one is negatively electrified.
    e. Thunder is heard.

12. Which of the following would be included as one of the four basic electrostatic laws?
    a. Archimedes' principle
    b. Conversion to magnetism
    c. Einstein's law
    d. Electric charge concentration
    e. Planck's law

13. An electrostatic force is created when a/an:
    a. Electrostatic charge exists.
    b. Neutron approaches a neutron.
    c. Neutron approaches an electron.
    d. Proton approaches a neutron.
    e. Proton approaches a proton.

14. A radiographic tube is operated at 500 mA. How many electrons per second is this?
    a. 3.2×10^9
    b. 3.2×10^{18}

c. 6.3×10^9
d. 6.3×10^{17}
e. 6.3×10^{18}

15. The unit of electrostatic force is the:
    a. Coulomb
    b. Electron volt
    c. Joule
    d. Newton
    e. Rad

16. Which of the following are *not* affected by electrostatically charged matter?
    a. Alpha particles
    b. Beta particles
    c. Electrons
    d. Protons
    e. X-rays

17. How many electrons are contained in 0.5 μC?
    a. 3.2×10^6
    b. 3.2×10^{12}
    c. 6.3×10^6
    d. 6.3×10^{12}
    e. 6.3×10^{18}

18. When a copper conductor becomes electrified:
    a. A kink in the wire will have higher surface electrification.
    b. Excess electrons are uniformly distributed throughout the wire.
    c. It becomes heated.
    d. Negative charges concentrate on the surface, and positive charges are distributed throughout.
    e. The distribution of protons on its surface is uniform.

19. The unit of electric potential is the:
    a. Ampere
    b. Coulomb
    c. Newton
    d. Ohm
    e. Volt

20. Two positive 0.5 C charges are positioned 1.0 m apart. The force acting between them is:
    a. Attractive
    b. Exponential
    c. Neutral
    d. Repulsive
    e. Variable

OHM'S LAW

Ohm's law: $V = IR$ where V is the electric potential in volts, I is the electric current in amperes, and R is the electric resistance in ohms (Ω).

SERIES CIRCUITS

Total resistance: $R_T = R_1 + R_2 + R_3 \ldots$
Total current: $I_T = I_1 + I_2 + I_3 \ldots$
Total voltage: $V_T = V_1 + V_2 + V_3 \ldots$

PARALLEL CIRCUITS

Total resistance: $\dfrac{1}{RT} = \dfrac{1}{R1} + \dfrac{1}{R2} + \dfrac{1}{R} + \ldots$

Total current: $I_T = I_1 + I_2 + I_3 + \ldots$
Total voltage: $V_T = V_1 = V_2 = V_3 \ldots$

EXERCISES

1. Which of the following is the best electric insulator?
   a. Aluminum
   b. Copper
   c. Nickel
   d. Water
   e. Wood

2. The ratio of the electric potential across a circuit element to the current flowing through that element is called:
   a. Current
   b. Energy
   c. Power
   d. Resistance
   e. Voltage

3. The electrical resistance of wire increases as the diameter of the:
   a. Insulator decreases.
   b. Insulator increases.
   c. Power supply increases.
   d. Wire decreases.
   e. Wire increases.

4. When an electric current flows through a wire with resistance (R), energy is:
   a. Absorbed as heat
   b. Absorbed as light
   c. Generated as heat
   d. Generated as x-rays
   e. Transformed to mass

5. When electrons move in a copper wire:
   a. Resistance to the electron flow exists.
   b. Ionization occurs.
   c. The condition is called electromagnetic force.
   d. The condition is called electrostatics.
   e. They move down the middle of the wire.

6. The number of volts required to cause a current of 40 A in a circuit having a resistance of 5 Ω is:
   a. 5 V
   b. 8 V
   c. 40 V
   d. 45 V
   e. 200 V

7. The unit of electric potential is the:
   a. Ampere
   b. Coulomb
   c. Joule
   d. Ohm
   e. Volt

8. Ohm's law states that:
   a. Electric current is the product of voltage and resistance.
   b. Electric power is equal to current squared times voltage.
   c. Electric power is equal to voltage times current.
   d. The electric potential is equal to current squared times resistance.
   e. The electric potential is the product of current and resistance.

9. The flow of 1 C/s in a conductor is equal to:
   a. 1 Ω
   b. 1 A
   c. 1 eV
   d. 1 kVp
   e. 1 V

10. In a series circuit:
    a. Ohm's law fails.
    b. Only three circuit elements are allowed.
    c. The total current is the sum of the individual currents.
    d. The total resistance is the sum of the individual resistances.
    e. The voltage drop across each circuit element is the same.

11. In electrodynamics, which of the following is a *correct* expression?
    a. I = Qt
    b. R = I²V
    c. R = IV
    d. V = IR
    e. V = I/R

12. Which of the following is normally measured in volts?
    a. Electric potential
    b. Electromagnetic force
    c. Electromagnetic potential
    d. Electromagnetic radiation
    e. Electrostatic force

13. Milliampere seconds (mAs) is a unit of:
    a. Electric current
    b. Electric potential
    c. Electromagnetic force
    d. Electromotive force
    e. Electrostatic charge

14. Electric insulators:
    a. Consist of materials like silicon and germanium
    b. Convert electric energy to electromagnetic energy

c. Convert electric energy to heat
d. Inhibit movement of electric charge
e. Permit movement of electric charge

15. 1 A is equal to:
    a. 1 Ω/s
    b. 1 C/s
    c. 1 eV/s
    d. 1 J/s
    e. 1 V/s

Match each of the following circuit elements with its appropriate symbol:
_____ 16. Battery
_____ 17. Capacitor
_____ 18. Resistor
_____ 19. Switch
_____ 20. Transformer

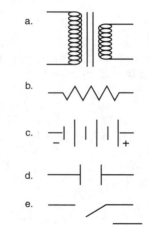

Match each of the following descriptions of circuit elements with the appropriate symbol:
_____ 21. Allows electrons to flow in only one direction
_____ 22. Increases or decreases voltage
_____ 23. Inhibits the flow of electrons
_____ 24. Measures electric current
_____ 25. Momentarily stores electric charge

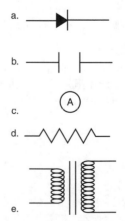

5-3 Alternating and Direct Currents

- Direct current (DC), which is usually provided by a battery, flows in one direction.
- Alternating current (AC) supplies power at 60 Hz.
- Electric power is measured in watts (W).

$$P = VI$$

Power (W) = Voltage (V) × Current (I)

and

$$P = I^2R$$

Power (W) = (Current [I]² × Resistance [R])

and

$$E = Pt$$

Electric energy (J) = Power (W) × Time (s)

EXERCISES

Exercises 1 to 6 refer to the following figure:

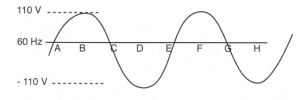

1. The length of time that elapses between A and E is:
   a. ½ s
   b. ⅟30 s
   c. ⅟60 s
   d. ⅟120 s
   e. ⅟240 s

2. One full cycle extends from:
   a. A to C
   b. B to F
   c. C to E
   d. D to E
   e. D to F

3. Considering the positive voltage pulse E to G, how many such pulses occur each second?
   a. 15
   b. 30
   c. 60
   d. 120
   e. 240

4. Given this waveform:
   a. The voltage at C is 60 Hz.
   b. The voltage at D is 60 Hz.
   c. The voltage at E is +110 V.
   d. The voltage at E is zero.
   e. The voltage at H is zero.

5. When one compares the figure segment from A to B with that from to B to C:
   a. Electron flow is fastest at B.
   b. Electrons are flowing faster from A to B than from B to C.
   c. Electrons are flowing in opposite directions at A and C.
   d. Electrons are speeding up from A to B and slowing down from B to C.
   e. The electric potential is higher at A than it is at C.

6. When one compares the segment from A to C with that from C to E:
   a. Electron flow is in opposite directions at B and D.
   b. Electrons are flowing more slowly between C and E.
   c. Electrons have more potential between A and C.
   d. Maximum electron velocity is at A, C, and E.
   e. The electromotive force is higher at B than it is at D.

7. The distinct difference between alternating current (AC) and direct current (DC) is that:
   a. DC can attain higher current.
   b. DC can attain higher voltage.
   c. DC electron flow is in one direction.
   d. DC electron flow varies in amplitude.
   e. DC has higher electrical resistance.

8. If a 60 W light bulb is operated at 120 V, the current flowing through the bulb is approximately:
   a. 0.5 A
   b. 1 A
   c. 50 A
   d. 100 A
   e. 500 A

9. An x-ray imaging system has a 30 kW generator. If the maximum tube voltage is 150 kV, what is the available tube current?
   a. 200 mA
   b. 400 mA
   c. 600 mA
   d. 2 A
   e. 5 A

10. If a sine curve is used to represent 60 Hz AC, then:
    a. During the negative half-cycle, there is no electron flow.
    b. The amplitude of the curve is directly related to wavelength.
    c. The time from a positive peak to the next negative valley is 8 ms.
    d. The time from zero crossing to maximum amplitude is one cycle.
    e. The time from zero crossing to maximum amplitude is one-half cycle.

11. When electricity exists as 60 Hz AC:
    a. Electrons flow in one direction in alternating bursts.
    b. Electrons flow randomly in both directions.
    c. The number of electrons is proportional to the voltage.
    d. The velocity of electron flow is proportional to the current.
    e. The velocity of electron flow is proportional to the voltage.

12. In the United States, normal household electric power is:
    a. 50 V, 120 Hz, three phase
    b. 60 V, 120 Hz, single phase
    c. 120 V, 50 Hz, three phase
    d. 120 V, 60 Hz, single phase
    e. 120 V, 60 Hz, three phase

13. The unit of electric power is the:
    a. Hertz
    b. Joule
    c. Newton
    d. Volt
    e. Watt

14. Electricity is purchased on the basis of the kilowatt hours one consumes. The kilowatt hour also can be expressed in the unit:
    a. Amperes per second
    b. Joule
    c. Newton
    d. Volt
    e. Watts per ampere

15. Which of the following equations can be used to calculate electric power (P) consumption?
    a. $P = I^2 V$
    b. $P = IR$
    c. $P = IV$
    d. $P = VR$
    e. $P = V/R$

16. A hair dryer is rated at 1000 W. Approximately what current will it produce on a normal 120 V, 60 Hz AC household supply?
    a. 8 A
    b. 10 A
    c. 80 A
    d. 110 A
    e. 800 A

WORKSHEET
5-4

Magnetism

- There are three states of magnetism: ferromagnetic, paramagnetic, and diamagnetic. Strongly magnetized material is ferromagnetic. Weakly magnetized material is paramagnetic. Nonmagnetic material is diamagnetic.
- The degree of magnetism increases as the number of unpaired electrons in an atom increases.
- Magnetic permeability is the property of a material to attract magnetic field lines.
- Magnetic susceptibility is the ease with which a material can be rendered magnetic.

EXERCISES

1. Which of the following is a physical property that we cannot sense?
   a. Acceleration
   b. Electric current
   c. Heat
   d. Magnetism
   e. Mass

2. An example of a magnetic domain is:
   a. A bar magnet
   b. A nucleus
   c. A permanent magnet
   d. An electromagnet
   e. The Earth

3. If a bar magnet were suspended in space and another bar of nonmagnetic material were brought close to it, what would happen?
   a. Nothing
   b. The bar magnet would be attracted.

   c. The bar magnet would become demagnetized.
   d. The bar magnet would rotate.
   e. The imaginary magnetic field lines would be deviated.

4. If two bar magnets suspended in space were brought together, what would happen?
   a. Nothing
   b. One would rotate.
   c. The north pole of one would point to the north pole of the other.
   d. They would rotate and attract.
   e. They would rotate and repel.

5. A lodestone is an example of:
   a. A magnetic domain
   b. A natural magnet
   c. An electromagnet
   d. Demagnetized matter
   e. Paramagnetism

6. Which of the following would likely be classified as ferromagnetic material?
   a. Air
   b. Glass
   c. Iron
   d. Lead
   e. Water

7. If two magnets are bought together, north-to-north poles will _____, whereas north-to-south poles will _____.
   a. Attract; attract
   b. Attract; repel

c. Not interact; interact
d. Repel; attract
e. Repel; repel

8. Most magnets:
   a. Are affected by another magnetic field
   b. Are diamagnetic
   c. Are naturally occurring if used in science and technology
   d. Have north, south, and neutral poles
   e. Have positive, negative, and neutral poles

9. Most magnetic materials are:
   a. Also radioactive
   b. Attracted to copper
   c. Bar shaped
   d. Shaped like a horseshoe
   e. Still magnetic when broken

10. A navigational compass:
    a. Has a north pole that is attracted to the equator
    b. Has a north pole that is attracted to the magnetic north pole of the Earth
    c. Has both a north and a south pole
    d. Is usually made of glass
    e. Will not work at the equator

11. Which of the following is a classification of magnetism?
    a. Coulombic
    b. Diploic
    c. Electromagnetism
    d. Paramagnetism
    e. Polar magnetism

12. The Earth's magnetic field is strongest:
    a. At the equator
    b. At the poles
    c. In deep space
    d. In near space
    e. In the atmosphere above the equator

13. The physical laws of magnetism:
    a. Include the conversion to electricity
    b. Include the conservation of magnetism
    c. Require that there be a south pole for every north pole
    d. Require that there be a south pole for every north pole but only for magnets of certain shapes
    e. Specify a force that increases with increasing distance from the magnet

14. Which of the following can create a magnetic field?
    a. A neutron at rest
    b. A quantum of visible light
    c. A spinning proton
    d. A stable atom
    e. An x-ray

15. The force between the poles of two bar magnets:
    a. Depends on the permeability of matter separating the magnets
    b. Is inversely proportional to the strength of each magnet
    c. Obeys a law similar in form to Planck's law
    d. Obeys the inverse square law
    e. Varies directly with the distance between them

16. When iron is fabricated into a magnet, magnetic domains:
    a. Align
    b. Cancel
    c. Disappear
    d. Induce
    e. Magnify

17. Magnetism has some properties similar to those of electrostatics, such as:
    a. Both can be converted to mass.
    b. Both can be sensed by touch.
    c. Both involve proton-type radiation.
    d. Both obey the inverse square law.
    e. Both refer to iron substances.

18. Magnetism:
    a. Can be converted to electricity
    b. Depends on monopolar atoms
    c. Is defined as a property that can attract glass, wood, or metal
    d. Is present in some naturally occurring ores
    e. Requires electricity

19. When a charged particle moves in a straight line, a magnetic field is:
    a. Created along the direction of particle motion
    b. Created and has the same sign as the particle
    c. Created perpendicular to the particle motion.
    d. Erased
    e. Reversed

20. Which of the following has an associated magnetic field?
    a. Helium atom
    b. Hydrogen atom
    c. Hydrogen nucleus
    d. Neutron
    e. Stationary electron

21. When iron is brought near a permanent magnet, the lines of the magnetic field are:
    a. Attracted to the iron
    b. Attracted to the magnet
    c. Repelled by the iron
    d. Repelled by the magnet
    e. Unaffected

A current-carrying coil of wire creates a magnetic field. If an iron core is inserted, the magnetic field becomes many times more intense because the magnetic permeability of iron is greater than that of air. Such a device is called an *electromagnet*. Electromagnets are used in some x-ray imaging systems as switches.

EXERCISES

1. An electron moving in a conductor:
   a. Causes the conductor to behave as a bar magnet
   b. Causes the conductor to bend
   c. Produces a magnetic field in the conductor
   d. Produces a magnetic field perpendicular to the conductor
   e. Produces light in the conductor

2. The voltaic pile:
   a. Consists of a magnet and a conductor
   b. Consists of a pile of charges
   c. Consists of zinc and copper plates sandwiched together
   d. Is a modern dry-cell battery
   e. Was invented by Faraday

3. Electromotive force (EMF):
   a. Is an electrical mechanical force
   b. Is expressed in joules
   c. Is expressed in volts
   d. Stands for electromagnetic field
   e. Was discovered by Hans Oersted

4. The experimental link connecting electric and magnetic forces was discovered by:
   a. Edison
   b. Faraday
   c. Lenz
   d. Oersted
   e. Volta

5. The device designed to measure electron flow in a conductor is known as a/an:
   a. Ammeter
   b. Choke coil
   c. Electromagnet
   d. Solenoid
   e. Voltmeter

6. The fact that an electric current is induced if the conductor is in a changing magnetic field:
   a. Is known as Faraday's law
   b. Is known as Ohm's law
   c. Is the statement of the second law of electromagnetics
   d. Was discovered by Lenz
   e. Was discovered by Volta

7. The term *electromagnetic induction* refers to the production of:
   a. A magnetic field
   b. A static charge
   c. An electric current
   d. An electromagnet
   e. Electromagnetic radiation

8. A difference between self-induction and mutual induction is that:
   a. Mutual induction is the basis for an electric motor and self-induction is the basis for a transformer.
   b. Mutual induction requires two coils and self-induction requires only one.
   c. Only self-induction can create EMF.
   d. Self-induction requires two coils and mutual induction requires only one.
   e. There is no difference.

9. The magnetic field produced by an electromagnet has:
   a. Alternating poles
   b. Neither a north nor a south pole
   c. Only a north pole
   d. Only a south pole
   e. Properties similar to a bar magnet

10. One law of electromagnetics states that:
    a. An electric current is induced in a circuit if some part of that circuit is in a magnetic field.
    b. Electrostatics can be converted to magnetism.
    c. The induced current flows in the opposite direction of the inducing action.
    d. The right-hand rule is used to determine the direction of the induced current.
    e. There are two basic types of induction: primary and secondary.

11. The magnetic field produced:
    a. By a solenoid is more intense than that produced by an electromagnet
    b. By AC is stronger than that produced by DC.
    c. By an AC source is constant
    d. In a transformer is based on mutual induction
    e. In an electromagnet is most intense in the plane perpendicular to its axis

12. An electromagnet:
    a. Cannot be turned off
    b. Has an air core
    c. Is a coil of wire wound around an iron core
    d. Produces a magnetic field with or without an electric current
    e. Produces a monopolar magnetic field

13. Given a closed loop of wire with no electron flow, an electric current can be induced if:
    a. A changing magnetic field is present.
    b. A constant magnetic field is present.
    c. No magnetic field is present.
    d. The loop is cycled open/close.
    e. The loop is opened.

14. When an AC source is connected to a coil of wire:
    a. A constant magnetic field is generated.
    b. A front EMF is produced.
    c. An opposite EMF is induced.
    d. Electromagnetic radiation is produced.
    e. Mutual induction occurs.

15. When an electric current is induced by mutual induction, such current flows:
    a. According to Faraday's law
    b. According to Lenz's law
    c. According to Oersted's law
    d. In the primary coil
    e. In the secondary coil

16. Which of the following scientists is associated with the early development of electromagnetism?
    a. Edison
    b. Faraday
    c. Marconi
    d. Planck
    e. Roentgen

17. A modern dry-cell battery is a source of:
    a. Coulomb per joule
    b. Joule per coulomb
    c. Newton per coulomb
    d. Ohm per volt
    e. Volt per ohm

18. When the right-hand rule is applied to a straight wire, the thumb indicates the direction of the:
    a. Circuit resistance
    b. Electric current
    c. Electric field
    d. Electric potential
    e. Magnetic field

19. The principal difference between a solenoid and an electromagnet is magnetic field:
    a. Homogeneity
    b. Intensity
    c. Penetrability
    d. Polarity
    e. Variability

20. Which of the following is based on electromagnetic induction?
    a. AC current
    b. Battery
    c. DC current
    d. Radio reception
    e. Solenoid

5-6

Electric Generators and Motors

 Electric generators and motors are electromechanical devices. The former converts mechanical energy to electric energy; the latter converts electric energy to mechanical energy.

Electric motors operate by passing an electric current through a loop of wire while in the presence of a magnetic field. The interaction between the electric current and the fixed magnetic field causes the loop to rotate, thereby producing mechanical energy. The induction motor, which is a type of electric motor, is used in all rotating anode x-ray tubes.

EXERCISES

1. Which of the following is *most* related to electromechanical devices?
   a. Edison's law of electromechanics
   b. Faraday's experiment
   c. Lenz's first law of electromagnetics
   d. Oersted's experiment on mutual induction
   e. The voltaic pile

2. In an electric generator:
   a. A coil of wire is rotated in a magnetic field.
   b. A transformer is charged.
   c. AC is changed to DC.
   d. Chemical energy is converted to electrical energy.
   e. Electrical energy is converted to mechanical energy.

3. The electric generator is *most* closely associated with experiments conducted by:
   a. Edison
   b. Faraday
   c. Lenz

   d. Oersted
   e. Volta

4. Which of the following statements about generators and motors is *true*?
   a. They are electromagnets.
   b. They both require commutators.
   c. They convert energy from one form into another.
   d. They have both primary and secondary windings.
   e. They require direct electric contact between primary and secondary coils.

5. In an electric motor:
   a. A coil of wire is mechanically rotated.
   b. A commutator ring is not necessary.
   c. AC is changed to DC.
   d. A transformer is discharged.
   e. Electric current is supplied to a coil of wire.

6. Which of the following would be classified as electromechanical devices?
   a. Generators and motors
   b. Generators and rectifiers
   c. Motors and rectifiers
   d. Transformers and electromagnets
   e. Transformers and rectifiers

7. The main difference between an AC and a DC electric generator is:
   a. The type of commutator ring
   b. A magnet
   c. A source of EMF
   d. A transformer
   e. A voltmeter

8. The electric current produced by an AC generator has:
   a. Alternating positive and negative intensity
   b. Constant negative intensity
   c. Constant positive intensity
   d. Pulsating negative intensity
   e. Pulsating positive intensity

9. An induction motor is used in an x-ray imaging system to:
   a. Control current
   b. Measure mAs
   c. Provide rectification
   d. Rotate the anode
   e. Vary voltage

10. In an induction motor, the only part to be rotated is the:
    a. Cathode
    b. Electromagnet
    c. Rotor
    d. Stator
    e. Wire loop

11. A fluoroscope is operated at 95 kVp, 2 mA. What is its power consumption?
    a. 47.5 W
    b. 190 W
    c. 47.5 kW
    d. 97 kW
    e. 190 kW

12. What power is required for a radiographic exposure at 76 kVp, 500 mA?
    a. 19 W
    b. 38 W
    c. 576 W
    d. 19 kW
    e. 38 kW

13. A 110 V heater requires 15 A. What is the power consumption?
    a. 15 W
    b. 110 W
    c. 125 W
    d. 1650 W
    e. 1800 W

14. How much current will a 60 W light bulb draw from a 120 V receptacle?
    a. 60 mA
    b. 500 mA
    c. 1 A
    d. 15 A
    e. 120 A

15. Electric current waveforms are graphs of:
    a. Electric current versus resistance
    b. Electric current versus time
    c. Electric voltage versus current
    d. Electric voltage versus resistance
    e. Electric voltage versus time

16. Theoretically, conduction electrons come to rest momentarily:
    a. At the peak of the waveform
    b. At the valley of the waveform
    c. At zero crossing
    d. Just before either a peak or a valley
    e. They never come to rest

17. Electric ranges, air conditioners, and furnaces require 220 V, 60 Hz AC. Therefore, compared with most household appliances, they require which of the following?
    a. A higher electric potential
    b. A higher operating frequency
    c. A lower electric potential
    d. Greater conductivity
    e. Greater semiconductivity

A transformer consists of two electromagnets with a common iron core. A voltage impressed on the primary coil will generate a voltage in the secondary coil, provided that the power is AC. The transformer law is as follows:

$$\frac{V_s}{V_p} = \frac{N_s}{N_p}$$

where the subscript s refers to the secondary coil, the subscript p refers to the primary coil, N is the number of turns of the coil, and V is the voltage. The ratio Ns/Np is known as the *turns ratio*.

In an x-ray imaging system, there are usually three transformers: the variable-voltage autotransformer, the high-voltage step-up transformer, and the step-down filament transformer.

EXERCISES

1. The transformer changes:
   a. Electric current to voltage
   b. Electric energy to electromagnetic energy
   c. Electric energy to mechanical energy
   d. Mechanical energy to electric energy
   e. The amplitude of the voltage

2. A transformer operates:
   a. On AC but not on DC
   b. On both DC and AC
   c. On DC but not on AC
   d. Only above its critical current
   e. Only on a constant voltage

3. If a transformer produces a large secondary current from a small primary current:
   a. Power will be increased.
   b. The turns ratio will be greater than 1.
   c. The turns ratio will be less than 1.
   d. The voltage will be larger on the secondary side than on the primary side.
   e. There will be more windings on the secondary side than on the primary side.

4. The symbol for a transformer is:

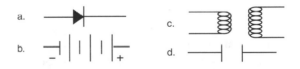

5. The principal application of a transformer in an x-ray imaging system is to:
   a. Change AC to DC
   b. Change DC to AC.
   c. Change frequency.
   d. Change voltage.
   e. Produce x-rays.

6. The output current in a step-up transformer is:
   a. Higher than the input current
   b. Independent of the input current
   c. Independent of the turns ratio
   d. Lower than the input current
   e. The same as the input current

7. A transformer with a turns ratio of 1000:1 is:
   a. A step-down transformer
   b. A step-up transformer
   c. An autotransformer
   d. Used to increase current
   e. Used to reduce voltage

8. When a step-up transformer is in use:
   a. The primary winding has more turns than the secondary winding.
   b. The secondary current is greater than the primary current.
   c. The secondary voltage is greater than the primary voltage.
   d. X-ray tube current is selected.
   e. The turns ratio is equal to 1.

9. When a transformer is designed, the change in current is:
   a. Dependent on the supply voltage
   b. Directly proportional to the voltage change
   c. In the same direction as the voltage change
   d. Inversely proportional to the turns ratio
   e. Proportional to the turns ratio

10. Which of the following is a transformer design used in x-ray imaging systems?
    a. Capacitor type
    b. Filament type
    c. Rectifier type
    d. Rotating type
    e. Shell type

11. An autotransformer:
    a. Contains a single coil that serves as both primary and secondary coils
    b. Controls x-ray tube current
    c. Is a shell type of transformer
    d. Is an electromechanical device
    e. Is used to control frequency

12. Which of the following statements about transformers is *correct*?
    a. If there were equal numbers of primary and secondary coil turns, the turns ratio would be zero.
    b. In the shell-type transformer, the primary and secondary coils are wound on different cores.
    c. Laminated transformer cores are more efficient than unlaminated ones.
    d. The autotransformer controls current.
    e. The high-voltage transformer in an x-ray imaging system is the autotransformer.

13. A transformer "transforms" or changes electric:
    a. Frequency
    b. Impedance
    c. Power
    d. Resistance
    e. Voltage

14. Transformers have iron cores to intensify the:
    a. Electric current
    b. Electric potential
    c. Electric power
    d. Electric voltage
    e. Magnetic field

15. Primary to secondary coupling in a transformer is enhanced by:
    a. 60 Hz
    b. AC
    c. An iron core
    d. DC
    e. EMF

16. If DC is applied to the primary coil of a step-up transformer, what is the result in the secondary coil?
    a. AC
    b. Increased current
    c. Increased magnetic field
    d. Increased voltage
    e. Nothing

17. The *turns ratio* is defined as:
    a. Number of secondary windings ÷ Primary windings
    b. Primary iron core ÷ Secondary iron core
    c. Primary voltage ÷ Secondary voltage
    d. Primary windings ÷ Number of secondary windings
    e. Secondary current ÷ Primary current

18. Which of the following accurately represents the transformer law?
    a. $I_s/I_p = N_p/N_s$
    b. $I_s/I_p = N_s/N_p$
    c. $I_s/I_p = V_s/V_p$
    d. $I_p/I_s = V_p/V_s$
    e. $I_p/I_s = N_p/N_s$

19. What is the transformer that looks like a square donut called?
    a. Auto
    b. Closed-core
    c. High-frequency
    d. Induction
    e. Shell-type

Nearly everything electric in a hospital operates on AC power. However, in radiology, the most important component of an x-ray imaging system, the x-ray tube, requires DC.

Circuit elements in the high-voltage generator of the x-ray imaging system, called **rectifiers**, transform the AC to DC. The process of conversion from AC to DC is called **rectification.**

Some types of x-ray imaging systems, primarily dental and portable systems, are capable of transforming AC into DC themselves, while simultaneously producing x-rays. Such a circuit is said to be **self-rectified.** Self-rectification results in half-wave rectification. **Full-wave rectification** is most often used in conventional x-ray imaging systems, and such a circuit requires a minimum of four rectifiers. To full-wave rectify **three-phase power,** a minimum of six rectifiers is required for a six-pulse unit, and 12 are required for a 12-pulse unit.

EXERCISES

1. Which of the following principles of rectification produces the maximum efficiency of x-ray production?
   a. Four-diode rectification
   b. Half-wave rectification
   c. High frequency
   d. Self-rectification
   e. Two-diode rectification

2. To generate three-phase, six-pulse power, at least how many rectifiers are necessary?
   a. 4
   b. 6
   c. 8
   d. 12
   e. 16

3. A semiconductor rectifier:
   a. Has a heated anode
   b. Has a heated cathode
   c. Is a solid-state device
   d. Is an electromechanical device
   e. Is used only for mammography

4. If a single rectifier is inserted into a circuit that conducts 60 Hz AC so that it suppresses the positive portion of the waveform, then the output waveform will contain:
   a. 60 negative pulses per second
   b. 60 positive pulses per second
   c. 120 negative pulses per second
   d. 120 positive pulses per second
   e. Variable pulses, depending on frequency

5. The voltage ripple associated with various x-ray generators is:
   a. 70.7% for single-phase, full-wave rectification
   b. 100% for self-rectification
   c. Higher for self-rectification than for half-wave rectification
   d. Highest with high frequency
   e. Less for single-phase than for three-phase power

6. A rectifier:
   a. Converts AC to DC
   b. Converts DC to AC
   c. Increases voltage

d. Refers to a type of electromagnetic device
e. Refers to a type of electromechanical device

7. Inspect the following circuit, and identify which diodes pass current at the same time:

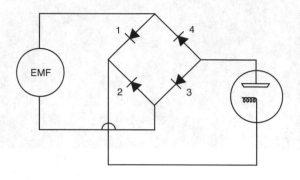

   a. 1 and 2
   b. 3 and 4
   c. 1 and 3
   d. 1 and 4

8. Near the p-n junction of a semiconductor diode, one will find:
   a. A filtered anode
   b. A heated anode
   c. A heated cathode
   d. A p type of material containing excess electrons
   e. An n type of material containing excess electrons

9. A semiconductor diode:
   a. Allows current to flow only from n type of material to p type
   b. Allows current to flow only from p type of material to n type
   c. Contains carriers that are also called proton traps
   d. Contains holes that are also called proton traps
   e. Is also called an electromechanical rectifier

10. In a circuit that contains a single rectifier:
   a. Electron flow is pulsed but uninterrupted.
   b. Electrons flow in one direction but not the other.
   c. The result is constant potential DC.
   d. Twice as many electrons flow in the output coil as in the input coil.
   e. Voltage is increased.

11. If 60 Hz AC power is full-wave rectified, output voltage consists of:
   a. 60 pulses per second
   b. 90 pulses per second

c. 120 pulses per second
d. 70% ripple
e. Zero ripple

12. The current from a common household wall receptacle in the United States is:
   a. 50 Hz AC
   b. 50 Hz DC
   c. 60 Hz AC
   d. 60 Hz DC
   e. Constant potential.

13. Thermionic emission refers to:
   a. Electron emission from a heated source
   b. Heat conduction
   c. Heat emission from an electric conductor
   d. Heat radiation
   e. Ionization with heat

14. Which of the following is the symbol for a diode?

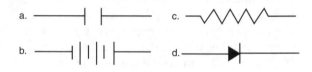

15. The main advantage of full-wave rectification over half-wave rectification is:
   a. Higher-energy x-rays
   b. Higher kVp
   c. Higher mA
   d. Less voltage ripple
   e. A greater number of x-rays per cycle

16. How many overlapping pulses are generated in 1 s for three-phase, six-pulse power?
   a. 60
   b. 120
   c. 360
   d. 720
   e. 2160

Match the approximate voltage ripple with each of the following. Some answers may be used more than once.

_____ 17. Full-wave rectified	a.	1%
_____ 18. High frequency	b.	4%
_____ 19. Three-phase, six-pulse	c.	13%
_____ 20. Three-phase, 12-pulse	d.	71%
_____ 21. Self-rectified	e.	100%

6-1

Control of Kilovolt Peak (kVp)

- Peak kilovoltage (kVp) is controlled by a series of electric taps on the autotransformer.
- The autotransformer has only one winding.
- The autotransformer can function in the step-up or the step-down mode.
- The transformer law can be used to calculate the secondary voltage:

$$\frac{V_s}{V_p} = \frac{N_s}{N_p}$$

where V_p refers to primary voltage, V_s is secondary voltage; N_p refers to the number of windings enclosed by primary taps, and N_s is the number of windings enclosed by secondary taps.

EXERCISES

1. Power to the primary side of the high-voltage transformer comes from the:
   a. Filament transformer
   b. Line-voltage compensator
   c. Primary side of the autotransformer
   d. Rectifier
   e. Secondary side of the autotransformer

2. The output voltage from the autotransformer is:
   a. Always less than the input voltage
   b. Always more than the input voltage
   c. Fed directly to the rectifiers
   d. Inversely proportional to the turns ratio
   e. Proportional to the turns ratio

3. The autotransformer converts:
   a. Chemical energy to electric energy
   b. Electric energy to chemical energy
   c. Electric energy to electric energy
   d. Magnetic energy to electric energy
   e. Mechanical energy to electric energy

4. The autotransformer operates on the principle of:
   a. Coulomb's law
   b. Edison's law
   c. Faraday's law
   d. Newton's law
   e. Oersted's law

5. The principal purpose of the high-voltage transformer is to do which of the following?
   a. Adjust voltage
   b. Increase voltage
   c. Rectify voltage
   d. Reduce voltage
   e. Stabilize voltage

6. The voltage supplied to an x-ray imaging system is 220 V. The voltage used by the x-ray tube is produced by which of the following?
   a. Autotransformer
   b. Exposure timer
   c. Filament transformer
   d. High-voltage transformer
   e. Rheostat

7. 220 V is supplied to 800 primary turns of an autotransformer. What will be the output voltage across 200 secondary turns?
   a. 27.5 V
   b. 55 V
   c. 880 V
   d. 1760 V
   e. 3520 V

8. The autotransformer has only one:
   a. Coil
   b. Meter
   c. Rectifier
   d. Switch
   e. Turns ratio

9. The principal purpose of the autotransformer is to:
   a. Adjust voltage
   b. Increase voltage
   c. Rectify voltage
   d. Reduce voltage
   e. Stabilize voltage

10. Which of the following is directly connected to the autotransformer?
    a. Filament
    b. kVp meter
    c. mA meter
    d. Rectifier
    e. X-ray tube

11. Taps on the windings of an autotransformer are used to select which of the following?
    a. Exposure time
    b. Focal spot
    c. Line compensation
    d. mA
    e. Rectification

12. 440 V is supplied to 1000 primary turns of an autotransformer. If the desired output voltage is 100 V, how many secondary turns must be tapped?
    a. 100
    b. 227
    c. 454
    d. 4400
    e. 10,000

13. The autotransformer can be used to do which of the following?
    a. Control exposure time
    b. Convert AC to DC
    c. Convert DC to AC
    d. Increase kVp
    e. Increase mA

14. If V stands for voltage and T for the number of turns enclosed between the taps of an auto-transformer, then the autotransformer law is which of the following?
    a. $V_p/V_s = T_p/T_s$
    b. $V_pT_p = T_sV_s$
    c. $V_pV_s = T_pT_s$
    d. $V_s/V_p = T_p/T_s$
    e. $V_s = V_p$

15. In the design of an autotransformer:
    a. A single coil serves as both the primary and the secondary coils.
    b. The exposure timer is on the primary side.
    c. The major kVp adjustment and the line-voltage compensator are on the secondary side.
    d. The major kVp adjustment is on the primary side and the minor kVp adjustment is on the secondary side.
    e. There are separate primary and secondary coils.

16. Selection of kVp:
    a. Involves two series of autotransformers
    b. Requires rectified voltage
    c. Requires that constant voltage be supplied to the autotransformer
    d. Uses meters and switches that are at high kVp
    e. Uses the step-up transformer

17. Line compensation:
    a. Adjusts the line frequency to 60 Hz
    b. Compensates for rectification
    c. Is necessary for proper exposure timing
    d. Is necessary to convert AC to DC
    e. Is required to stabilize voltage

18. Which of the following is used to determine the voltage before exposure?
    a. A filament transformer
    b. A postreading voltmeter
    c. A prereading voltmeter
    d. A step-up transformer
    e. An autotransformer

6-2

Control of Milliamperage (mA)

The x-ray tube current is controlled by an electric filament circuit that is separate from that of the high-voltage circuit. The circuit elements of importance for supplying and controlling the tube mA are the autotransformer, the precision resistors, the filament transformer, and the filament.

The mA meter, although physically located on the operating console, is electrically connected to the secondary side of the high-voltage transformer through a center tap to electrical ground. This allows for direct measurement of the tube current without the possibility of electric shock.

EXERCISES

1. One coulomb per second (C/s) is equivalent to 1 A, and 1 C is equal to 6.3×10^{18} electrons. Therefore, operation at 100 mA would result in a current of:
   a. 6.3×10^{16} electrons
   b. 6.3×10^{16} electrons/s
   c. 6.3×10^{17} electrons
   d. 6.3×10^{17} electrons/s
   e. 6.3×10^{18} electrons

2. The filament transformer:
   a. Has four windings
   b. Increases current
   c. Increases voltage
   d. Is an autotransformer
   e. Must have precision resistors

3. The filament transformer is usually:
   a. A part of the autotransformer
   b. Located with the high-voltage generator
   c. An autotransformer
   d. Located in the operating console
   e. A step-down transformer

4. A PA chest requires a technique of 125 kVp at 4 mAs. The total number of electrons used to make the exposure is:
   a. 2.5×10^{15}
   b. 2.5×10^{16}
   c. 2.5×10^{17}
   d. 6.3×10^{16}
   e. 6.3×10^{17}

5. The filament circuit:
   a. Begins at the filament and ends at the filament transformer
   b. Begins at the autotransformer and ends at the filament
   c. Controls kVp
   d. Is located entirely in the operating console
   e. Is located in all three of the major components of an x-ray imaging system: the console, the high-voltage generator, and the x-ray tube

6. A filament transformer has a turns ratio of 1:20. What current must be supplied to the primary windings if 5 A is required by the filament?
   a. 125 mA
   b. 200 mA
   c. 250 mA
   d. 50 A
   e. 100 A

7. The filament transformer in the previous question is supplied with 150 V to the primary side. What is the secondary voltage?
   a. 750 mV
   b. 3000 mV
   c. 1.5 V
   d. 7.5 V
   e. 30 V

8. The unit mAs:
   a. Could be expressed in coulombs
   b. Could be expressed in coulombs/second.
   c. Is a unit of electric current
   d. Is a unit of electromotive force (EMF)
   e. Is electron/s

9. An exposure technique of 100 mA at 100 ms compared with 50 mA at 50 ms results in:
   a. Eight times the total number of electrons
   b. Fewer projectile electrons
   c. Four times the total number of electrons
   d. Three times the total number of electrons
   e. Twice the total number of electrons

10. The control of focal spot size depends on:
    a. The filament that is energized
    b. The mA station selected
    c. The secondary taps of the autotransformer
    d. The target angle selected
    e. The turns ratio of the filament transformer

11. The meter that monitors x-ray tube current is:
    a. Connected to the autotransformer
    b. Connected to the secondary side of the step-down transformer
    c. Grounded to the primary center tap of the step-up transformer
    d. Physically located on the control console
    e. The same as the filament current monitor

12. X-ray tube current is usually measured in which of the following?
    a. Amperes (A)
    b. Ampere-seconds (As)

c. Microamperes (μA)
d. Milliamperes (mA)
e. Milliampere-seconds (mAs)

13. A filament current of 5 A is necessary for thermionic emission. What electron flow is this?
    a. 3.2×10^{15} electrons/s
    b. 3.2×10^{16} electrons/s
    c. 3.2×10^{17} electrons/s
    d. 3.2×10^{18} electrons/s
    e. 3.2×10^{19} electrons/s

14. The filament transformer is designed:
    a. As a step-up transformer
    b. To operate on DC power
    c. With a turns ratio less than 1
    d. With a turns ratio greater than 1
    e. With an mA meter grounded to the center tap

15. Which of the following would be *correct* to use for expressing x-ray tube current?
    a. Coulombs
    b. Coulombs/second
    c. Electron volts
    d. Kilovolt peak
    e. Kilovolts/second

16. The design of fixed mA stations requires the use of which of the following?
    a. A center-tapped meter
    b. DC power
    c. Major and minor taps
    d. Precision resistors
    e. Primary and secondary windings

17. Operation at 100 mA for 1 s results in which of the following?
    a. 6.3×10^{16} electrons
    b. 6.3×10^{17} electrons/s
    c. 6.3×10^{17} electrons
    d. 6.3×10^{18} electrons/s
    e. 6.3×10^{18} electrons

18. A filament transformer has 800 primary windings and is supplied with 200 mA. If the secondary coil has 100 windings, what will be the secondary current?
    a. 25 mA
    b. 100 mA
    c. 400 mA
    d. 1600 mA
    e. 3200 mA

19. If a filament transformer has turns ratio of 0.05 and 200 mA is supplied to the primary side of the transformer, what will be the secondary current?
    a. 100 mA
    b. 400 mA
    c. 1 A
    d. 4 A
    e. 6 A

20. mA is a unit of electric current, and mAs is a unit of:
    a. Electric charge
    b. Electric potential
    c. Reciprocal kVp
    d. X-ray beam quality
    e. X-ray beam quantity

6-3

Exposure Timers

Exposure timers are precision devices that start and stop x-ray production. There are four basic types of exposure timers:

1. **Mechanical timers:** These operate by spring action, similarly to a hand-wound alarm clock. These timers are not very accurate, and they are not used on modern equipment.
2. **Synchronous timers:** These timers use a synchronous motor that operates at 60 rps. Their shortest possible exposure time is $\frac{1}{60}$ s.
3. **Electronic timers:** This type of timer operates on an electronic resistive-capacitive circuit based on the time required to charge a capacitor. These timers are accurate, allow exposures as short as 1 millisecond (ms), and can be used for serial radiography.
4. **mAs timers:** These timers are electronic timers that monitor the product of mA and time and terminate the exposure when the proper mAs is reached.

Automatic exposure control (AEC) incorporates a radiation-measuring device that terminates the x-ray exposure when enough radiation has reached the image receptor.

EXERCISES

1. A radiographic technique calls for a 50 ms exposure, but the exposure control has only fractional notation. Which of the following should be selected?
   a. $\frac{1}{60}$ s
   b. $\frac{1}{40}$ s
   c. $\frac{1}{20}$ s
   d. $\frac{1}{10}$ s
   e. $\frac{1}{4}$ s

2. A radiographic technique calls for a 400 mA, $\frac{1}{20}$ s exposure. What is the mAs?
   a. 5 mAs
   b. 10 mAs
   c. 20 mAs
   d. 40 mAs
   e. 80 mAs

3. If an x-ray imaging system is operated at 600 mA, 50 ms, the total mAs will be which of the following?
   a. 6 mAs
   b. 30 mAs
   c. 60 mAs
   d. 300 mAs
   e. 600 mAs

4. A radiographic technique of 100 mA at $\frac{1}{4}$ s has been used. If one changes to the 500 mA station, the appropriate exposure time for the same mAs is which of the following?
   a. $\frac{1}{4}$ s
   b. $\frac{3}{20}$ s
   c. $\frac{1}{20}$ s
   d. $\frac{1}{5}$ s
   e. $\frac{1}{10}$ s

5. Operation at 300 mA for $\frac{1}{20}$ s is equivalent to operation at 900 mA for:
   a. 8 ms
   b. 17 ms
   c. 60 ms

d. 200 ms
e. 500 ms

6. The control of exposure time is always:
   a. Automatically set
   b. Determined by kVp
   c. On the primary side of the autotransformer
   d. On the primary side of the high-voltage transformer
   e. On the secondary side of the filament circuit

7. The exposure timer on a three-phase radiographic imaging system will:
   a. Be automatic
   b. Be electronic
   c. Be synchronous
   d. Limit exposure to $\frac{1}{60}$ s or longer
   e. Limit exposure to 8 ms and no shorter

8. An automatic exposure control (AEC) device:
   a. Can use a photomultiplier tube on the entrance side of the patient
   b. Can use an ionization chamber between the patient and the image receptor
   c. Cannot control exposures shorter than $\frac{1}{120}$ s.
   d. Does not require a manual timer
   e. Works only with three-phase and high-frequency power

9. With an automatic exposure control (AEC) device:
   a. Exposures less than 100 ms are not possible.
   b. It is not necessary to depress the exposure control.
   c. The exposure starts and stops automatically.
   d. Technique selection is not necessary.
   e. A backup timer is required.

10. The shortest exposure possible with single-phase equipment is $\frac{1}{120}$ s. How many milliseconds is that?
    a. 8 ms
    b. 17 ms
    c. 35 ms
    d. 50 ms
    e. 120 ms

11. Mammography sometimes requires exposures as long as 1.5 s. This is equivalent to which of the following?
    a. 15 ms
    b. 100 ms
    c. 150 ms
    d. 1000 ms
    e. 1500 ms

12. The shortest exposure possible with three-phase equipment is 1 ms. What fraction of a second is that?
    a. $\frac{1}{50}$
    b. $\frac{1}{100}$
    c. $\frac{1}{120}$
    d. $\frac{1}{500}$
    e. $\frac{1}{1000}$

13. There are 30 video frames each second for a fluoroscopic CRT dynamic image. What is the length for each frame?
    a. 1 ms
    b. 10 ms
    c. 16 ms
    d. 33 ms
    e. 60 ms

14. The human eye cannot visualize faster than approximately five views each second. What is the integration time of the human eye?
    a. 1 ms
    b. 10 ms
    c. 20 ms
    d. 100 ms
    e. 200 ms

15. A radiographic technique calls for 86 kVp/200 mAs using the 800 mA station. What is the exposure time?
    a. 10 ms
    b. 25 ms
    c. 100 ms
    d. 250 ms
    e. 500 ms

6-4

High-Voltage Generation and Rectification

The high-voltage section of the x-ray imaging system contains the following:

- The **high-voltage transformer** ($N_s/N_p > 1$), which converts low voltage from the autotransformer to the required kVp.
- The **filament transformer** ($N_s/N_p > 1$), which reduces the voltage from the autotransformer to

about 10 V for heating the filament. At the same time, the filament current is regulated to the range of 4 to 10 A.

- A **rectifier circuit** that converts the alternating voltage into a direct voltage before use by the x-ray tube.

The accompanying figure shows the change in voltage waveform at each stage of generation.

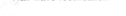

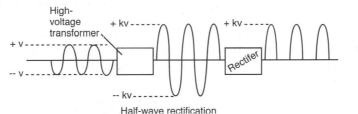

Half-wave rectification

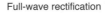

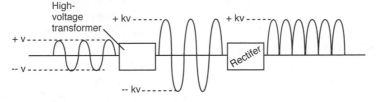

Full-wave rectification

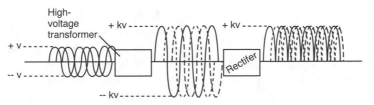

Three-phase rectification

Voltage Waveform	Pulses per Second	Percentage Ripple
Half-wave	60	100
Full-wave	120	100
Three-phase, six-pulse	360	13
Three-phase, 12-pulse	720	4
High frequency	Up to 1000	1

EXERCISES

1. Which of the following is contained in a typical high-voltage generator?
   a. Diode rectifiers
   b. Autotransformer
   c. Exposure switch
   d. kVp meter
   e. mA meter

2. A change in the voltage waveform from the primary side to the secondary side of the high-voltage transformer produces a change in:
   a. Amplitude
   b. Frequency
   c. Phase
   d. Velocity
   e. Wavelength

3. In half-wave rectification, each inverse half-cycle in the primary circuit corresponds to how many voltage pulses across the x-ray tube?
   a. None
   b. One
   c. Two
   d. Four
   e. Twelve

4. Which of the following is higher for a single-phase high-voltage generator than for a three-phase high-voltage generator?
   a. kVp
   b. Purchase price
   c. Rotor speed
   d. Voltage ripple
   e. X-ray quality

5. Which of the following is a disadvantage of three-phase power compared with single-phase power?
   a. Higher capital cost
   b. Higher electrical operating costs
   c. Limited kVp
   d. Longer minimum exposure time
   e. Softer radiation

6. The disadvantage of a self-rectified circuit is:
   a. Its complexity
   b. Its cost
   c. Its limitation of use to dental imaging systems
   d. Its limited exposure time
   e. Its requirement of DC power

7. An exposure of $\frac{1}{10}$ s:
   a. At 50 mA is 50 mAs
   b. At 100 mA is 1000 mAs
   c. Is 120 ms
   d. Produces six pulses in full-wave rectification
   e. Produces twice as much radiation if full-wave rectified than if half-wave–rectified

8. Full-wave rectification:
   a. Has less ripple compared with half-wave rectification
   b. Is one example of self-rectification
   c. Produces higher kVp than half-wave rectification
   d. Requires at least four rectifiers
   e. Requires at least twelve rectifiers

9. A rectifier:
   a. Can be a semiconductor
   b. Converts DC to AC
   c. Increases current
   d. Increases voltage
   e. Increases x-ray intensity

10. Concerning the transformers used in the x-ray circuit:
    a. The filament transformer is also an auto-transformer.
    b. The filament transformer usually is located in the console.
    c. The high-voltage transformer is a step-up device.
    d. They convert AC to DC.
    e. They operate only on DC.

11. Which of the following is an advantage of three-phase power over single-phase power?
    a. Improved spatial resolution
    b. Increased kVp
    c. Increased mAs
    d. Increased x-ray intensity per mAs
    e. Lower capital cost

12. Oil is used in the high-voltage section of an x-ray imaging system for which of the following functions?
    a. Electrical insulation
    b. Reduction of rotor friction
    c. Reduction of voltage ripple
    d. Thermal conduction
    e. Voltage rectification

13. Which power supply should provide the highest-quality x-ray beam?
    a. Full-wave rectified
    b. High-frequency

c. Self-rectified
d. Three-phase, six-pulse
e. Three-phase, 12-pulse

Match the following high-voltage power supplies with the appropriate voltage ripple (answers may be used more than once):

_____	14. Full-wave rectified power	a. 1%
_____	15. Half-wave rectified power	b. 4%
_____	16. High-frequency power	c. 13%
_____	17. Three-phase, six-pulse power	d. 71%
_____	18. Three-phase, 12-pulse power	e. 100%

ACROSS

1. Rectification is accomplished through the use of _____.

2. The phototimer used by most manufacturers incorporates a flat, parallel plate ____ation chamber.

3. One advantage of the high-frequency generator is _____.

4. Inverter circuits convert DC into a series of _____ pulses.

5. For any given radiographic examination, the number of x-rays that reach the image receptor is directly related to current and _____.

6. The penetrating quality of an x-ray beam is expressed by kVp or _____ layer.

7. The incorporation of automatic exposure control is often called photo _____.

8. A filament transformer is a _____ -down transformer.

9. The number of x-rays or the intensity of the beam is usually expressed in mR or mR per mAs and is called the _____ of the x-ray beam.

10. The piece of equipment designed to supply precise voltage to the filament circuit and to the high-voltage circuit of the x-ray imaging system is _____.

11. In a full-wave–rectified circuit, the negative half-cycle that corresponds to the inverse voltage is _____ d so that a positive voltage is always directed across the x-ray tube.

12. The continual variation in mAs during an exposure to minimum exposure time is called a _____ load mA.

13. Variation in _____ voltage results in variation in the x-ray beam.

14. As a filament's current increases, the filament becomes hotter, and electrons are released through _____ ionic emission.

DOWN

1. Because transformers operate only on alternating current, the voltage waveform on both sides of a high-voltage transformer is _____oidal.

2. One way in which the autotransformer differs from the conventional transformer is that it has a _____ winding.

3. A phototimer measures the quantity of radiation that reaches the _____ receptor.

4. A _____-wave–rectified circuit usually contains two diodes, although some contain one or more.

5. The autotransformer works on the principle of _____ induction.

6. The penetrating quality of the x-ray beam, expressed in kVp, refers to the _____ of the x-ray beam.

7. High-frequency voltage generation uses _____ circuits.

8. In controlling the voltage supplied to the high-voltage transformer, it is much safer and easier to vary _____ voltage and then increase it than to increase low voltage to the kilovolt level and then vary its magnitude.

9. Half-wave rectification refers to a condition in which the voltage is not allowed to swing _____ during the negative half of its cycle.

10. The number of electrons emitted by a filament is determined by the filament's _____.

11. Tube _____ is monitored with an mA meter that must be placed in the tube circuit.

12. The voltages an autotransformer receives and provides relate directly to the number of _____s of the transformer enclosed by the respective connections.

13. X-ray tube current is controlled through the _____ circuit.

14. Voltage _____ is the variation in peak voltage waveform.

15. Synchronous timers cannot be used for _____ exposures.

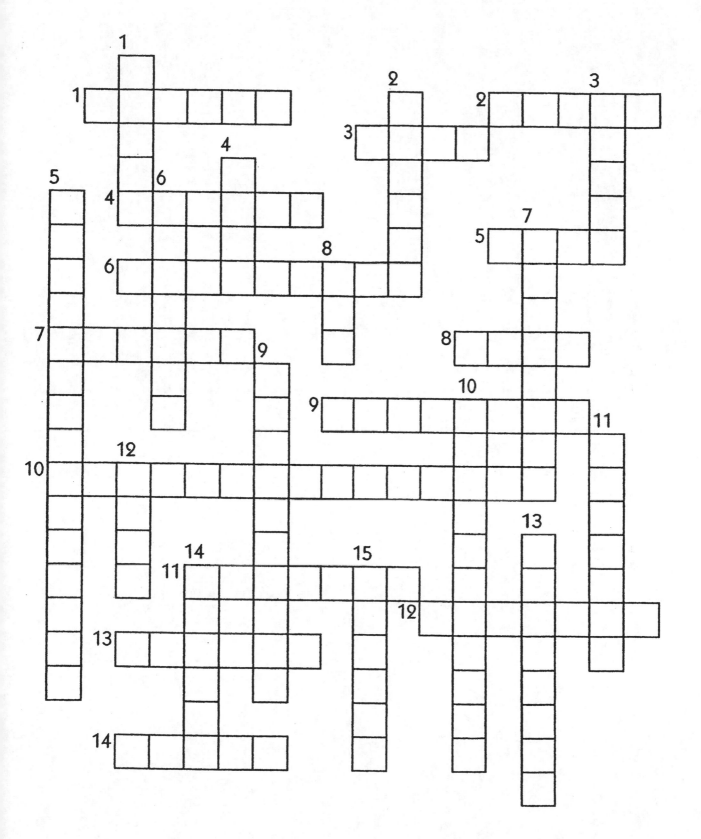

The cathode is the negative side of the x-ray tube. Its major components are the **filament** and the **focusing cup.** The filament is a small coil of wire, usually of thoriated tungsten, that provides electrons for the production of x-rays. The focusing cup directs the beam of electrons to the target on the anode.

EXERCISES

1. The three principal parts of an x-ray imaging system are:
   a. Anode, cathode, and focusing cup
   b. Anode, cathode, and high-voltage generator
   c. X-ray tube, control console, and high-voltage generator
   d. X-ray tube, high-voltage generator, and image receptor
   e. X-ray tube, protective housing, and high-voltage generator

2. The primary purpose of the glass envelope of an x-ray tube is to:
   a. Control leakage radiation
   b. Control off-focus radiation
   c. Cool the tube
   d. Ensure against electric shock
   e. Provide a vacuum

3. The protective housing of an x-ray tube is designed to:
   a. Control isotropic x-ray emission
   b. Control scatter radiation
   c. Limit operation to 100 kVp or less
   d. Reduce the hazard of leakage radiation
   e. Reduce the hazard of scatter radiation

4. A diagnostic x-ray tube is an example of which of the following?
   a. Cathode
   b. Diode
   c. Tetrode
   d. Anode
   e. Electrode

5. The large filament is used during radiography when the heat load is:
   a. High, and visibility of detail is important
   b. High, and visibility of detail is less important
   c. Low, and high kVp is required
   d. Low, and visibility of detail is important
   e. Low, and visibility of detail is less important

6. In most x-ray tubes, there are two filaments to:
   a. Ensure saturation current
   b. Produce higher-energy x-rays
   c. Provide two electrodes
   d. Provide two focal spots
   e. Reduce space charge effects

7. The focusing cup:
   a. Is on the positive side of the x-ray tube
   b. Is slightly positive with respect to the filament
   c. Is the grid in a grid-controlled x-ray tube
   d. Is usually made of thoriated tungsten
   e. Selects the filament

8. Once filament temperature becomes adequate, a further small rise in filament temperature will cause tube current to:
   a. Decrease just a bit
   b. Decrease very much
   c. Increase just a bit
   d. Increase very much
   e. Not change

9. The cathode beam of an x-ray tube is the:
   a. Current that heats the filament
   b. Focused electron beam within the tube
   c. Off-focus radiation
   d. Primary x-ray beam
   e. Secondary radiation

10. The x-ray tube current:
    a. Controls x-ray energy
    b. Flows through both filaments at the same time
    c. Is controlled by the filament current
    d. Is the current that flows through the filament
    e. Usually varies from 50 to 1000 A

11. Most x-ray tubes used for radiography:
    a. Are dual-focus tubes
    b. Do not emit leakage radiation
    c. Have a fixed anode
    d. Operate in the space charge–limited mode
    e. Use tungsten filaments that do not vaporize

12. The cathode is:
    a. A diode
    b. Designed to supply heat
    c. One of the two parts of a diode
    d. Part of the target
    e. Positively charged

13. When a filament burns out:
    a. It should be replaced within 30 days.
    b. The filament current goes to maximum.
    c. The filament current goes to zero.
    d. The tube current is maximum.
    e. The x-ray intensity is maximum.

14. The space charge effect:
    a. Is more pronounced at high kVp
    b. Is more pronounced at low mA
    c. Limits kVp
    d. Occurs in the vicinity of the anode
    e. Occurs in the vicinity of the cathode

15. The x-ray tube filament:
    a. Conducts approximately 5 A
    b. Conducts current only when an exposure is made
    c. Is a diode
    d. Is the space charge
    e. Is usually copper

16. If saturation is achieved and the filament current is fixed, tube current:
    a. Decreases with use
    b. Falls with increasing kVp
    c. Remains fixed
    d. Rises with increasing exposure time
    e. Rises with increasing kVp

17. X-ray tube current:
    a. Depends on exposure time
    b. Depends on voltage
    c. Increases when the kVp is decreased
    d. Is measured in milliamperes rather than amperes
    e. Is zero when filament current is below thermionic emission

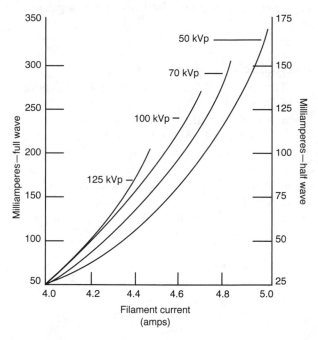

Examine the filament emission chart above and answer Exercises 18 and 19.

18. What is the full-wave tube current when the filament current is 4.6 A and the tube voltage is 70 kVp?

19. To obtain 125 mA half-wave–rectified x-ray tube current at 100 kVp, what must the filament current be?

7-2

The X-Ray Tube Anode

The x-ray tube anode serves four principal functions: (1) **electrical conduction** of the x-ray tube current, (2) **mechanical support** for the target, (3) **thermal conduction** of heat, and (4) **x-ray production.** The active portion of the anode, in which x-rays are produced, is the target. Almost all targets are made of tungsten (usually alloyed with rhenium). However, some that are used exclusively for mammography have molybdenum or rhodium targets.

The area of the target on which the projectile electrons interact is the **focal spot.** All diagnostic x-ray tubes have an inclined anode to take advantage of the **line-focus principle.**

EXERCISES

1. A stationary-anode x-ray tube:
   a. Incorporates the line-focus principle
   b. Is used to produce very short exposures
   c. Limits leakage radiation
   d. Provides for greater heat dissipation
   e. Usually has a very small focal spot

2. The heel effect occurs because of:
   a. A focusing cup
   b. Reduced tube current
   c. The shape charge effect
   d. The shape of the filament
   e. X-ray absorption in the anode

3. The main reason for using the line-focus principle is to:
   a. Increase heat capacity
   b. Increase x-ray intensity
   c. Reduce exposure time
   d. Reduce focal-spot size
   e. Reduce heel effect

4. Rotating anode x-ray tubes:
   a. Have a copper target embedded in a tungsten anode
   b. Have a tungsten target embedded in a copper anode
   c. Have target angles that are less than 10 degrees
   d. Incorporate the line-focus principle
   e. Produce higher-energy x-rays

5. X-ray intensity is higher on the cathode side than on the anode side because of which of the following?
   a. The focusing cup
   b. The line-focus principle
   c. The space charge effect
   d. X-ray absorption in the anode
   e. X-ray deflection from the anode

6. Which of the following target angles is characteristic of a rotating anode x-ray tube?
   a. 1 degree
   b. 10 degrees
   c. 20 degrees
   d. 50 degrees
   e. 100 degrees

7. Small target angles result in which of the following?
   a. Better collimation
   b. Increased heat capacity
   c. Less heel effect

d. Small focal-spot size
e. Small space charge

8. Molybdenum is used for anode stem material because of which of the following?
   a. It has a high atomic number.
   b. It has a shiny surface and reflects electrons well.
   c. It has longer life.
   d. It is a good heat conductor.
   e. It is a good heat insulator.

9. Tungsten is the choice material for x-ray anodes because of its:
   a. High atomic number
   b. High rpm
   c. High x-ray intensity
   d. Low atomic number
   e. Low rpm

10. The effective focal spot is:
    a. Larger than the actual focal spot
    b. Largest on the anode side of the central axis
    c. Smaller than the actual focal spot
    d. Smallest on the cathode side of the central axis
    e. The same size as the actual focal spot

11. The heel effect:
    a. Is more pronounced when large target angles are used
    b. Is reduced with a focusing cup
    c. Occurs only with rotating anode x-ray tubes
    d. Requires that the cathode be positioned to the thicker anatomy
    e. Suggests that the cathode be up during PA chest radiography

12. What is a prominent engineering difficulty in the manufacture of high-speed rotating anodes?
    a. Balance of the rotor
    b. Control of space charge effects
    c. Marriage to the focusing cup
    d. Proper target angle
    e. Target-face polish

13. Which of the following is a component of an electromagnetic induction motor?
    a. Cathode
    b. Filament
    c. Stator
    d. Target angle
    e. Target disc

14. Necessary properties of x-ray target material include which of the following?
    a. High melting point
    b. High rotation speed
    c. Low atomic number
    d. Low coefficient of friction
    e. High electrical resistance

15. Which of the following is an advantage of the rotating anode tube over the stationary anode tube?
    a. Higher heat capacity
    b. Higher kVp capacity
    c. Longer exposure time
    d. Reduced heel effect
    e. The line-focus principle

16. The anode angle of an x-ray tube is increased to give which of the following?
    a. Smaller focal spot
    b. Higher heat capacity
    c. Proper focusing of the electron beam
    d. Proper reflection
    e. Uniform x-ray intensity

17. Which of the following components of a diagnostic x-ray tube is on the positive side of the tube?
    a. The cathode
    b. The filament
    c. The focusing cup
    d. The grid
    e. The stator

18. As the anode target angle increases:
    a. Effective focal-spot size increases.
    b. Heel effect becomes more pronounced.
    c. kVp increases.
    d. Radiation intensity on the central ray increases.
    e. Target rotating speed increases.

19. A stationary anode will *most* likely be used in which of the following?
    a. Chest radiography
    b. Dentistry
    c. General radiography
    d. Interventional radiology
    e. Mammography

20. Which of the following is *not* a function of the anode?
    a. Conduction of electricity
    b. Mechanical support
    c. Thermal conduction
    d. Thermionic emission
    e. X-ray production

21. Which of the following is the principal hurdle in the design of an x-ray anode for high-capacity radiologic techniques?
    a. Heat dissipation
    b. Radiation quality
    c. Radiation quantity
    d. Rotating speed
    e. X-ray intensity

The three types of tube rating charts are the radiographic rating chart, the anode cooling chart, and the housing cooling chart.

The **radiographic rating chart** shows which single radiographic techniques are within the safe limits of operation for a particular x-ray tube. The **anode cooling chart** displays the thermal capacity of the anode and the time required for the heated anode to cool. The **housing cooling chart** gives the maximum heat capacity of the x-ray tube housing, as well as the time required for that housing to cool. Thermal energy absorbed by the anode is measured in **heat units (HU)**.

$$HU = kVp \times mA \times \text{Seconds for single-phase}$$
$$\text{power} = 0.7 \text{ J}$$

$$HU = 1.4 \text{ kVp} \times mA \times \text{Seconds for three-phase}$$
$$\text{and high-frequency power} = 1.0 \text{ J}$$

EXERCISES

Use the charts on page 106 to answer questions 1 through 21.

1. The high-speed rotor (10,000 rpm) permits longer exposure times than the low-speed rotor at single-phase operation (3400 rpm).
   a. True
   b. False

2. If the intersection of time and kVp falls on an mA curve, that mA is safe.
   a. True
   b. False

3. Most of the troublesome heat generated in an x-ray tube occurs at the filament.
   a. True
   b. False

4. Generally, a small focal spot allows longer exposure times than a large focal spot.
   a. True
   b. False

5. The radiographic rating chart reports the time that should elapse between exposures.
   a. True
   b. False

6. It is *not* possible to exceed the heat capacity of the housing without first exceeding that of the anode.
   a. True
   b. False

7. A tube can become "gassy" because of anode overheating and the release of gas.
   a. True
   b. False

8. The radiographic rating chart is designed primarily to protect the filament.
   a. True
   b. False

9. Rotor speed does *not* influence heat capacity.
   a. True
   b. False

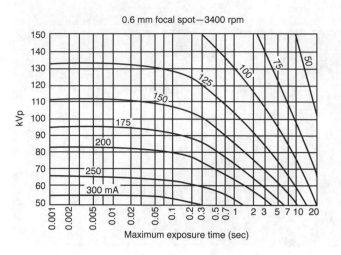

0.6 mm focal spot—3400 rpm

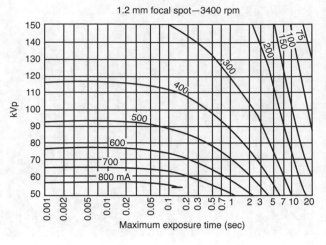

1.2 mm focal spot—3400 rpm

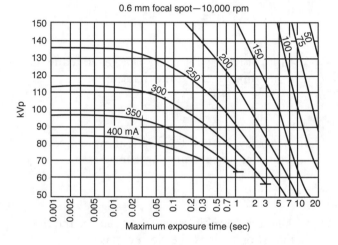

0.6 mm focal spot—10,000 rpm

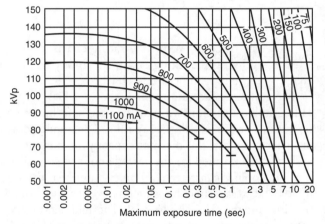

1.2 mm focal spot—10,000 rpm

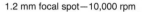

10. Heat units (HU) can be expressed as exposure rate in R/min (Gy_a/min).
    a. True
    b. False

Which of the following conditions of exposure are safe, and which are unsafe?

11. 100 kVp, 150 mA, 500 ms; 3400 rpm, 0.6 mm focal spot
    a. Safe
    b. Unsafe

12. 100 kVp, 150 mA, 500 ms; 3400 rpm, 1.2 mm focal spot
    a. Safe
    b. Unsafe

13. 100 kVp, 150 mA, 500 ms; 10,000 rpm, 0.6 mm focal spot
    a. Safe
    b. Unsafe

14. 100 kVp, 150 mA, 500 ms; 10,000 rpm, 1.2 mm focal spot
    a. Safe
    b. Unsafe

15. 100 kVp, 700 mA, 1000 ms; 10,000 rpm, 1.2 mm focal spot
    a. Safe
    b. Unsafe

16. 60 kVp, 200 mA, 100 ms; 3400 rpm, 0.6 mm focal spot
    a. Safe
    b. Unsafe

17. 120 kVp, 200 mA, 700 ms; 10,000 rpm, 0.6 mm focal spot
    a. Safe
    b. Unsafe

18. 80 kVp, 300 mA, 2000 ms; 3400 rpm, 0.6 mm focal spot
    a. Safe
    b. Unsafe

19. 120 kVp, 150 mA, 10 ms; 3400 rpm, 0.6 mm focal spot
    a. Safe
    b. Unsafe

20. 105 kVp, 700 mA, 100 ms; 10,000 rpm, 1.2 mm focal spot
    a. Safe
    b. Unsafe

21. How many heat units are produced by the following radiographic technique: 100 kVp, 150 mA, 500 ms, single phase, 3400 rpm, 0.6 mm focal spot.

Use the following charts to answer questions 22 through 25.

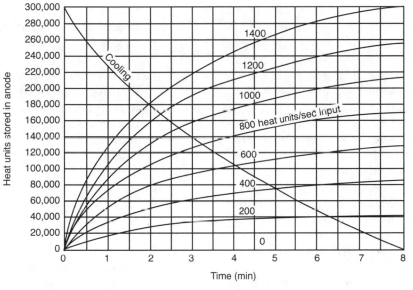

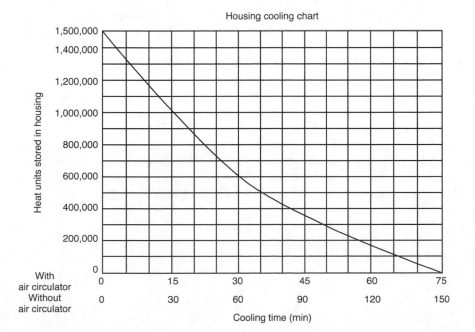

22. What is the maximum number of heat units that the anode can absorb?
23. How long would it take the tube to cool down completely from maximum heat as determined in the previous question?
24. If an anode absorbs 200,000 HU, how long will it take to cool completely?
25. If an anode absorbs 180,000 HU, how long will it be before another 180,000 HU can be absorbed?

Select the *one* correct answer from the following:

26. To determine whether any set of tube rating charts is applicable for a given x-ray tube, one should:
    a. Check to see that the operating console will allow operation at 150 kVp because this is the maximum indicated on all radiographic rating charts.
    b. Determine whether the operating console allows all of the mA settings indicated for the radiographic rating chart.
    c. Identify the type of tube, the anode rotation, the focal-spot size, and the type of generator to make certain that all of these match the specifications on the chart.
    d. Make an exposure at a radiographic technique that exceeds the maximum permitted by the charts, and check to see whether the interlock circuit prevents the exposure.
    e. Warm the tube with five rapid exposures.

27. Which of the following would be allowed according to the 1.2 mm/10,000 rpm radiographic rating chart on page 106?
    a. 68 kVp/800 mA/500 ms
    b. 82 kV/1000 mA/200 ms
    c. 88 kV/1000 mA/50 ms
    d. 90 kVp/800 mA/500 ms
    e. 108 kVp/600 mA/1000 ms

28. If a single exposure were made with factors *slightly* exceeding those permitted by the appropriate radiographic rating chart, which of the following would be the *most* probable result?
    a. The anode would pit or crack.
    b. The glass envelope would crack.
    c. The rotor would freeze and stop.
    d. The tube filament would burn out.
    e. The useful life of the tube would be reduced.

29. If a single exposure were made with factors *greatly* exceeding those permitted by the appropriate radiographic rating chart, which of the following would be the *most* probable result?
    a. The anode would pit or crack.
    b. The glass envelope would crack.
    c. The rotor would freeze and stop.
    d. The tube filament would break.
    e. The tube would become gassy.

30. Which of the following conditions will *not* damage an x-ray tube?
    a. Exceeding the anode heat storage capacity
    b. Exceeding the heat storage capacity of the tube housing
    c. Exceeding the instantaneous filament emission rate
    d. Exceeding the prescribed SID
    e. Successive high-intensity exposures

31. In the design of a rotating anode x-ray tube:
    a. Dual-focus tubes require two high-voltage, step-up transformers.
    b. Dual-focus tubes require two separate anodes.
    c. Dual-focus tubes require two target materials.
    d. Most anodes rotate at 3400 or 10,000 rpm.
    e. The disc can be made thicker so that the rpm can be increased.

32. Regarding the tube rating charts on page 107:
    a. "Heat units per second" refers to the fluoroscopic use of the x-ray tube.
    b. The anode thermal characteristics chart is for fluoroscopic use only.
    c. The filament chart is used to select exposure times.
    d. The housing cooling chart can be applied only to fluoroscopy.
    e. The maximum radiographic exposure time is shown on the anode cooling chart.

33. A fluoroscopic examination at 85 kVp and 4 mA, single phase, requires 4 min. The number of anode heat units produced would be approximately:
    a. 1360
    b. 1836
    c. 40,800
    d. 81,600
    e. 96,400

34. According to the anode thermal characteristics chart on page 107:
    a. If 180,000 HU is generated, the time required for complete cooling is approximately 4 min.
    b. Maximum capacity is 180,000 HU.
    c. The low HU capacity indicates that this is a three-phase operation.
    d. The maximum fluoroscopy time at 80 kVp and 2 mA is approximately 6.5 min.
    e. The maximum fluoroscopy time at 80 kVp and 2 mA is unlimited.

35. The formula for heat units (HU) in a single-phase high-voltage generator is:
    a. $kVp \times mA \times s$
    b. $kVp \times mA \times s^2$
    c. $kVp \times mAs \times s$
    d. $kVp \times mAs \times s^2$
    e. $kVp \times mA \times s^{-1}$

In characteristic x-ray production, the projectile electron ionizes a target atom through the removal of a tightly bound inner-shell electron. The hole created in the inner electron shell of the target atom is filled by an outer-shell electron or a free electron falling into the hole. This transition of an electron from an outer shell to an inner shell is accompanied by the emission of an x-ray of energy equal to the difference between the binding energies of the two electron shells involved.

Energy of characteristic x-ray =
BE_K shell electron − BEL shell electron
(Binding energy   (Binding energy of
of ejected electron)   replacement electron)

Approximate Electron Binding Energy, keV		
Shell	Molybdenum (Mo)	Tungsten (W)
K	20.0	69.0
L	3.0	12.0
M	0.5	2.0
N	—	1.0
O	—	0.1

EXERCISES

1. If mass is expressed in kilograms and velocity in meters per second, kinetic energy will be expressed in:
   a. Coulombs
   b. Electron volts
   c. Ergs
   d. Joules
   e. Newtons

2. The kinetic energy of the projectile electron in an x-ray tube:
   a. Causes excitation in the vacuum of the x-ray tube
   b. Causes ionization in the vacuum of the x-ray tube
   c. Is about 1% efficient in the production of x-rays
   d. Is converted to mass
   e. Is totally converted to x-ray energy

3. The shift of the characteristic x-ray spectrum to higher energy occurs because of which of the following?
   a. A decrease in voltage ripple
   b. A decrease in kVp
   c. A higher atomic number filter
   d. An increase in kVp
   e. An increase in target atomic number

4. Useful characteristic x-rays are produced in tungsten:
   a. By excitation of a K-shell electron
   b. By removal of a K-shell electron
   c. By ionization of an L-shell electron
   d. When a valence electron is removed
   e. When the projectile electron interacts with an outer-shell electron

5. An L-shell electron (binding energy 26 keV) is removed from an atom that has M-shell binding energy of 4 keV and N-shell binding energy of 1 keV. If a free electron fills the vacancy in the L-shell, the characteristic x-ray produced will have energy of:
   a. 1 keV
   b. 4 keV
   c. 22 keV
   d. 25 keV
   e. 26 keV

6. What is produced when the projectile electron excites an outer-shell electron?
   a. Bremsstrahlung x-ray
   b. Characteristic x-ray
   c. Energy
   d. Heat
   e. Photoelectric x-ray

7. The energy of characteristic x-rays increases with increasing:
   a. Filtration
   b. Atomic mass of target material
   c. Atomic number of target material
   d. kVp
   e. Voltage waveform

8. X-rays are produced when:
   a. Electric current flows through the x-ray tube filament.
   b. Projectile electrons bounce off the cathode.
   c. Projectile electrons interact with target atoms.
   d. The target angle is sufficiently large.
   e. The x-ray tube filament is heated to thermionic emission.

9. Characteristic x-rays:
   a. Are characteristic of target Z
   b. Are characteristic of the filter material
   c. Are characteristic of the voltage waveform
   d. Have velocity varying from zero to the speed of light
   e. Vary in energy as kVp is varied

10. When a tungsten-targeted x-ray tube is operated at 68 kVp:
    a. K-shell characteristic x-rays cannot be produced.
    b. L-shell x-rays cannot be produced.
    c. One possible K-shell characteristic x-ray will have 12 keV of energy.
    d. Some projectile electrons may have 68 keV of energy.
    e. Some projectile electrons may have 75 keV of energy.

11. According to the table on page 111:
    a. The farther from the nucleus, the higher the electron binding energy.
    b. The K-shell characteristic x-rays of molybdenum are lower in energy than the L-shell characteristic x-rays of tungsten.
    c. The L-shell characteristic x-rays of molybdenum are of higher energy than the L-shell characteristic x-rays of tungsten.
    d. Tungsten obviously has a lower atomic number than molybdenum.
    e. Tungsten obviously has a greater number of electrons than molybdenum.

12. When characteristic x-rays are produced, the energy is characteristic of:
    a. The atomic number of the filter
    b. The atomic number of the target
    c. The electron binding energy
    d. The mass of filtration
    e. The orientation of the target

13. Gold is sometimes used as target material in special types of radiation-producing systems. Its electron-binding energies are as follows: K-shell: 81 keV; L-shell: 14 keV; M-shell: 3 keV; and N-shell: 1 keV. Which of the following characteristic x-rays would be produced with operation at 90 kVp?
    a. 12 keV
    b. 67 keV
    c. 76 keV
    d. 87 keV
    e. 90 keV

14. The kinetic energy of a projectile electron can be measured in:
    a. Amperes
    b. Coulombs
    c. Joules
    d. Newtons
    e. Rads

15. The efficiency of x-ray production is:
    a. Approximately 5%
    b. Greater than that of heat production
    c. In excess of 5%
    d. Independent of tube current
    e. Independent of tube voltage

Bremsstrahlung x-rays are produced when a projectile electron from the cathode passes close enough to the nucleus to be influenced by the nucleus. As the projectile electron passes the nucleus, the electron slows and its direction changes. Therefore, it leaves the electron with reduced kinetic energy.

The loss in kinetic energy reappears as an x-ray. These are bremsstrahlung x-rays. They can have energy ranging from zero to a maximum that is equal to the projectile electron energy. The most frequent bremsstrahlung x-ray energy is approximately one third of the maximum energy of the projectile electron.

EXERCISES

1. In a tungsten-targeted x-ray tube operated at 90 kVp, the *most* abundant x-ray would be a:
   a. 10 keV characteristic x-ray
   b. 12 keV characteristic x-ray
   c. 30 keV bremsstrahlung x-ray
   d. 69 keV bremsstrahlung x-ray
   e. 90 keV bremsstrahlung x-ray

2. Which of the following electron transitions results in the *most* useful bremsstrahlung x-ray?
   a. L to K
   b. M to K
   c. M to L
   d. O to K
   e. None of the above

3. Bremsstrahlung radiation is produced by:
   a. Conversion of projectile electron kinetic energy to electromagnetic energy
   b. Conversion of target electron kinetic energy to electromagnetic energy
   c. Intrashell electron transitions
   d. Projectile electron–target electron interaction
   e. Target electron–nuclear interaction

4. When a bremsstrahlung x-ray is produced:
   a. A projectile electron is absorbed.
   b. A projectile electron loses energy.
   c. A target electron is displaced.
   d. A target electron is excited.
   e. A target electron is ionized.

5. In bremsstrahlung x-ray production:
   a. The projectile electron is bound to tungsten.
   b. The projectile electron is from the cathode.
   c. The target electron exists as a free electron.
   d. The target electron is from the cathode.
   e. The target electron is ionized.

6. If an average radiographic technique is used:
   a. Excitation of the target is approximately 50%.
   b. Ionization of the target is almost complete.
   c. Maximum-energy x-ray is the electron binding energy.
   d. Most x-rays are bremsstrahlung.
   e. Most x-rays are characteristic.

7. Bremsstrahlung x-rays are produced only at:
   a. Discrete energies
   b. Energies above characteristic x-rays
   c. Energies below characteristic x-rays
   d. Energies up to projectile electron energy
   e. Projectile electron kinetic energy

8. If radiographic technique is 74 kVp/80 mAs:
   a. Bremsstrahlung x-ray energy increases if the voltage is increased to 84 kVp.
   b. Bremsstrahlung x-rays are emitted at discrete energies.
   c. Bremsstrahlung x-rays have a maximum energy of 80 keV.
   d. Characteristic x-ray energy increases if the voltage is increased to 84 kVp.
   e. Characteristic x-rays are emitted only at 74 keV.

9. If radiographic technique in a tungsten target at 60 kVp/80 mAs is changed to 80 kVp/80 mAs:
   a. Additional filtration is required.
   b. Bremsstrahlung x-ray intensity remains unchanged.
   c. Characteristic x-ray intensity remains unchanged.
   d. The number of projectile electrons increases.
   e. The number of x-rays produced increases.

10. Bremsstrahlung x-rays produced in a tungsten-targeted x-ray tube:
    a. Are all diagnostically useful
    b. Are generally less useful than characteristic x-rays
    c. Are less intense than characteristic x-rays
    d. Are less intense than if produced in molybdenum
    e. Outnumber characteristic x-rays

11. When a bremsstrahlung x-ray is emitted:
    a. A projectile electron is absorbed.
    b. An inner-shell electron is removed from the target atom.
    c. An outer-shell electron is removed from the target atom.
    d. This results from the conversion of kinetic energy.
    e. The target atom is ionized.

12. The wavelength of an x-ray:
    a. Becomes longer as projectile electron kinetic energy is reduced
    b. Becomes longer with increasing projectile electron energy
    c. Is longer than that of ultraviolet light
    d. Is longest when the projectile electron loses all its kinetic energy
    e. Is proportional to its frequency

13. When projectile electron energy is increased:
    a. Characteristic x-ray energy decreases.
    b. Characteristic x-ray energy increases.
    c. More bremsstrahlung x-rays are produced.
    d. More bremsstrahlung x-rays are produced, but only at high energies.
    e. More bremsstrahlung x-rays are produced, but only at low energies.

14. The efficiency of bremsstrahlung x-ray production increases with increasing:
    a. Collimation
    b. Filtration
    c. mA
    d. SID
    e. Target atomic number

15. The output intensity of an x-ray tube:
    a. Increases when filtered
    b. Is limited by the K-shell binding energy
    c. Is monoenergetic
    d. Often is measured in curies (becquerels)
    e. Is primarily due to bremsstrahlung x-rays

16. Which of the following projectile electron-target interactions results in x-ray emission?
    a. Excitation of inner-shell electron
    b. Excitation of outer-shell electron
    c. Removal of inner-shell electron
    d. Removal of nucleus
    e. Removal of outer-shell electron

17. When a projectile electron enters a target atom and interacts with the nuclear force field:
    a. It decreases in velocity.
    b. It increases in velocity.
    c. It ionizes the atom.
    d. It ionizes the nucleus.
    e. It removes an inner-shell electron.

8-3

X-Ray Emission Spectrum

 An x-ray emission spectrum is a graph of the relative number of x-rays plotted as a function of the energy of each x-ray.

The characteristic x-ray emission spectrum represents monoenergetic x-rays emitted after ionization of the target atom. It consists of vertical lines at fixed energies and is called a **discrete** x-ray emission spectrum.

The bremsstrahlung x-ray emission spectrum results from x-rays created by the bremsstrahlung process and has energy ranging from zero to the maximum projectile electron energy. This spectrum is the **continuous** emission spectrum, and its maximum amplitude occurs at an energy that is approximately one third of the maximum energy.

EXERCISES

1. The area under the curve of the x-ray emission spectrum represents:
   a. The average energy of the x-rays
   b. The average number of x-rays per unit of energy
   c. The total energy of the x-rays
   d. The total number of x-rays
   e. Total exposure (mGy_a)

2. Normally, the x-ray emission spectrum contains:
   a. Both characteristic and bremsstrahlung x-rays
   b. Both photoelectric and Compton x-rays
   c. Only bremsstrahlung x-rays
   d. Only characteristic x-rays
   e. Only discrete lines

3. The characteristic x-ray emission spectrum principally depends on which of the following?
   a. Filtration
   b. kVp
   c. mAs
   d. Projectile electron energy
   e. Target material

4. The continuous x-ray emission spectrum principally depends on which of the following?
   a. Exposure time
   b. Filtration
   c. mAs
   d. Projectile electron energy
   e. Target material

5. Which of the following factors explains the low number of x-rays produced at low energy?
   a. Added filtration
   b. The glass envelope of the x-ray tube
   c. The kVp
   d. The mAs enclosing the x-ray tube
   e. The product of tube current and exposure time

6. The x-ray emission spectrum represents:
   a. Projectile electron energy
   b. Atomic mass and number of the target atom
   c. Electron binding energy of target material
   d. Total x-ray beam filtration
   e. X-rays emitted from the x-ray tube

7. Both the shape and the position of the characteristic x-ray emission spectrum:
   a. Are described by the number of projectile electrons
   b. Represent projectile electron energy
   c. Can be described as continuous
   d. Correspond to target electron binding energies
   e. Result from nuclear interaction

8. A diagnostic x-ray beam contains:
   a. Bremsstrahlung only
   b. Mostly bremsstrahlung x-rays, with some characteristic x-rays
   c. Mostly Compton x-rays, few bremsstrahlung x-rays, and some pair production x-rays
   d. Some Compton x-rays, some bremsstrahlung x-rays, and no pair production x-rays
   e. Some photoelectric x-rays

9. The x-ray emission spectrum is a plot of:
   a. mAs versus kVp
   b. The number of electrons versus energy
   c. The number of x-rays versus energy
   d. X-rays and electrons emitted from cathode atoms
   e. X-rays and electrons emitted from target atoms

10. The amplitude of the bremsstrahlung x-ray emission spectrum:
    a. Approaches maximum at an energy equal to the kVp
    b. Approaches maximum at zero energy
    c. Has maximum value at energy approximately one third of the kVp
    d. Has maximum value at energy equal to the kVp
    e. Is enhanced with filtration

11. If an x-ray emission spectrum represented operation at 85 kVp with a tungsten target:
    a. At 85 keV, the number of projectile electrons would be maximum.
    b. Bremsstrahlung x-rays would be most intense at 85 keV.
    c. The K-characteristic x-ray emission would occur at 69 keV.
    d. X-rays representing maximum frequency would occur at 69 keV.
    e. X-rays representing minimum wavelength would occur at 0 keV.

12. If an x-ray emission spectrum represented operation at 26 kVp with a molybdenum target:
    a. K-characteristic x-rays would not be produced.
    b. More characteristic bremsstrahlung x-rays are emitted.
    c. The characteristic radiation would have an energy of approximately 19 keV.
    d. Maximum-frequency x-rays would have an energy of 17 keV.
    e. Minimum-wavelength x-rays would have an energy of 20 keV.

13. Which of the following factors principally accounts for the reduced x-ray intensity at low energy?
    a. Added filtration
    b. Beam collimation
    c. Atomic number of the target material
    d. Energy spectrum of the projectile electrons
    e. Voltage waveform

14. Characteristic x-radiation is related to the:
    a. Difference between K- and L-shell binding energy
    b. Energy required to eject K-shell electrons
    c. Energy to eject L-shell electrons
    d. Number of electrons
    e. Number of K-shell electrons

15. Molybdenum has a lower atomic number than tungsten; therefore, the molybdenum x-ray emission spectrum:
    a. Extends to higher energies
    b. Extends to lower energies
    c. Has higher amplitude
    d. Has higher-energy characteristic x-rays
    e. Has lower amplitude

16. To construct an x-ray emission spectrum, one must know the:
    a. kVp and mAs
    b. mAs and x-ray frequency
    c. Number of x-rays at each energy interval
    d. Projectile electron number and energy interval
    e. Target element and filtration

X-ray emission sometimes is shown as a function of x-ray wavelength rather than energy. Because x-ray energy and wavelength are inversely proportional, the highest x-ray energy corresponds to the shortest x-ray wavelength, which is also called the minimum wavelength.

Planck's equation is:

$$E = h\nu$$

where

$$\nu = c/\lambda$$

Therefore:

$$E = \frac{hc}{\lambda}$$

$$E = \frac{(4.14 \times 10^{-15} \text{eVs}) \, (3 \times 10^8 \text{ m/s})}{\lambda}$$

$$E = \frac{12.4 \times 10^{-7} \text{ eV m}}{\lambda} \frac{1 \text{ keV}}{10^3 \text{ eV}}$$

$$E = \frac{12.4 \times 10^{-10} \text{ keV m}}{\lambda}$$

This equation can be rearranged to solve for λ, which is the wavelength of an x-ray having energy E in keV:

$$\lambda = \frac{12.4 \times 10^{-10} \text{ keV m}}{E}$$

$$\lambda_{min} = \frac{12.4 \times 10^{-10} \text{ keV m}}{\text{kVp}}$$

$$\lambda_{min}(\text{nm}) = \frac{1.24}{\text{kVp}}$$

EXERCISES

1. Which characteristic is reduced as x-ray energy increases?
   a. Filtration
   b. Projectile electron energy
   c. Target electron energy
   d. X-ray frequency
   e. X-ray wavelength

2. The wavelength of an x-ray is:
   a. Determined by filter thickness
   b. Determined by the number of projectile electrons
   c. Determined by the number of target electrons
   d. Directly proportional to its energy
   e. Inversely proportional to its energy

3. The product of Planck's constant (h) and the velocity of light (c) has units of:
   a. Jm^2
   b. Jm
   c. J/m
   d. Js
   e. J/s

4. The product of Planck's constant (h) and the velocity of light (c) equals:
   a. 12.4 eVm
   b. 12.4 keVm
   c. 12.4×10^{-7} eVm

d. 12.4×10^{-10} eVm
e. 12.4×10^{-15} eVm

5. If one knows the minimum wavelength of a given x-ray beam, the kVp of operation can be determined if one also knows:
a. Planck's constant
b. That nothing more is needed
c. The mA
d. The mAs
e. The speed of light

6. Indicate which of the following figures represents an x-ray emission spectrum:

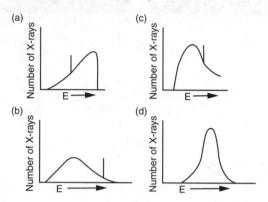

7. The relationship of minimum wavelength to maximum x-ray energy is sometimes called the:
a. Duane-Hunt Law
b. Faraday Law
c. Haus-Hendrick Law
d. Hurter-Driffield curve
e. Quantum theory of Planck

8. Minimum wavelength is related to:
a. Nuclear charge.
b. The atomic number of the target material
c. The degree of collimation of the x-ray beam
d. The kinetic energy of the projectile electron
e. The total filtration in the x-ray beam

9. That region of the x-ray emission spectrum associated with minimum wavelength is the:
a. Highest-energy bremsstrahlung x-ray
b. Highest-energy characteristic line
c. Intersection of the two axes
d. Lowest-energy bremsstrahlung x-ray
e. Lowest-energy characteristic line

10. If one knows the minimum wavelength of an x-ray emission spectrum, one can calculate:
a. Filter atomic number
b. Filtration thickness
c. mA

d. mAs
e. Maximum projectile electron energy

11. To calculate minimum x-ray wavelength, one must know the value of:
a. Filtration
b. kVp
c. mA
d. mAs
e. Phase

12. How would the total emission spectrum be affected by operation at 80 kVp/400 mA/100 ms? The relative position of the spectrum would:
a. Remain the same
b. Remain the same, but the amplitude would decrease
c. Remain the same, but the amplitude would increase
d. Shift to the left, and the amplitude would be lower
e. Shift to the right

13. How would the emission spectrum be affected by the addition of 2 mm Al filtration? The relative position of the spectrum would:
a. Remain the same
b. Remain the same, but the amplitude would decrease
c. Remain the same, but the amplitude would increase
d. Shift to the left, and the amplitude would be lower
e. Shift to the right, and the amplitude would be lower

14. How would the emission spectrum be affected if the power supply were changed from single phase to three phase? The relative position of the spectrum would:
a. Not change, but the energy of the characteristic lines would increase
b. Remain the same
c. Remain the same, the amplitude would increase, and the characteristic lines would increase in height
d. Shift to the left, the amplitude would increase, and the characteristic lines would increase in height
e. Shift to the right, the amplitude would increase, and the characteristic lines would increase in height

8-5

Factors That Affect the X-Ray Emission Spectrum

The shape of the emission spectrum and its relative position vary with changes in kVp, mAs, filtration, target material, and voltage waveform. Higher amplitude in the emission spectrum represents greater x-ray intensity (beam quantity), whereas a shift of the spectrum to the right along the energy axis represents greater penetrability (beam quality).

In general, the following relationships apply:

- Increasing kVp increases the height of the x-ray emission spectrum and extends it to the right along the energy axis.
- Increasing mAs increases the height of the x-ray emission spectrum.
- Increasing filtration decreases the height of the x-ray emission spectrum and shifts the shape to the right along the energy axis.
- Changing to a higher atomic number x-ray target increases the x-ray emission spectrum amplitude, shifts the spectrum to the right, and results in higher-energy characteristic lines.
- Changing from half-wave to full-wave rectification doubles the height of the spectrum.
- Changing from single-phase to three-phase power results in greater amplitude and a shift to the right on the energy axis.

EXERCISES

1. Which of the following statements applies to the x-ray emission spectrum?
   a. Adding filtration affects characteristic x-ray energy.
   b. Adding filtration affects minimum wavelength.
   c. Adding filtration increases entrance skin exposure.
   d. The target material affects the amplitude of bremsstrahlung x-rays.
   e. The target material affects the minimum wavelength.

2. An increase in mAs results in an increase in:
   a. Average x-ray energy.
   b. Both characteristic and bremsstrahlung x-rays
   c. Minimum wavelength
   d. Only the bremsstrahlung x-rays
   e. Only the characteristic x-rays

3. An increase in kVp results in an increase in:
   a. Characteristic x-ray energy.
   b. Only the bremsstrahlung x-ray emission spectrum
   c. Only the characteristic x-ray emission spectrum
   d. Radiation quality
   e. Minimum wavelength

4. The intensity of x-ray exposure is best represented by:
   a. The amplitude of the bremsstrahlung x-ray emission spectrum
   b. The amplitude of the characteristic x-ray emission spectrum
   c. The amplitude of the highest emission spectrum
   d. The area under the emission spectrum
   e. The energy range of the emission spectrum

Examine the following figure, and answer questions 5 through 7:

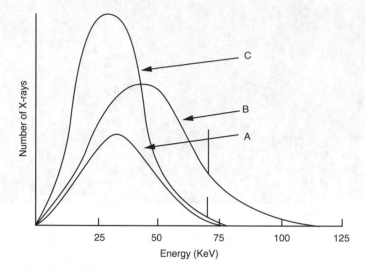

5. Which of these curves have equal minimum wavelength and equal maximum energy?
   a. A, B, and C
   b. A and B
   c. A and C
   d. B and C
   e. None of the above

6. Of the three curves represented:
   a. A and B represent two different targets.
   b. A and C were produced at the same kVp.
   c. A and C were produced at the same mAs.
   d. A is single phase and C is three phase.
   e. C and B represent two different targets.

7. Of the three spectra:
   a. A is more penetrating than B.
   b. A is more penetrating than C.
   c. B is more penetrating than C.
   d. C is more penetrating than A.
   e. C is more penetrating than B.

8. Which of the following factors primarily affects the low-energy side of the x-ray emission spectrum?
   a. Exposure time
   b. Filtration
   c. Tube current
   d. Tube voltage
   e. Voltage waveform

9. In general, when changes are made that affect the x-ray emission spectrum and the:
   a. Amplitude increases, the radiation quantity decreases

   b. Line spectrum moves, voltage waveform has changed
   c. Spectrum shifts to the left, a higher-quality beam is emitted
   d. Spectrum shifts to the left, more filtration was used
   e. Spectrum shifts to the right, a more penetrating beam is emitted

Answer the remaining questions about an emission spectrum that represents a diagnostic imaging system operated at 80 kVp/200 mA/100 ms with a tungsten target.

10. How would the bremsstrahlung spectrum change if operation at 80 kVp/200 mA/100 ms were changed to 64 kVp/200 mA/100 ms?
    a. It would remain the same, but the amplitude would decrease.
    b. It would remain the same, but the amplitude would increase.
    c. It would shift to the left, and the amplitude would be lower.
    d. It would shift to the left, and the amplitude would be higher.
    e. It would shift to the right, and the amplitude would be higher.

11. How would the characteristic spectrum change if operation were at 64 kVp/200 mA/20 ms? The characteristic x-ray spectrum would:
    a. Decrease in height
    b. Disappear
    c. Increase in height
    d. Shift slightly to the left
    e. Shift slightly to the right

The intensity of x-rays in the useful beam is measured in roentgens (R) or mGy_a and milliroentgens (mR), and is referred to as *x-ray quantity*. At 70 kVp, the output intensity (or quantity) of a radiographic tube ranges from about 3 to 10 mR/mAs at 100 cm source-to-image receptor distance (SID). This wide range of x-ray quantity exists because of differences in tube design, filtration, and voltage generation.

Three adjustable factors affect x-ray quantity:

1. mAs: X-ray quantity is directly proportional to milliampere-seconds (mAs):

$$\frac{I_1}{I_2} = \frac{mAs_1}{mAs_2}$$

2. kVp: X-ray quantity varies approximately as the square of the change in kilovolt peak (kVp):

$$\frac{I_1}{I_2} = (kVp_1/kVp_2)^2$$

3. Distance: X-ray quantity varies inversely with the square of the distance from the target (the inverse square law):

$$I_1/I_2 = (d_2/d_1)^2$$

When these factors are viewed collectively, x-ray exposure of a patient can be estimated at a reasonable approximation with the use of the following equation:

$$X\text{-ray quantity (mR)} = \frac{k\ (mAs)\ (kVp)^2}{d^2}$$

where d is the source-to-skin distance (SSD) in centimeters. The constant k will vary from approximately 10 to 30, depending on many factors, including voltage, voltage ripple, filtration, and field size.

EXERCISES

1. When the mAs is increased, x-ray quantity:
   a. Decreases as the square of the mAs
   b. Decreases proportionately
   c. Increases as the square of the mAs
   d. Increases proportionately
   e. Remains the same

2. When the kVp is increased, x-ray quantity:
   a. Decreases in proportion to kVp^2
   b. Decreases proportionately
   c. Increases in proportion to kVp^2
   d. Increases proportionately
   e. Remains the same

3. When distance is increased, x-ray quantity at that distance:
   a. Decreases in proportion to distance squared
   b. Decreases proportionately
   c. Increases in proportion to distance squared
   d. Increases proportionately
   e. Remains the same

4. When x-ray tube filtration is increased, x-ray quantity:
   a. Decreases
   b. Decreases proportionately
   c. Increases
   d. Increases proportionately
   e. Remains the same

5. In general, x-ray quantity will increase with a/an:
   a. Decrease in exposure time
   b. Decrease in tube current
   c. Increase in distance
   d. Increase in filtration
   e. Increase in kVp

6. X-ray quantity usually is measured as which of the following?
   a. Absorbed dose in rad
   b. Absorbed dose in roentgens
   c. Dose equivalent in roentgens
   d. Exposure in rad
   e. Exposure in roentgens

7. A tungsten-targeted x-ray imaging system is operated at 66 kVp/150 mAs and has an output intensity of 600 mR. Therefore:
   a. Characteristic x-rays will be prominent.
   b. If the mAs is increased to 200, the minimum wavelength will be increased.
   c. Most electron–target atom interactions will result in x-ray emission.
   d. No useful bremsstrahlung radiation will be produced.
   e. The most frequent x-ray emission will be in the 20 to 25 keV range.

8. X-ray quantity can be measured in which of the following?
   a. Bq
   b. Gy_a
   c. Gy_t
   d. Rem
   e. Sv

9. Another meaning of "x-ray quantity" is x-ray:
   a. Energy
   b. Filtration
   c. Intensity
   d. Penetrability
   e. Quality

10. Which of the following does *not* affect x-ray quantity?
    a. Filtration
    b. kVp
    c. mA
    d. Radioactivity
    e. Time

11. To maintain a constant optical density, what percentage increase in kVp should be accompanied by a reduction of one half in mAs?
    a. 5%
    b. 10%
    c. 15%
    d. 30%
    e. 50%

12. An extremity radiograph requires 5 mAs and results in an exposure of 18 mR. What will be the exposure if the technique is changed to 7 mAs?
    a. 18 mR
    b. 19 mR
    c. 22 mR
    d. 25 mR
    e. 36 mR

13. An abdominal view is taken at 82 kVp and results in a patient exposure of 132 mR. To improve contrast and density, the kVp is reduced to 74 with no change in mAs. What is the new patient exposure?
    a. 108 mR
    b. 119 mR
    c. 134 mR
    d. 146 mR
    e. 162 mR

14. A portable chest x-ray is taken at 90 cm SID, and the patient exposure is 28 mR. What will the exposure be if the distance is increased to 180 cm and there is no accompanying technique change?
    a. 7 mR
    b. 12 mR
    c. 17 mR
    d. 63 mR
    e. 142 mR

15. The output intensity for an x-ray imaging system operated at 70 kVp/400 mA and 50 ms is 70 mR. If the mA selector is changed to 600 mA and the exposure time is increased to 80 ms, what will be the output intensity?
    a. 105 mR
    b. 112 mR
    c. 168 mR
    d. 210 mR
    e. 234 mR

An x-ray beam that easily penetrates soft tissue and bone is said to be of high quality, whereas a beam that is easily absorbed is of low quality. X ray quality therefore is a measure of the penetrating ability of an x-ray beam or the energy of the x-ray beam.

- As the voltage of operation is increased, the energy of the x-ray beam is increased; therefore, penetrating ability and quality also increase.
- When filtration is added to the beam, it becomes lower quantity, higher energy, and more penetrating, and therefore of greater quality.
- Tube current (mA), exposure time (s), and distance (SID) do not influence the quality of an x-ray beam.
- X-ray beam quality usually is measured by the **half-value layer (HVL)**.
- The HVL is that thickness of an absorber that will reduce the x-ray intensity to one half of its original value.

EXERCISES

1. Which of the following is the *most* appropriate measure of x-ray beam quality?
   a. Added filtration
   b. HVL
   c. kVp
   d. mAs
   e. Total filtration

2. The quality of an x-ray beam is principally a function of which of the following?
   a. Field size
   b. Filtration
   c. kVp
   d. mAs
   e. SID

3. The HVL is affected principally by a change in which of the following?
   a. Filter thickness
   b. kVp
   c. mAs
   d. SID
   e. X-ray intensity

4. When filtration is added to an x-ray tube, which of the following increases?
   a. Radiation output
   b. Radiation quality
   c. Radiation quantity
   d. SID
   e. SSD

5. Which of the following is the probable HVL of a radiographic x-ray beam at 70 kVp?
   a. 0.5 cm Al
   b. 5.0 cm Al
   c. 0.5 cm soft tissue
   d. 5.0 cm soft tissue
   e. 10 cm soft tissue

6. As filtration is added to an x-ray beam:
   a. All x-rays are removed about equally from the useful beam.
   b. High-energy x-rays are removed more readily than low-energy x-rays.
   c. Low-energy x-rays are removed more readily than high-energy x-rays.

d. No x-rays are removed, but their average energy is increased.

e. No x-rays are removed, but their average energy is reduced.

7. An increase in mAs will increase which of the following?
a. Exposure time
b. HVL
c. Total filtration
d. X-ray quality
e. X-ray quantity

8. It is often stated that mAs controls quantity and kVp controls:
a. Collimation
b. Filtration
c. Output
d. Quality
e. SID

9. However, it should be clear that mAs controls quantity and kVp controls:
a. Filtration and quality
b. Output and filtration
c. Quality and quantity
d. SID and quality
e. SID and SSD

10. If the mA during fluoroscopy is increased by 25%:
a. kVp should be reduced by 4.
b. The effective energy of the beam is increased.
c. The scatter exposure to the operator is increased by 25%.
d. The scatter exposure to the operator is reduced by 25%.
e. The x-ray output is reduced by 25%.

11. A minimum HVL is required for diagnostic x-ray beams because:
a. A greater HVL would mean lower than average x-ray energy.
b. A higher HVL would result in an increased absorbed dose to the patient with no improvement in image quality.
c. A lower HVL would result in an increased absorbed dose to the patient with no improvement in image quality.
d. A lower HVL would result in reduced subject contrast.
e. It protects the operator from excessive scatter.

12. An x-ray beam can be made to have higher effective energy if which of the following occurs?
a. Filtration is added.
b. Filtration is removed.
c. mAs is increased.
d. SID is increased.
e. SSD is increased.

13. According to the data below, which were obtained at 26 kVp, which of the following is closest to the HVL?

mm Al	0	0.2	0.4	0.6	1.0
mR	94	69	52	39	30

a. 0.1 mm Al
b. 0.2 mm Al
c. 0.3 mm Al
d. 0.5 mm Al
e. 1.0 mm Al

14. Which of the following will enhance x-ray beam quality?
a. Collimation
b. Filtration
c. mA
d. mAs
e. SID

15. Reducing kVp will do which of the following?
a. Harden the x-ray beam
b. Increase the x-ray quality
c. Increase the x-ray quantity
d. Require removal of filtration
e. Soften the x-ray beam

16. Adding filtration to an x-ray beam will do which of the following?
a. Decrease x-ray quality
b. Increase inherent filtration
c. Increase x-ray quality
d. Increase x-ray quantity
e. Reduce scatter radiation

17. A radiographic tube has 0.5 mm Al inherent filtration, 1.0 mm Al added filtration, and 1.0 mm Al filtration in the light-localizing collimator. Therefore, the total filtration is:
a. 0.5 mm Al
b. 1.0 mm Al
c. 2.0 mm Al
d. 2.5 mm Al
e. 4.0 mm Al

18. A representative radiographic tube has 0.5 mm Al inherent filtration and 2.0 mm Al added filtration. Therefore:
    a. An additional 1.0 mm Al filtration will harden the x-ray beam.
    b. An additional 1.0 mm Al will increase the x-ray quantity.
    c. An additional 1.0 mm Al will increase total filtration to 3.0 mm Al.
    d. An additional 1.0 mm Al will reduce scatter radiation.
    e. The total filtration is 1.5 mm Al.

19. Which of the following is the softest radiation?
    a. Diagnostic x-rays
    b. Grenz rays
    c. Megavoltage x-rays
    d. Orthovoltage x-rays
    e. Supervoltage x-rays

20. The HVL is defined as:
    a. A thickness of attenuator that will double x-ray quantity
    b. A thickness of attenuator that will halve x-ray quantity
    c. Half the required shielding
    d. The mAs value required to double quantity
    e. Twice the required shielding

21. To measure HVL, which of the following is required?
    a. A collimator
    b. A densitometer
    c. A penetrameter
    d. A sensitometer
    e. Aluminum absorbers

22. As the HVL of a beam increases, its penetrability:
    a. Decreases
    b. Decreases as Z^2
    c. Increases
    d. Increases as Z^2
    e. Is unchanged

23. If increasing the kVp increases the HVL, x-ray quantity will:
    a. Decrease
    b. Decrease by kVp^2
    c. Increase
    d. Increase by kVp^2
    e. Not change

24. If the HVL is increased by the addition of 1 mm Al, x-ray quantity will:
    a. Decrease
    b. Decrease by $(mm\ Al)^2$
    c. Increase
    d. Increase by $(mm\ Al)^2$
    e. Not change

25. At 70 kVp, the x-ray beam is attenuated in soft tissue approximately:
    a. 0.05%/cm
    b. 0.5%/cm
    c. 5%/cm
    d. 25%/cm
    e. 50%/cm

Examine the following illustration and answer Exercises 26 and 27:

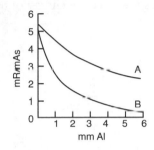

26. The approximate HVL of curve A is closest to:
    a. 1 mm Al
    b. 2 mm Al
    c. 3 mm Al
    d. 4 mm Al
    e. 6 mm Al

27. The approximate HVL of curve B is closest to:
    a. 1 mm Al
    b. 2 mm Al
    c. 3 mm Al
    d. 4 mm Al
    e. 6 mm Al

28. There is a 75% chance that an x-ray will be attenuated by 2 mm lead. The HVL is:
    a. 0.5 mm Pb
    b. 1.0 mm Pb
    c. 1.5 mm Pb
    d. 2.0 mm Pb
    e. 4.0 mm Pb

29. What occurs when the small rather than the large cathode coil is energized?
    a. Increased cathode heating
    b. Increased x-ray quality

c. Longer exposures needed
d. Lower HVL
e. Smaller effective focal spot

30. Added filtration affects the x-rays beam in what way?
    a. Higher beam quantity
    b. Higher patient dose
    c. Increased beam hardening
    d. Poorer beam quality
    e. Reduced kVp

31. An aluminum filter:
    a. Decreases the intensity of all energies of the x-ray beam
    b. Increases skin dose
    c. Is not necessary below 50 kVp
    d. Of at least 1 cm is required
    e. Reduces the effective energy of the beam

32. If patient thickness is 6 HVLs, what is the approximate intensity at the midline of the patient?
    a. 1%
    b. 5%
    c. 12%
    d. 50%
    e. 75%

33. A diagnostic x-ray beam has an HVL of approximately 3 cm soft tissue. What percentage of the beam is absorbed by a 21 cm abdomen?
    a. 0 to 10
    b. 10 to 20
    c. 20 to 60
    d. 60 to 90
    e. >90

Three types of x-ray beam filtration exist:
• **Inherent filtration**—This results from the glass or metal envelope of the x-ray tube and the window in the x-ray tube housing. It is usually equivalent to approximately 0.5 mm Al.
• **Added filtration**—This is the result of placing an absorber in the path of the x-ray beam. The absorber, usually 1 to 3 mm Al, is positioned between the collimator and the tube housing.
• **Compensating filter**—This has nothing to do with patient dose; compensating filters are used specifically for shaping the x-ray intensity over the beam area, so that radiation that reaches the image receptor is more uniform and produces more uniform optical density.

EXERCISES

1. The inherent filtration in a general purpose radiographic x-ray tube is usually equivalent to:
   a. 0 mm Al
   b. 0.1 mm Al
   c. 0.5 mm Al
   d. 1.0 mm Al
   e. 2.5 mm Al

2. The equivalent added filtration provided by a conventional light-localizing, variable-aperture collimator is closest to:
   a. 0 mm Al
   b. 0.5 mm Al
   c. 1.0 mm Al
   d. 2.0 mm Al
   e. 2.5 mm Al

3. The purpose of a wedge filter in diagnostic radiology is to produce:
   a. A harder beam
   b. A softer beam
   c. A uniform x-ray beam intensity at the image receptor
   d. A uniform x-ray beam intensity at the patient
   e. An x-ray beam to fit the image receptor

4. The primary purpose of adding filtration to an x-ray beam is to:
   a. Cause high-energy x-rays to Compton scatter
   b. Protect the film from low-energy x-rays
   c. Remove low-energy electrons
   d. Remove low-energy x-rays
   e. Remove penetrating x-rays

5. An x-ray beam filter has the *greatest* effect on dose reduction to the:
   a. Gonads
   b. Lens
   c. Skin
   d. Thyroid
   e. Whole body

6. X-rays of higher maximum energy can be obtained by doing which of the following?
   a. Increasing filtration
   b. Increasing kVp
   c. Increasing mAs
   d. Reducing inherent filtration
   e. Using a higher Z target

7. The light-localizing, variable-aperture collimator contributes:
   a. No filtration when its light is off
   b. No filtration when its light is on
   c. Scatter x-rays
   d. To added filtration
   e. To inherent filtration

8. If 5 mm Al filtration is added to the x-ray tube:
   a. Contrast resolution will improve.
   b. Motion unsharpness will decrease.
   c. Optical density will decrease.
   d. Patient dose will increase.
   e. Radiographic contrast will increase.

9. An x-ray beam can be made harder by increasing which of the following?
   a. Filtration
   b. mA
   c. mAs
   d. SID
   e. SSD

10. When filtration is added to a normally filtered x-ray beam, the x-ray emission spectrum will:
    a. Decrease in amplitude
    b. Have higher-energy discrete lines
    c. Have lower-energy discrete lines
    d. Increase in amplitude
    e. Shift to the left

11. Added filtration:
    a. Increases x-ray quantity
    b. Is expensive
    c. Is usually thinner than inherent filtration
    d. Protects the patient from unnecessary radiation exposure
    e. Reduces x-ray quality

12. Inherent filtration:
    a. Consists of sheets of aluminum
    b. Helps harden the x-ray beam
    c. Is approximately 2.0 mm Al
    d. Is mainly due to the light localizer
    e. Tends to decrease with tube age

13. To produce low inherent filtration in an x-ray beam:
    a. A thin section of glass is used.
    b. Insulating oil is placed around the tube.
    c. kVp should be reduced.
    d. The collimator should be removed.
    e. Windows made of copper are used.

14. Wedge filters are:
    a. Always better than uniform filters because they attenuate a greater number of x-rays
    b. Used for lateral skull examinations
    c. Used to image a knee
    d. Used to match the image receptor
    e. Used to obtain uniform optical density

15. During mammography:
    a. Added filtration is removed to enhance x-ray quality.
    b. Aluminum is the usual filter.
    c. Low total filtration is desirable.
    d. No filtration is required.
    e. The total filtration should be between 2 and 3 mm Al.

16. When added filtration is increased:
    a. kVp must be reduced.
    b. mAs must be reduced.
    c. Effective x-ray energy is reduced.
    d. X-ray quality is enhanced.
    e. X-ray quantity is increased.

17. If a radiographic tube has 0.5 mm Al inherent filtration and 2.0 mm Al added filtration, which of the following is *true*?
    a. Adding 1.0 mm Al will harden the x-ray beam.
    b. Adding 1.0 mm Al will increase the total filtration to 2.5 mm Al.
    c. Adding 1.0 mm Al will increase the x-ray quantity.
    d. Removing 1.0 mm Al will increase HVL.
    e. The total filtration is 1.5 mm Al.

18. Inherent filtration is:
    a. Dependent on the type of aluminum used
    b. Increased when kVp is raised
    c. Increased with patient thickness
    d. Increased with tube age
    e. Produced by slowing down electrons

19. An x-ray tube has a total filtration of 3.0 mm Al and an HVL of 2.5 mm Al, and emits 180 mR. Therefore:
    a. The addition of 1.0 mm Al filtration will increase the quantity of the beam.
    b. The addition of 1.0 mm Al will enhance the quality of the beam.
    c. The addition of 2.5 mm Al will reduce the output intensity to 100 mR.
    d. The addition of 2.5 mm Al will reduce the output intensity to 135 mR.
    e. The output is also 7.2 mR/mAs.

X-ray interaction with loosely bound electrons of tissue atoms is responsible for scatter radiation. The incident x-ray interacts with an outer-shell electron of a tissue atom and transfers some of its energy to the electron. After the interaction, the electron is ejected from the atom (the atom is ionized) and the x-ray is scattered. Because the incident x-ray imparts some of its energy to the Compton electron, it loses energy.

The probability that an x-ray will undergo a Compton interaction decreases with increasing x-ray energy. The occurrence of the Compton effect is independent of the atomic number of the absorber. In conventional radiography, more than 70% of the incident x-rays undergo Compton interactions; this interaction contributes to the radiographic noise that reduces contrast.

EXERCISES

1. Which of the following is *not* one of the five basic x-ray interactions with matter?
   a. Bremsstrahlung
   b. Classical scattering
   c. Compton scattering
   d. Photodisintegration
   e. Photoelectric effect

2. Which of the following x-rays would be *most* likely to undergo classical scattering?
   a. 5 keV
   b. 15 keV
   c. 35 keV
   d. 66 keV
   e. 85 keV

3. Which of the following interactions contributes to image noise?
   a. Bremsstrahlung
   b. Characteristic
   c. Compton scattering
   d. Photodisintegration
   e. Photoelectric effect

4. Which of the following occurs in a Compton interaction?
   a. An atom is excited.
   b. An atom is ionized.
   c. The secondary electron has kinetic energy equal to the difference between the energy of the incident x-ray and the electron binding energy.
   d. The secondary electron has kinetic energy equal to the incident x-ray.
   e. The secondary photon has wavelength equal to the primary x-ray.

5. If Ei = incident x-ray energy, E_s = scattered x-ray energy, E_b = electron binding energy, and E_{KE} = secondary electron kinetic energy, then which of the following is *true*?
   a. $E_i = E_s + E_b + E_{KE}$
   b. $E_i = E_s - E_b - E_{KE}$

c. $E_i = E_s - E_b + E_{KE}$
d. $E_i = E_s + (E_b - E_{KE})$
e. $E_i = E_{KE} - (E_b + E_s)$

6. If E_i = incident x-ray energy, E_s = scattered x-ray energy, E_b = electron binding energy, and E_{KE} = secondary electron kinetic energy, then which of the following is *true*?
   a. $E_s = E_b + E_{KE} + E_i$
   b. $E_s = E_b - (E_{KE} + E_i)$
   c. $E_s = E_{KE} - (E_b + E_i)$
   d. $E_s = E_i - (E_b + E_{KE})$
   e. $E_s = E_{KE} + E_i - E_b$

7. During the Compton effect, *most* of the incident x-ray energy is given to which of the following?
   a. Characteristic radiation
   b. Excitation
   c. Electron binding energy
   d. Electron mass
   e. Scattered x-ray

8. After Compton scattering, the scattered x-ray has:
   a. Higher energy
   b. Higher frequency
   c. Less mass
   d. Longer wavelength
   e. Lower velocity

9. Compton interaction affects the image by increasing which of the following?
   a. Contrast resolution
   b. Latitude
   c. Noise (fog)
   d. Spatial resolution
   e. Speed

10. The probability that an x-ray will interact with an outer-shell electron is influenced principally by:
    a. The atomic number of the absorber
    b. The binding energy of the electron
    c. The energy of the incident x-ray
    d. The kinetic energy of the electron
    e. The x-ray production mode

11. The Compton effect is:
    a. Independent of Z
    b. Inversely proportional to Z

c. Proportional to E
d. Proportional to Z
e. Proportional to Z^2

12. The Compton effect is:
    a. Also called classical scattering
    b. The principal source of image noise (fog)
    c. The same as Rayleigh scattering
    d. The same as the Thomson effect
    e. The source of static marks on film

13. If a 45 keV x-ray interacts with the K-shell electron in an atom of molybdenum (E_b = 20 keV) and ejects it with 8 keV energy, what will be the energy of the scattered x-ray?
    a. 12 keV
    b. 17 keV
    c. 25 keV
    d. 37 keV
    e. 45 keV

14. The probability that an x-ray will undergo Compton interaction:
    a. Decreases with increasing x-ray energy
    b. Increases with decreasing electron energy
    c. Increases with increasing electron energy
    d. Increases with increasing x-ray energy
    e. Increases with increasing Z of the target atom

15. The Compton interaction involves so-called "unbound" electrons because:
    a. Excitation occurs.
    b. Free electrons are ejected.
    c. Ionization occurs.
    d. K-shell electrons are not involved.
    e. They have a very low binding energy.

16. Which of the following is the x-ray interaction that does *not* cause ionization?
    a. Classical scattering
    b. Compton scattering
    c. Pair production
    d. Photodisintegration
    e. Photoelectric effect

17. Compton-scattered x-rays:
    a. Are helpful in diagnostic radiology
    b. Have lower energy than the incident x-ray
    c. Improve contrast resolution
    d. Produce image artifacts
    e. Result from bremsstrahlung

The photoelectric effect occurs when an incident x-ray imparts all its energy to an orbital electron of a tissue atom, usually a K-shell electron. The x-ray disappears, and the orbital electron is ejected from the atom. This electron is a **photoelectron,** and it escapes with kinetic energy equal to the difference between the incident x-ray energy and its binding energy.

The probability that a given x-ray will undergo a photoelectric interaction is **inversely** proportional to the third power of the photon energy ($1/E^3$) and **directly** proportional to the third power of the atomic number (Z^3) of the absorber.

Photoelectric effect results in image contrast. Contrast agent studies incorporating barium or iodine are successful because the atomic number of these atoms is much higher than that of the atoms of surrounding tissue.

EXERCISES

1. If E_i = incident x-ray energy, E_s = scattered x-ray energy, E_b = electron binding energy, and E_{KE} = photoelectric kinetic energy, then which of the following is *true?*
   a. $E_i = E_s + E_b + E_{KE}$
   b. $E_i = E_s - (E_b + E_{KE})$
   c. $E_i = E_b + E_{KE}$
   d. $E_i = E_b - E_{KE}$
   e. $E_i = E_{KE} - E_b$

2. If E_i = incident x-ray energy, E_s = scattered x-ray energy, E_b = electron binding energy, and E_{KE} = photoelectric kinetic energy, then which of the following is *true?*
   a. $E_{KE} = E_i - E_b$
   b. $E_{KE} = E_i/E_b$
   c. $E_s = E_i - (E_b + E_{KE})$
   d. $E_s = (E_b + E_{KE}) E_i$
   e. $E_i = E_s + E_b + E_{KE}$

3. The photoelectric effect is principally associated with which of the following?
   a. Absorption of an x-ray
   b. Bremsstrahlung x-ray production
   c. Characteristic x-ray production
   d. Electron excitation
   e. Scattering of an x-ray

4. A 50 keV x-ray has a 0.02 chance of photoelectric interaction with muscle (Z = 7.4). What is its chance of interacting with bone (Z = 13.8)?
   a. 0.01
   b. 0.04
   c. 0.07
   d. 0.14
   e. 0.37

5. Which of the following has the lowest effective atomic number?
   a. Air
   b. Bone
   c. Fat
   d. Lung
   e. Muscle

6. Photoelectric interaction with soft tissue is *most* likely with which of the following x-rays?
   a. 0.3 keV
   b. 3.0 keV
   c. 30 keV
   d. 300 keV
   e. 3000 keV

7. During photoelectric interaction:
   a. An electron is emitted from the atom.
   b. An x-ray is emitted from the atom.
   c. Electron excitation results.
   d. The atom is made radioactive.
   e. The incident x-ray reappears with reduced energy.

8. During operation at 80 kVp, which of the following photoelectric interactions is *most* probable?
   a. 30 keV x-ray and bone
   b. 30 keV x-ray and fat
   c. 50 keV x-ray and lung
   d. 70 keV x-ray and bone
   e. 70 keV x-ray and fat

9. The radiographic image is formed principally by which of the following?
   a. Classical scattering
   b. Compton scattering
   c. Off-focus radiation
   d. Photoelectric interactions
   e. Uniform distribution of remnant x-rays

10. A 35 keV x-ray *most* likely will undergo K-shell photoelectric interaction with which of the following?
    a. Barium (E_b = 37 keV)
    b. Calcium (E_b = 4 keV)
    c. Iodine (E_b = 33 keV)
    d. Muscle (E_b < 1 keV)
    e. Tungsten (E_b = 69 keV)

11. The probability of photoelectric effect varies as what function of x-ray energy (E)?
    a. E^{-3}
    b. E^{-2}
    c. E
    d. E^2
    e. E^3

12. As a result of photoelectric interaction:
    a. An electron is absorbed.
    b. An electron leaves the atom.
    c. The incident x-ray is scattered.
    d. The incident x-ray leaves the atom with more energy.
    e. The incident x-ray leaves the atom with reduced energy.

13. The photoelectric effect is:
    a. A partially exciting event
    b. A partially ionizing event
    c. A radiation-scattering event
    d. The complete absorption of an electron with the subsequent emission of an x-ray
    e. The complete absorption of an x-ray with the subsequent emission of an electron

14. Lead has a K-shell electron binding energy of 88 keV. Therefore:
    a. An 84 keV x-ray can undergo photoelectric interaction with the K-shell electron.
    b. An 84 keV x-ray can undergo photoelectric interaction with the L-shell electron.
    c. An 87 keV x-ray is more likely to undergo photoelectric interaction with a K-shell electron than is an 84 keV x-ray.
    d. An 87 keV x-ray is more likely to undergo photoelectric interaction with an L-shell electron than is an 84 keV x-ray.
    e. An 87 keV x-ray will be replaced by a 1 keV electron.

15. A 39 keV x-ray interacts through photoelectric effect with a K-shell electron of barium (binding energy 37 keV). Therefore:
    a. The photoelectron will have 2 keV energy.
    b. The photoelectron will have 37 keV energy.
    c. The photoelectron will have 39 keV energy.
    d. The scattered x-ray will have 2 keV energy.
    e. The scattered x-ray will have 37 keV energy.

16. The probability of photoelectric effect varies as what function of target atomic number (Z)?
    a. Z^{-3}
    b. Z^{-2}
    c. Z
    d. Z^2
    e. Z^3

10-3 Differential Absorption

- • Only two interactions of the incident x-ray are important to diagnostic x-ray imaging: Compton scattering and the photoelectric effect. The photoelectric effect predominates when low-energy x-rays interact with atoms that have a high atomic number.
- • Compton scattering predominates at high voltage, where it accounts for most of the interactions between x-rays and tissue.
- • Both interactions are equally proportional to mass density.
- • However, the ratio of Compton scattering to photoelectric effect increases with increasing x-ray energy.
- • The pattern of absorption and scatter of the incident x-ray beam caused by atomic number, mass density, and thickness of tissue is called **differential absorption**.

EXERCISES

1. Anatomic structures that readily transmit x-rays:
   a. Are called *radiolucent*
   b. Are called *radiopaque*
   c. Have a high effective atomic number
   d. Have a high probability for photoelectric effect
   e. Usually have high mass density

2. Differential absorption, although a complicated process, is basically the result of differences between:
   a. Compton scattering and photoelectric effect
   b. Compton scattering and transmission
   c. High-E and low-E x-rays
   d. High-Z and low-Z tissue
   e. Photoelectric effect and transmission

3. When a radiograph is taken:
   a. High kVp is preferred for maximum differential absorption.
   b. Low kVp is necessary when soft tissue is imaged because it leads to high Compton effect.
   c. Low kVp is necessary when soft tissue is imaged because it leads to high photoelectric effect.
   d. The most probable interaction is no interaction.
   e. With increasing kVp, differential absorption increases.

4. At what approximate x-ray energy is the probability of a photoelectric interaction in soft tissue equal to the probability of a Compton interaction?
   a. 10 keV
   b. 20 keV
   c. 40 keV
   d. 80 keV
   e. 120 keV

5. Which of the following has the greatest mass density?
   a. Blood
   b. Bone
   c. Fat
   d. Lung
   e. Muscle

6. The colon is imaged during a barium enema examination principally because of differences in:
   a. Beam energy
   b. Beam intensity
   c. Subject atomic number
   d. Subject mass density
   e. Subject mass number

7. Air-contrast studies such as a colon examination are successful principally for which of the following reasons?
   a. High-kVp technique is used.
   b. Low-kVp technique is used.
   c. There are differences in effective atomic number.
   d. There are differences in mass density.
   e. X-rays are produced with a continuous-energy spectrum.

8. To optimize x-ray mammography:
   a. High kVp is required to minimize Compton effect.
   b. High kVp should be used with adequate filtration.
   c. Low kVp is necessary to take advantage of the Compton effect.
   d. Low kVp is required because of high Z of microcalcifications.
   e. The main x-ray interaction should be the photoelectric effect.

9. Differential absorption between bone and soft tissue occurs principally for which of the following reasons?
   a. There is a difference in effective atomic number.
   b. There is a difference in mass density.
   c. There is a difference in reflectance.
   d. The x-ray beam is monoenergetic.
   e. The x-ray beam is polyenergetic.

10. Angiography with iodinated compounds:
    a. Requires high kVp for high contrast
    b. Works because of Compton effect
    c. Works principally because of differences in effective atomic number
    d. Works principally because of differences in mass density
    e. Would not be possible with monoenergetic x-rays

11. Differential absorption is:
    a. Better with increasing Compton interaction
    b. Better with increasing kVp
    c. Better with thicker anatomy

d. The difference between those x-rays that are absorbed and those that are reflected
e. The difference between those x-rays that are absorbed and those that are transmitted

12. As kVp increases, the relative number of x-rays:
    a. That are reflected decreases
    b. That are transmitted decreases
    c. That interact by way of Compton effect increases
    d. That interact by way of the photoelectric effect increases
    e. That interact with tissue decreases

13. In which of the following tissues does differential absorption *most* depend on differences in mass density?
    a. Fat and bone
    b. Lung and bone
    c. Lung and fat
    d. Muscle and bone
    e. Muscle and fat

14. The SI unit of mass density is which of the following?
    a. m^3/g
    b. g/m^3
    c. kg/m^3
    d. joule
    e. newton

15. How is photoelectric interaction with tissue related to the mass density (ρ) of the tissue?
    a. It is inversely proportional.
    b. It is inversely proportional to ρ^3.
    c. It is proportional.
    d. It is proportional to ρ^3.
    e. It is unrelated.

16. Lungs are imaged on a chest radiograph principally because of differences in which of the following?
    a. Beam energy
    b. Beam intensity
    c. Tissue atomic number
    d. Tissue mass density
    e. Tissue mass number

17. Differential absorption between lung and soft tissue occurs principally because of which of the following?
    a. The difference in effective atomic numbers (Z)
    b. The difference in mass density
    c. The x-ray beam is filtered.

d. The x-ray beam is homogeneous.

e. The x-ray beam is polyenergetic.

18. The reduction in intensity of an x-ray beam after it passes through tissue is called:

a. Absorption

b. Attenuation

c. Exponential

d. Interaction

e. Scattering

19. X-ray transmission decreases exponentially, which also means that:

a. Beam intensity is reduced abruptly.

b. The number of x-rays is never reduced to zero.

c. The x-ray beam becomes more penetrating.

d. There is a finite thickness for 100% absorption.

e. X-ray scattering increases.

20. Which of the following plots represents x-ray attenuation in matter?

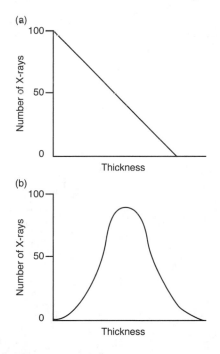

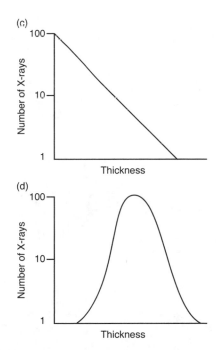

21. Which process contributes *most* to the radiographic image?

a. Classical scattering

b. Compton scattering

c. Pair production

d. Photodisintegration

e. Photoelectric effect

22. High kVp in chest radiography will:

a. Increase contrast

b. Increase patient dose

c. Increase penumbra

d. Reduce patient dose

e. Reduce shadowing from rib

23. Increasing kVp in x-ray imaging will:

a. Increase contrast

b. Increase filtration

c. Reduce screen sensitivity

d. Reduce SID

e. Reduce skin dose

24. In high-kVp chest radiography, contrast depends *most* upon:

a. Atomic number

b. mAs

c. Mass density

d. Mass number

e. SID

25. Microcalcifications are imaged on mammograms principally because of:

a. Atomic number

b. Atomic mass

c. Electron density

d. Mass density

e. Optical density

26. More contrast is present from a barium examination than from an iodine examination because:
    a. Barium has a higher atomic number.
    b. Barium has a higher concentration.
    c. Barium has a higher mass attenuation coefficient.
    d. The K edge of Ba is higher.
    e. The luminal size is greater for colon than for ureter.

27. Photoelectric effect is proportional to:
    a. $E^{-1/2}$
    b. $E^{1/2}$
    c. E^3
    d. $Z^{1/2}$
    e. Z^3

28. What will increase the energy of bremsstrahlung radiation?
    a. Filament current
    b. Exposure time
    c. SID
    d. Target material
    e. X-ray tube voltage

29. What is the ideal kVp for a given K edge?
    a. Approximately three times the K edge
    b. Much higher than the K edge
    c. Much lower than the K edge
    d. Slightly higher than the K edge
    e. Slightly lower than the K edge

30. Compton interaction occur with outer-shell electrons and results in:
    a. Auger electron + Photon of lower energy
    b. Conversion electron + Photon of lower energy
    c. Electron capture + Characteristic x-ray
    d. Recoil electron + Photon of lower energy
    e. Reduced gray scale

31. At 60 keV in soft tissue, what predominates?
    a. Classical scattering
    b. Compton scattering
    c. Pair production
    d. Photodisintegration
    e. Photoelectric effect

11-1

Film Construction

The physical characteristics of radiographic film make it perhaps the strongest link in the radiographic imaging system. Radiographic film consists of two principal parts: the base and the emulsion. The manufacture of each is precisely controlled.

The base is made of polyester and is somewhat rigid—not flexible, like photographic film. This rigidity allows a radiograph to be easily handled and positioned on a viewbox. This property of the base is known as *dimensional stability.*

The emulsion is a homogenous mixture of gelatin and silver halide crystals. The silver halide is the ingredient that is sensitive to x-ray or light exposure. The concentration and crystal size distribution give the emulsion speed and contrast characteristics.

EXERCISES

1. An easily observable difference between x-ray film and photographic film is:
   a. The archival quality
   b. The processing requirements
   c. The speed of the film
   d. The thickness and rigidity of the base
   e. The thickness of the emulsion

2. The principal characteristic of the emulsion that makes it particularly x-ray sensitive is its:
   a. Atomic mass
   b. Atomic number
   c. Mass density
   d. Optical density
   e. Sensitivity center

3. Average silver halide crystal surface size in radiographic film is approximately:
   a. 0.1 μm
   b. 1.0 μm
   c. 10 μm
   d. 100 μm
   e. 1000 μm

4. The radiographic film base appears blue:
   a. Because of added hardeners
   b. Because of the sensitivity centers
   c. Because of the silver halide crystals
   d. So that image viewing is more comfortable
   e. To match the light emitted by intensifying screens

5. Which of the following has been used as a radiographic film base?
   a. Cellulose nitrate
   b. Cellulose triacetate
   c. Gadolinium oxysulfide
   d. Gelatin
   e. Silver halide

6. The emulsion that is commonly used in x-ray film consists of which of the following?
   a. Cellulose acetate and silver halide
   b. Gelatin and cellulose acetate
   c. Gelatin and silver nitrate
   d. Silver halide and gelatin
   e. Silver nitrate and cellulose acetate

7. A common base of contemporary x-ray film is:
   a. Polyester
   b. Polyethylene
   c. Polyurethane

d. Silver bromide
e. Silver nitrate

8. In the manufacture of radiographic film:
   a. Direct-exposure film contains a thicker emulsion layer with a greater number of silver halide crystals.
   b. Screen-film is made before direct-exposure film.
   c. Single-emulsion type is most frequently produced.
   d. The emulsion layer is thicker than the base.
   e. X-ray interaction accounts for approximately one half of the latent-image centers in screen-film exposure.

9. The adhesive layer of radiographic film:
   a. Ensures uniform adhesion of the emulsion to the base
   b. Ensures uniform adhesion of the protective layer to the emulsion
   c. Is approximately 200 μm thick
   d. Is between 5 and 25 μm thick
   e. Serves as the protective layer

10. Which of the following are the two basic parts of radiographic film?
    a. Base and emulsion
    b. Emulsion and phosphor
    c. Emulsion and supercoating
    d. Phosphor and base
    e. Phosphor and density

11. The overcoat usually consists of which of the following?
    a. Cellulose
    b. Gelatin
    c. Phosphor
    d. Polyester
    e. Silver halide

12. Dimensional stability is the property of maintaining the size and shape of which of the following?
    a. Base
    b. Emulsion
    c. Image
    d. Phosphor
    e. Supercoiling

13. When polyester is compared with cellulose tri-acetate as a base, which of the following does *not* apply to polyester?
    a. Better dimensional stability
    b. Less warping with age

c. Nonflammable
d. Stronger
e. Thicker

14. The principal purpose of gelatin in the emulsion is to:
    a. Facilitate image processing
    b. Produce film that is lucent
    c. Provide dimensional stability to the film
    d. Provide for easier roller transport
    e. Support the silver halide crystals uniformly

15. Which of the following properties of silver halide is *most* important in the production of a latent image?
    a. Atomic number
    b. Dimensional stability
    c. Mass
    d. Mass density
    e. Optical density

16. X-ray film is sensitive to which of the following?
    a. All x-rays and gamma rays, visible light, and radio waves
    b. Only electromagnetic radiation
    c. Only x-rays and gamma rays
    d. Only x-rays, gamma rays, and visible light
    e. Only x-rays

17. X-ray film used with radiographic intensifying screens usually has which of the following?
    a. A base made of cellulose nitrate
    b. A clear base
    c. A phosphor coat on the surface
    d. A treatment to make the film especially sensitive to x-rays
    e. An emulsion coat on both sides of the base

18. Which of the following is usually thinner than 5 μm?
    a. Base
    b. Emulsion
    c. Film
    d. Overcoat
    e. Phosphor

19. Which of the following is a principal component of the emulsion?
    a. Bromine nitrate
    b. Cellulose nitrate
    c. Cellulose triacetate
    d. Silver bromide
    e. Silver nitrate

Formation of Latent Image

The interaction of electromagnetic radiation (light or x-rays) with the radiographic film emulsion results in a latent image. The latent image is the invisible change in the silver halide crystals of the emulsion.

The latent image is made visible by processing. Six steps are necessary for processing a radiograph: (1) wetting, (2) development, (3) stop bath, (4) fixation, (5) washing, and (6) drying. All are important, but the two most critical steps are development and fixation. During development, the latent image is made visible. During fixation, that visibility is made permanent (archival quality).

EXERCISES

1. The latent image actually is formed in the:
   a. Base
   b. Bromine atom
   c. Gelatin
   d. Protective layer
   e. Silver halide crystal

2. During the photographic process, metallic silver accumulates at the:
   a. Base
   b. Bromine ion
   c. Gelatin contaminant
   d. Secondary electron
   e. Sensitivity center

3. The latent image at the crystal level:
   a. Is a collection of bromine atoms
   b. Is a collection of silver atoms
   c. Is present regardless of whether that crystal was irradiated

d. Is visible with a microscope
e. Requires x-ray interaction

4. The term *latent image* actually refers to which of the following?
   a. A processed image
   b. An unprocessed image
   c. Film inertia
   d. Image intensification
   e. Reciprocity law failure

5. The sensitivity center is usually silver:
   a. Atoms
   b. Bromide
   c. Iodide
   d. Ions
   e. Sulfide

6. In the manufacture of the emulsion, which of the following molecules is particularly sensitive to visible light?
   a. $AgBr$
   b. $AgNO_3$
   c. $CaWO_4$
   d. KBr
   e. KNO_3

7. When the latent image is processed, what type of image does it become?
   a. Crystal
   b. Dimensional
   c. Excited
   d. Induced
   e. Manifest

8. What do we call the radiation exiting the patient that is responsible for latent image formation?
   a. Image-forming
   b. Leakage
   c. Remnant
   d. Scatter
   e. Useful beam

9. When x-rays interact directly with film, which of the following *most* likely is involved?
   a. Bromine
   b. Gelatin
   c. Iodine
   d. Silver
   e. Tungsten

10. An ion is an atom:
    a. That has electric charge
    b. That is neutral
    c. That is radioactive
    d. With a sensitivity center
    e. With too many nucleons

11. The interstitial atoms in a crystal of silver halide include which of the following?
    a. Bromine, iodine, and gelatin
    b. Gelatin, silver, and bromine
    c. Iodine, gelatin, and silver
    d. Silver, bromine, and iodine
    e. Silver, sulfide, and gelatin

12. X-ray interaction with silver halide can result in formation of all *except* which of the following?
    a. A charged electron
    b. A latent-image center
    c. A radioactive atom
    d. A secondary electron
    e. An ion

13. After irradiation, a secondary electron *most* likely will interact with a silver ion to form:
    a. A positive ion
    b. A sensitivity center
    c. A silver atom
    d. A silver bromide crystal
    e. A silver halide crystal

14. In a silver halide crystal, which of the following is missing an electron?
    a. Bromine
    b. Gelatin
    c. Iodine
    d. Silver
    e. Sulfide

15. Which of the following statements about processing is *true*?
    a. It includes AgBr formation.
    b. It includes gelatin ionization.
    c. It includes neutral silver migration.
    d. It is required for latent-image formation.
    e. It is required for manifest-image formation.

16. The latent-image center:
    a. Consists of halide crystals
    b. Consists of migrating electrons
    c. Consists of silver ions
    d. Forms at the sensitivity center
    e. Forms on the surface of a crystal

17. The formation of a latent image follows which interaction with the emulsion?
    a. Classical scattering
    b. Pair production
    c. Photodisintegration
    d. Photoelectric effect
    e. Thomson scattering

18. If one observes a film immediately after exposure, what is seen?
    a. A distributed image
    b. A latent image
    c. A manifest image
    d. A visible image
    e. Nothing

19. Which of the following theories best explains the photographic effect?
    a. Duane-Hunt
    b. Gurney-Mott
    c. Haus-Hendrick
    d. Hurter-Driffield
    e. Planck-Bohr

Radiologic imaging has advanced so far technologically that it is imperative that the radiologic technologist be aware of the various image receptors available and the bases for differences among radiographic films.

- **Contrast, speed,** and **spectral characteristics** are three exceedingly important parameters by which a radiologic technologist should select film.
- Proper matching of film emulsion with screen phosphor is also essential.
- Proper darkroom safelight protection is absolutely essential.
- Storage in a climate-controlled environment is necessary for the ultimate production of acceptable images.

EXERCISES

1. The *most* commonly used radiographic image receptor is which of the following?
   a. Direct-exposure film
   b. Electrostatic plate
   c. Nonscreen film
   d. Screen-film
   e. Single-emulsion film

2. Which of the following is *not* a characteristic the radiographer should consider when selecting film?
   a. Contrast
   b. Latitude
   c. Light absorption
   d. Light emission
   e. Sensitivity

3. The contrast of radiographic film is:
   a. Directly proportional to dose
   b. Directly proportional to its sensitivity
   c. Highest at high dose
   d. Important to archival quality
   e. Inversely proportional to its latitude

4. High-contrast film has:
   a. A thinner base
   b. A wide range of grain size
   c. Larger grain size
   d. Less silver halide
   e. Uniform grain size

5. The difference between fast film and slow film is silver halide crystal:
   a. Charge
   b. Concentration
   c. Shape
   d. Size
   e. Size distribution

6. The spectral response of an emulsion refers to:
   a. Its ability to detect x-rays
   b. Its absorption of visible light
   c. Its emission of visible light
   d. Its sensitivity to x-rays
   e. Its transmission of viewbox light

7. Calcium tungstate screens emit which of the following?
   a. Blue light
   b. Green light
   c. Infrared light
   d. Red light
   e. Yellow light

8. Which of the following will *not* fog film?
   a. A darkroom light leak
   b. Background radiation
   c. Fringe magnetic fields from an MRI
   d. Gamma radiation from an adjacent nuclear medicine laboratory
   e. X-radiation from the adjacent x-ray room

9. Orthochromatic film is sensitive to which of the following?
   a. Green light
   b. Infrared light
   c. Red light
   d. Visible light
   e. Yellow light

10. Which of the following is the principal result of using rare Earth screens with green-sensitive film?
    a. Darkroom fog
    b. Fewer artifacts
    c. Higher contrast
    d. Increased patient dose
    e. Reduced patient dose

11. When rare earth screens are in use, what type of safelights are required?
    a. Amber
    b. Blue
    c. Green
    d. None
    e. Red

12. Mammography film:
    a. Has a thick emulsion
    b. Has a thin base
    c. Is coarse-grain, double-emulsion
    d. Is used with a screen
    e. Must be viewed in the dark

13. When comparing 35-mm cine film with 16-mm film, the 35-mm film can be seen to have:
    a. Better resolution
    b. Four times the area
    c. Higher contrast
    d. Less patient dose
    e. Twice the area

14. Most rare Earth screens emit which of the following?
    a. Blue light
    b. Green light
    c. Infrared light
    d. Ultraviolet light
    e. Violet light

15. If film is stored near steam pipes, the *most* likely result will be which of the following?
    a. Artifacts
    b. Loss of contrast
    c. Loss of latitude
    d. Loss of speed
    e. The appearance of radiopaque artifacts

16. Which of the following is *most* likely to fog film?
    a. 0.2 mR
    b. An improper safelight filter
    c. High humidity
    d. High temperature
    e. Storage of film for longer than 1 month

17. Which of the following are acceptable storage conditions for film?
    a. 16°C and 10% humidity
    b. 20°C and 90% humidity
    c. 32°C and 50% humidity
    d. 36°C and 60% humidity
    e. 50°C and 50% humidity

18. Which of the following darkroom conditions is *not* acceptable?
    a. Blue-sensitive film, amber safelight
    b. Green-sensitive film, amber safelight
    c. Orthochromatic film, red safelight
    d. Silver halide emulsion, amber safelight
    e. Silver halide emulsion, red safelight

19. Which of the following is the *least* important characteristic of screen-film?
    a. Contrast
    b. Cost
    c. Light absorption
    d. Light emission
    e. Sensitivity

20. Which of the following would be considered an image artifact?
    a. A pressure mark
    b. A smudge mark on the viewbox diffuser
    c. An unexposed but processed film
    d. Developer depletion
    e. Film identification mark

21. If other factors are equal, which of the following emulsions is fastest?
    a. Blue sensitive
    b. Green sensitive
    c. Large grain
    d. Small grain
    e. Uniform grain size

Automatic processing uses three principal chemistries, each contained in a separate tank of the processor.

- The **developer** contains developing agents, activators, hardeners, preservatives, and water.
- The **fixer** contains clearing agents, activators, preservatives, and hardeners.
- The third chemistry is **water,** which is used in copious amounts at high flow rates to wash the film clear of unused chemistries.

EXERCISES

1. At what stage in automatic processing is the latent image made visible?
   a. Developing
   b. Drying
   c. Fixation
   d. Stop bath
   e. Wetting

2. Which of the following is the component of the developer that helps to keep unexposed crystals from the developing agent?
   a. Hydroquinone (developing agent)
   b. Phenidone (developing agent)
   c. Potassium bromide (restrainer)
   d. Silver halide (crystal)
   e. Sodium carbonate (buffer)

3. What stage of processing involves a synergistic reaction?
   a. Development
   b. Drying
   c. Fixation
   d. Washing
   e. Wetting

4. Aerial oxidation is controlled by which of the following?
   a. The activator
   b. The concentrator
   c. The fixer
   d. The preservative
   e. The restrainer

5. The hardeners in a fixer:
   a. Cause swelling and softening of the emulsion
   b. Cause the emulsion to swell
   c. Clean the rollers of the transport system
   d. Ensure archival quality
   e. Remove excess hypo from the emulsion

6. Which of the following is the *most* common result of inadequate washing?
   a. A damp film
   b. Excess hypo retention
   c. Incomplete development
   d. Incomplete fixing
   e. Loss of archival quality

7. Conversion of the latent image to a visible image occurs:
   a. In less than 10 seconds
   b. In the developer
   c. In the fixer
   d. In the gelatin portion of the emulsion
   e. When silver bromide is cleared

8. Which of the following ingredients of the developer is responsible for producing the blackest parts of a radiograph?
   a. Glutaraldehyde
   b. Hydroquinone

   c. Phenidone
   d. Potassium bromide
   e. Sodium sulfite

9. During development, silver:
   a. Atoms are changed to ions.
   b. Atoms are ionized.
   c. Ions are changed to atoms.
   d. Ions are oxidized.
   e. Is removed

10. The archival quality of a radiograph is principally:
   a. Controlled by developer concentration
   b. Controlled by the activator
   c. Controlled by the developing agent
   d. Established during development
   e. Established during fixing

11. Which of the following terms does *not* belong?
   a. Clearing agent
   b. Fixer
   c. Hypo
   d. Stop bath
   e. Thiosulfate

12. Which of the following is *not* a separate stage in automatic processing?
   a. Development
   b. Drying
   c. Fixation
   d. Washing
   e. Wetting

13. Which of the following is the preservative normally used in both the developer and the fixer?
   a. Glutaraldehyde
   b. Potassium alum
   c. Silver sulfide
   d. Sodium carbonate
   e. Sodium sulfite

14. Which of the following is a reducing agent?
   a. Hydroquinone
   b. Glutaraldehyde
   c. Potassium bromide
   d. Silver sulfite
   e. Sodium sulfite

15. Which of the following ingredients in the fixer functions as a stop bath?
   a. The activator
   b. The clearing agent
   c. The hardener

   d. The preservative
   e. The silver sulfide

16. *Hypo retention* refers to which of the following?
   a. Improved archival quality
   b. Replenishment of a clearing agent
   c. The formation of silver sulfide
   d. The formation of sodium sulfite
   e. Thiosulfate left in the emulsion

17. Development fog will increase when which of the following is abnormally low in the developer?
   a. Glutaraldehyde
   b. Hydroquinone
   c. Potassium bromide
   d. Silver sulfide
   e. Sodium sulfite

18. Which of the following is the component of the developer that is *most* responsible for archival quality?
   a. Glutaraldehyde
   b. Hydroquinone
   c. Silver sulfide
   d. Sodium carbonate
   e. Sodium sulfite

19. The wetting agent used in automatic processors is usually which of the following?
   a. Acetic acid
   b. Glutaraldehyde
   c. Silver halide
   d. Silver sulfide
   e. Water

20. The temperature of the wash water should be approximately:
   a. 5°C below the developer
   b. 5°C below the fixer
   c. 5°F below the developer
   d. 5°F below the fixer
   e. The same temperature as the fixer

21. Which of the following is sometimes used as a developing agent?
   a. Glutaraldehyde
   b. Phenidone
   c. Silver sulfide
   d. Sodium sulfite
   e. Water

The time from insertion of the exposed radiograph into the processor to the appearance of the processed radiograph in the receiving bin—the dry-to-drop time—is 90 seconds. This type of automatic processor is an electromechanical device that consists of four main systems: (1) the transport system, (2) the circulation system, (3) the replenishment system, and (4) the dryer system.

The transport system is a series of rollers, racks, and drive chains that takes the exposed radiograph and automatically feeds it through the four stations of the processor: (1) the developing tank, (2) the fixing tank, (3) the wash tank, and (4) the drying chamber.

The circulation system is powered by pumps that continuously circulate the chemistries in each tank to ensure complete chemistry mixing and uniform temperature of solution. The circulation system in the developing tank and the fixing tank is a closed loop, whereas the wash tank is a single-pass, flow-through system.

The replenishment system consists of a small pump, tubing, and a microswitch control. As the film is fed into the receiving tray of the automatic processor, the microswitch activates the pump to feed a measured amount of developer into the developing tank, and fixer into the fixing tank.

EXERCISES

1. Which of the following is an assembly that consists of one master roller, several planetary rollers, and two guide shoes?
   a. A crossover rack
   b. A detector assembly
   c. A roller subassembly
   d. A transport rack
   e. A turnaround assembly

2. Replenishment of which tank in the processing system is *most* important?
   a. Developer
   b. Dryer
   c. Fixer
   d. Wash
   e. Wetter

3. When a film is inserted into an automatic processor:
   a. A microswitch grips it.
   b. Guide shoes grip it.
   c. It should be centered on the feed tray.
   d. The long dimension should be against the rail.
   e. The short dimension should be against the rail.

4. Adequate drying is necessary to:
   a. Complete development
   b. Complete fixation
   c. Obtain adequate contrast
   d. Reduce artifacts
   e. Strengthen the base

5. The fastest automatic processors can process a film in:
   a. 30 seconds
   b. 90 seconds
   c. 180 seconds
   d. 5 minutes
   e. 7 minutes

6. Between the fixing tank and the wash tank, the film passes through a:
   a. Crossover rack
   b. Drying chamber
   c. Receiving bin
   d. Transportation rack
   e. Turnaround rack

7. Which of the following is *not* one of the major systems of an automatic processor?
   a. The development system
   b. The drying system
   c. The electrical system
   d. The replenishment system
   e. The transport system

8. The principal purpose of the circulation system is to:
   a. Agitate the chemistry.
   b. Agitate the film.
   c. Control chemistry concentration.
   d. Control chemistry temperature.
   e. Replenish the chemistry.

9. Which segment of the circulation system is *most* important to archival quality?
   a. Developing
   b. Drying
   c. Fixation
   d. Washing
   e. Wetting

10. Underreplenishment of the developer will result in:
    a. A decrease in contrast
    b. A reduction in spatial resolution
    c. An improvement in spatial resolution
    d. An increase in contrast
    e. No change in contrast

11. Replenishment tanks should have close-fitting floating lids primarily:
    a. For control of replenishment rate
    b. For control of temperature
    c. To control aerial oxidation
    d. To easily monitor fluid level
    e. To reduce splash hazard

12. *Dry-to-drop time* refers to
    a. Development time
    b. Exposure-to-viewbox time
    c. Passbox-to-receiving bin time
    d. Time from feed tray to receiving bin
    e. Time in the passbox

13. The segment of the circulation system that is *most* likely to contain a filter is the:
    a. Developer
    b. Dryer
    c. Fixer
    d. Wash cycle
    e. Wetting cycle

14. If the power of the drive motor is transferred through a chain, the connecting device is usually a:
    a. Gear
    b. Pulley
    c. Roller
    d. Spring
    e. Sprocket

15. Control of the replenishment system is accomplished by a:
    a. Drive motor
    b. Float valve
    c. Microswitch
    d. Timer
    e. Transport rack

16. The approximate developer conditions in a 90-second processor are:
    a. 85°C, 22 s
    b. 85°C, 45 s
    c. 85°F, 45 s
    d. 95°C, 25 s
    e. 95°F, 22 s

17. The transport system includes all *except* which of the following?
    a. Drive motor
    b. Drying chamber
    c. Guide shoes
    d. Rollers
    e. Transport racks

18. The 3-inch master roller is a part of a:
    a. Guide shoe
    b. Microswitch
    c. Planetary roller
    d. Replenishment system
    e. Turnaround assembly

An unwanted optical density on a radiograph is an artifact. Artifacts are undesirable because they may obscure a meaningful optical density and thereby reduce diagnostic accuracy.

Artifacts are identified according to three general classifications: (1) processing artifacts, (2) exposure artifacts, and (3) handling and storage artifacts.

To minimize the generation of artifacts, a program of quality control must be implemented.

EXERCISES

1. Which of the following artifacts is associated with inadequate processing?
   a. A kink
   b. A smudge
   c. Crown static
   d. Grid lines
   e. Pi lines

2. If a radiograph turns yellow during storage, this is *most* likely the result of which of the following?
   a. Developer retention
   b. Incomplete washing
   c. Presence of sodium sulfite
   d. Radiation fog
   e. Wet pressure sensitization

3. A radiographic image shows the central region exposed and the sides unexposed. The probable cause is:
   a. A laterally positioned grid
   b. An off-center grid
   c. An upside-down grid
   d. Improper SID
   e. Patient motion

4. Which of the following *best* describes an example of preventive maintenance?
   a. Changing motor oil every 3000 miles
   b. Quitting smoking
   c. Repairing a flat tire
   d. Rotating intensifying screens
   e. Using gonadal shields in radiology

5. What is the limiting factor when an extremely fast image receptor is used?
   a. Contrast resolution
   b. Noise
   c. Screen blur
   d. Screen-film contact
   e. Spatial resolution

6. Which of the following artifacts is *most* likely to occur before processing?
   a. A small blur on an otherwise sharp radiograph
   b. Chemical fog
   c. Dichroic stain
   d. Image yellowing
   e. Wet pressure sensitization

7. What is the likely result of excessively high developer temperature?
   a. Increased base density
   b. Increased fog density
   c. Increased graininess
   d. Reduced quantum mottle
   e. Reduced speed

8. In a 90-second processor, immersion time in the developer is approximately:
   a. 10 s
   b. 20 s
   c. 30 s
   d. 40 s
   e. 60 s

9. Most facilities would be sure that the automatic processor was:
   a. Cleaned weekly
   b. Maintained annually
   c. Monitored hourly
   d. Replaced biannually
   e. Replenished daily

10. The classification of artifacts includes all of the following *except:*
    a. Exposure artifacts
    b. Handling artifacts
    c. Location artifacts
    d. Processing artifacts
    e. Storage artifacts

11. Which of the following would be identified as a handling artifact?
    a. Curtain effect
    b. Double exposure
    c. Kink marks
    d. Motion
    e. Radiation fog

12. Motion blur is usually caused by too:
    a. High a kVp
    b. Long an SID
    c. Long an exposure time
    d. Short an SID
    e. Short an exposure time

13. Processor cleaning:
    a. Does not require disassembly
    b. Is unnecessary unless artifacts appear
    c. Should be done monthly
    d. Should be scheduled for a 4-hour interval
    e. Takes no longer than a few minutes

14. Which of the following would be considered a storage artifact?
    a. Pi lines
    b. Radiation fog
    c. Tree static

d. Warped cassette
e. Wrong screen-film match

15. Failure of a system or subsystem of an automatic processor will result in which of the following?
    a. Equipment replacement
    b. High retake rate
    c. Nonscheduled maintenance
    d. Preventive maintenance
    e. Scheduled maintenance

16. Pi lines are so called because they have which of the following characteristics?
    a. They look like a slice of pie.
    b. They look like parallel lines.
    c. They occur at 3.1416-inch intervals.
    d. They occur at intervals of p times the roller diameter.
    e. They occur at principal intervals.

17. Which of the following artifacts is the *most* distinctive and identifiable?
    a. Chemical fog
    b. Light leaks
    c. Pi lines
    d. Poor screen-film contact
    e. Radiation fog

18. Artifacts caused by wet pressure sensitization usually occur:
    a. After drying
    b. Before processing
    c. In the developing tank
    d. In the drying chamber
    e. In the fixing tank

19. Where will guide shoe artifacts be found on a radiograph?
    a. Center
    b. Leading and trailing edges
    c. Leading edge
    d. Side
    e. Trailing edge

20. Archival quality is a term that refers to
    a. Long-term storage of film
    b. Organization of the film file room
    c. The lucency of unexposed film
    d. The range of optical densities on an image
    e. Unintended radiation exposure

13-1

Screen Construction
Luminescence
Screen Characteristics

- Radiographic intensifying screens are used principally to reduce patient radiation dose.
- The radiographic intensifying screen is constructed by pasting a phosphor on a base material with a reflective layer in between.

$$\frac{I_1}{I_2} = \frac{mAs_1}{mAs_2}$$

EXERCISES

1. Radiographic intensifying screen speed increases with increasing:
   a. Atomic mass
   b. Base thickness
   c. mAs
   d. Optical density
   e. Phosphor thickness

2. Direct-exposure, nonscreen technique:
   a. Produces less noise
   b. Reduces scatter radiation
   c. Results in better contrast resolution
   d. Results in better spatial resolution
   e. Results in less motion blur

3. Afterglow is a property of intensifying screens that:
   a. Enhances resolution
   b. Improves contrast
   c. Is enhanced at high kVp
   d. Reduces screen speed
   e. Results in image blur

4. The resolution achievable with radiographic intensifying screens is approximately:
   a. 1 lp/mm
   b. 2 lp/mm
   c. 5 lp/mm
   d. 15 lp/mm
   e. 20 lp/mm

5. Which of the following factors controlled by the radiologic technologist affects radiographic screen speed the *most*?
   a. Exposure time
   b. kVp
   c. mAs
   d. Processor temperature
   e. Room temperature

6. When screen-film is the image receptor, image quality is a trade-off among speed, spatial resolution, and noise. In general:
   a. As noise increases, spatial resolution improves.
   b. As quantum mottle increases, spatial resolution improves.
   c. As speed increases, so does noise.
   d. As speed increases, spatial resolution improves.
   e. Low-noise systems have fewer artifacts.

7. At x-ray energies below the K-shell electron binding energy:
   a. Another rapid reduction in photoelectric absorption occurs with increasing x-ray energy.
   b. The incident photon does not have sufficient energy to ionize K-shell electrons.

c. The two K-shell electrons become available for photoelectric interaction.

d. There is an abrupt increase in the probability of photoelectric absorption.

e. None of the above

8. The intensification factor:
   a. Decreases with increasing kVp
   b. Increases with increasing temperature
   c. Is greater for detail screens than for par speed screens
   d. Is greater for rare Earth screens than for calcium tungstate screens
   e. Is less at high mAs

9. A phosphor currently used in radiographic intensifying screens is:
   a. Barium fluorochloride
   b. Barium platinocyanide
   c. Cadmium tungstate
   d. Calcium sulfate
   e. Cesium iodide

10. Screen blur:
    a. Is greater with detail screens than with par speed screens
    b. Is less with rare Earth screens
    c. Is reduced with fast screens
    d. Is the loss of sharpness of an image when screens are used
    e. Occurs because the light emitted is not properly focused on the film

11. With regard to luminescence, which of the following statements is *true*?
    a. Fluorescence lasts longer than phosphorescence.
    b. Luminous watch dials that fade in the dark are fluorescent devices.
    c. Materials that luminesce are called *lumenites*.
    d. Phosphorescence occurs only when a stimulus is applied.
    e. There are two types: fluorescence and phosphorescence.

12. Radiographic intensifying screens are used with radiographic film principally to:
    a. Allow for shorter exposures
    b. Improve contrast resolution

c. Improve spatial resolution
d. Increase radiographic latitude
e. Reduce patient radiation exposure

13. Radiographic intensifying screens are used with radiographic film to:
    a. Increase the latitude of the imaging system
    b. Increase the spatial resolution of the imaging system
    c. Lower the necessary kVp
    d. Reduce image noise
    e. Reduce motion blur

14. Which of the following properties principally determines screen blur?
    a. Antihalation dye
    b. Phosphor concentration
    c. Phosphor crystal size
    d. Reflective layer
    e. Type of phosphor

15. Luminescence is a process that:
    a. Absorbs light
    b. Always requires x-ray absorption
    c. Always requires x-ray attenuation
    d. Involves inner-shell electrons
    e. Involves outer-shell electrons

16. Because x-ray interaction with a phosphor produces light *isotropically*:
    a. A base is required.
    b. A protective layer is required.
    c. The light is focused.
    d. The light is parallel.
    e. The light spreads out.

17. Mammography conducted with detail screens results in entrance skin exposures (ESE) as low as 300 mR (3 mGy$_a$). The intensification factor for these screens is about 30. If such an examination were conducted as a nonscreen procedure, what would be the ESE?
    a. 100 mR
    b. 900 mR
    c. 1000 mR
    d. 9000 mR
    e. 1200 mR

Screen-Film Combinations
Screen Care
Fluoroscopic Screens

Most radiographic intensifying screens are described as rare Earth because the phosphors are compounds that incorporate the rare Earth elements gadolinium (Gd), lanthanum (La), and yttrium (Y).

The principal advantage of rare earth screens is speed. They are much faster than an earlier standard—calcium tungstate screens. **The principal disadvantage is quantum mottle, a source of image noise.** Rare Earth screens have spatial resolution equal to that of calcium tungstate screens.

The increased speed of rare Earth screens results from their ability to absorb a greater number of x-rays and to convert more of the x-ray energy to light.

EXERCISES

1. Which of the following is a rare Earth element?
   a. Gadolinium
   b. Nobelium
   c. Thallium
   d. Thulium
   e. Palladium

2. In the formula $La_2O_2S:Tb$, the Tb:
   a. Improves contrast resolution.
   b. Improves luminescence.
   c. Improves spatial resolution.
   d. Reduces noise.
   e. Stands for *tungsten bromide*.

3. The principal advantage of rare Earth screens over calcium tungstate screens is:
   a. Better contrast resolution
   b. Better spatial resolution
   c. Faster speed
   d. Lower cost
   e. Reduced noise

4. Rare Earth screens exhibit higher x-ray absorption than calcium tungstate screens:
   a. Because of their thickness
   b. Only at high x-ray energy range
   c. Only at low x-ray energy
   d. Only over an intermediate x-ray energy range
   e. Regardless of the x-ray energy

5. Which of the following elements has the highest atomic number?
   a. Gadolinium
   b. Lanthanum
   c. Molybdenum
   d. Tungsten
   e. Yttrium

6. Which of the following principally contributes to the increased speed of rare Earth screens?
   a. Conversion efficiency
   b. Higher atomic number
   c. Longer wavelength emission
   d. Phosphor thickness
   e. Screen-film contact

7. Which of the following spectra is discrete?
   a. Bremsstrahlung
   b. Calcium tungstate emission
   c. Orthochromatic absorption
   d. Panchromatic absorption
   e. Rare Earth emission

8. Compared with calcium tungstate, rare Earth screens:
   a. Are faster because of scatter radiation
   b. Have better spatial resolution
   c. Have higher rates of absorption for x-rays greater than 80 keV
   d. Have higher rates of absorption for x-rays less than 25 keV
   e. Have higher rates of x-ray absorption in the diagnostic range

9. When diagnostic x-rays interact with rare Earth phosphors:
   a. K-shell interaction will not occur at energies less than 70 keV.
   b. Light is not emitted isotropically.
   c. The lower the x-ray energy, the more probable is photoelectric absorption.
   d. The number of x-rays absorbed is approximately the same as that for calcium tungstate.
   e. With increasing x-ray energy, an abrupt decrease in x-ray absorption will occur.

10. When rare Earth intensifying screens are used:
    a. All rare Earth elements have higher K-shell electron binding energy than tungsten.
    b. As x-ray energy increases up to the K-shell binding energy, absorption also increases.
    c. Contrast resolution is improved.
    d. There is an abrupt increase in absorption at an energy equal to the K-shell binding energy.
    e. There is an abrupt reduction in x-ray absorption at an energy equal to the K-shell binding energy.

11. Compared with calcium tungstate, when an x-ray is absorbed in a rare Earth screen:
    a. It will be absorbed, never scattered.
    b. More energy will be transferred.
    c. More light will be emitted.
    d. Shorter-wavelength light will be emitted.
    e. The ratio of visible light emitted to x-ray energy absorbed will be less.

12. Compared with calcium tungstate screens, rare Earth screens:
    a. Absorb one to two times as many x-rays
    b. Absorb three to five times as many x-rays
    c. Emit higher-energy light
    d. Emit shorter-wavelength light
    e. Have less internal absorption

13. Compared with calcium tungstate screens, rare Earth screens:
    a. Do not need grids
    b. Emit light in the blue-violet region
    c. Emit more intense light per x-ray interaction
    d. May require a new darkroom
    e. Should be used with blue-sensitive radiographic film

14. Compared with calcium tungstate screens, rare Earth radiographic intensifying screens:
    a. Have better spatial resolution
    b. Have less noise
    c. Have less quantum mottle
    d. Require less screen-film contact
    e. Result in lower patient dose

15. Which of the following statements about radiographic intensifying screens is *true*?
    a. All have conversion efficiencies greater than one.
    b. Calcium tungstate screens emit green-yellow light.
    c. Par-speed screens emit green light.
    d. Rare Earth screens must be used in carbon fiber cassettes.
    e. They are used to reduce patient dose.

16. What is the principal limitation of the rare earth radiographic intensifying screen?
    a. Increased exposure factor
    b. Increased quantum mottle
    c. Patient dose
    d. Reduced contrast resolution
    e. Reduced spatial resolution

17. In the proper design and use of a radiographic cassette:
    a. Scratches on the front cover indicate that replacement is necessary.
    b. The back cover should be made of high-Z material so that it can function as a primary barrier for personnel protection.
    c. The back cover should be made of high-Z material to reduce scatter radiation.
    d. The back cover should be made of low-Z material to protect unexposed film while it is in the passbox.
    e. The front cover should be made of low-Z material to minimize x-ray attenuation.

18. Carbon fiber is particularly useful in x-ray imaging because of its:
    a. Dimensional stability
    b. Flexibility
    c. Increased x-ray absorption
    d. Low atomic number
    e. Low mass density

19. The routine care of radiographic intensifying screens requires that they be:
    a. Periodically calibrated
    b. Periodically cleaned
    c. Periodically exchanged
    d. Reinforced against radiation fatigue
    e. Replaced because of radiation fatigue

20. Quantum detection efficiency (QDE) refers to:
    a. Atomic number
    b. Light absorption
    c. Light emission
    d. Mass density
    e. X-ray absorption

21. Phosphor afterglow:
    a. Improves contrast resolution
    b. Is also called *conversion efficiency*
    c. Is also called *lag*
    d. Is helpful
    e. Results from fluorescence

22. The patient exposure for a direct-exposure chest x-ray examination is 210 mR (2.1 mGy_a). If par-speed screens are used, the exposure required is 15 mR (0.15 mGy_a). The intensification factor is:
    a. 0.07
    b. 7
    c. 14
    d. 740
    e. 3150

23. A direct-exposure radiograph requires 650 mR (6.5 mGy_a). If the intensification factor of rare Earth screens was 200, what would be the patient exposure if such screens were used?
    a. 3.25 mR
    b. 6.5 mR
    c. 130 mR
    d. 200 mR
    e. 1300 mR

ACROSS

1. Each of the rare Earth screens has an absorption curve characteristic of the phosphor that determines the speed of the screen and how it changes with ____.
2. A disadvantage of some of the fastest rare Earth screens is the noticeable effects of ____ ____.
3. When a luminescent material is stimulated, the ____-shell electrons are raised to an excited energy state.
4. When an outer-shell electron is raised to an excited state and returns to its ____ ____ with the emission of a light photon, luminescence occurs.
5. An example of a good material for a compression device to be placed between each screen and the cassette to maintain close film-screen contact is ____.
6. An intensifying screen base must not ____ with the phosphor layer; it must be chemically inert.
7. For x-ray absorption to be high, the intensifying screen should have a phosphor with a ____ ____ number.
8. If you were to x-ray an intensifying screen in a darkened x-ray room, the luminescence would be visible because many ____ photons are released with each x-ray interaction.
9. For mammography, a ____ screen is used on the far side of the emulsion to reduce screen blur.
10. In a calcium tungstate screen, it is the ____ atom that determines its absorption properties.
11. As x-ray energy increases, the probability of absorption ____ rapidly until the x-ray energy is equal to the binding energy of the K-shell electrons.

DOWN

1. When an incident x-ray has energy equal to the ____ electron binding energy, photoelectric absorption is maximum for those electrons.
2. Phosphorescence becomes objectionable, which is referred to as *afterglow*, when it occurs in an ____ screen.
3. One of the most common causes of poor screen-film contact is ____ latches or hinges.
4. An example of a transitional, rare Earth phosphor found in low abundance in nature is ____ ____.
5. One advantage of screen-film over direct-exposure film use is a decrease in x-ray tube ____.
6. Reduction in spatial resolution is ____ when phosphor layers are thick or when crystal size is large.
7. Use of rare Earth screens results in lower patient dose and less ____ stress on the x-ray tube.
8. Adequate x-ray conversion efficiency requires that the phosphor emit a large amount of light per ____ of x-ray photons.
9. The presence of a reflective layer in an intensifying screen increases x-ray ____-____ conversion efficiency but also increases image blur.
10. Rare Earth screens obtain their ____ sensitivity through higher x-ray absorption and more efficient conversion of x-ray energy into light.
11. A disadvantage of intensifying screens is a lower ____ resolution compared with direct-exposure radiographs.
12. Resolution usually is measured by the ____ pairs per millimeter that can be detected on the radiograph.
13. Carbon fiber was useful in the early days of the space program because of its high strength and ____ resistance.
14. The light emitted by calcium tungstate screens is readily absorbed if the radiographic film is ____trally matched.

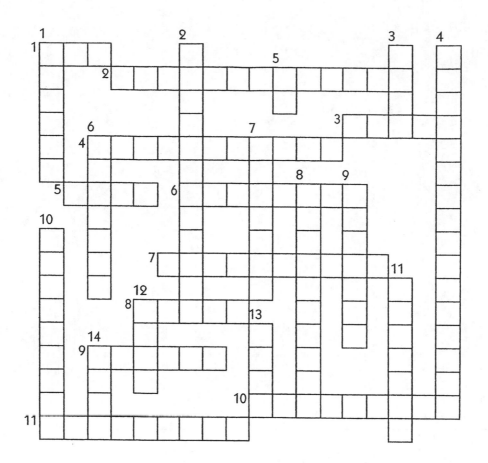

14-1

Production of Scatter Radiation

Scatter radiation results from Compton interaction with patient tissue and reduces image contrast. Three principal factors influence the quantity of scatter radiation. Two of these can be manipulated by the radiologic technologist.

- **Kilovoltage (kVp):** Increasing kVp also increases the proportion of scatter radiation because the Compton effect predominates at higher energies.
- **Field size:** Scatter radiation increases with increasing field size because more tissue is exposed.
- **Patient thickness:** Scatter radiation increases as patient thickness increases. X-ray beam collimation and tissue compression reduce scatter radiation and therefore improve image contrast.

EXERCISES

1. Remnant x-rays are those that:
   a. Are absorbed within the patient
   b. Do not interact with the patient or the image receptor
   c. Exit the patient
   d. Interact with the patient and are scattered away
   e. Scatter back toward the source

2. Which of the following factors that affect scatter radiation can be controlled by the radiologic technologist?
   a. Added filtration
   b. Field size
   c. Inherent filtration
   d. mAs
   e. Patient thickness

3. As kVp increases, scatter radiation will:
   a. Decrease because of less Compton interaction
   b. Decrease because of less photoelectric interaction
   c. Increase because of more Compton interaction
   d. Increase because of more photoelectric interaction
   e. Remain unchanged

4. What is the approximate percentage of x-rays that are transmitted through a patient?
   a. 0.1%
   b. 1%
   c. 5%
   d. 10%
   e. 20%

5. At high kVp (e.g., 125 kVp), most x-rays are:
   a. Backscattered.
   b. Not transmitted through the body
   c. Remnant x-rays
   d. Transmitted through the body with interaction
   e. Transmitted through the body without interaction

6. When kVp is increased with a compensating reduction in mAs, which of the following is reduced?
   a. Optical density
   b. Patient dose
   c. Remnant radiation
   d. Scatter proportion
   e. Spatial resolution

7. If a constant optical density is maintained while kVp is increased:
   a. Collimation should be enlarged.
   b. Collimation should be reduced.
   c. Contrast resolution will improve.
   d. Patient dose will decrease.
   e. Patient dose will increase.

8. As field size is increased, scatter radiation:
   a. Increases
   b. Is reduced
   c. Is removed
   d. Is reversed
   e. Remains constant

9. Which of the following is *not* a device designed to reduce the level of scatter radiation that reaches the image receptor?
   a. A beam restrictor
   b. A collimator
   c. A compression device
   d. A diaphragm
   e. A test pattern

10. Scatter radiation reduces radiographic quality by changing:
   a. Blurring
   b. Contrast
   c. Distortion
   d. Mass density
   e. Optical density

11. X-rays that the technologist would like to have interact with the image receptor are those that are:
   a. Absorbed in the body
   b. Attenuated in the body
   c. High energy
   d. Scattered in the body
   e. Transmitted in the body

12. As kVp is increased from 70 to 80:
   a. Contrast resolution will improve.
   b. The mAs must be increased.
   c. The SID must be increased.
   d. There will be a higher proportion of scatter radiation.
   e. There will be a lower proportion of scatter radiation.

13. Image-forming x-rays consist of which type that emerge from the patient in the direction of the image receptor?
   a. Absorbed x-rays
   b. Backscattered x-rays
   c. Emitted x-rays
   d. Intercepted x-rays
   e. Transmitted x-rays

14. As kVp increases from 70 to 90, if all other factors remain constant:
   a. Contrast resolution will improve.
   b. The number of absorbed x-rays will decrease.
   c. The number of transmitted x-rays will decrease.
   d. The ratio of absorbed to transmitted x-rays will increase.
   e. The ratio of scattered to transmitted x-rays will increase.

15. What increases as the field size of the x-ray beam increases?
   a. Heel effect
   b. kVp
   c. mAs
   d. Scatter radiation
   e. Total filtration

16. In general, as the thickness of the anatomy for which radiographs are made increases:
   a. Contrast resolution improves.
   b. kVp is increased.
   c. mAs is increased.
   d. Patient exposure is unaffected.
   e. Total filtration is increased.

17. Which of the following processes is most responsible for the production of scatter radiation?
   a. Bremmstrahlung interaction
   b. Characteristic interaction
   c. Compton effect
   d. Photoelectric effect
   e. Transmission

14-2 Control of Scatter Radiation

 Beam-restricting devices are used in radiology to limit the volume of tissue irradiated to reduce patient dose and scatter radiation. Three types of beam-restricting devices exist:

- **Aperture diaphragm:** A fixed-aperture device that consists of a lead or lead-lined metal diaphragm attached to the head of the x-ray tube.
- **Cones and cylinders:** Fixed-aperture devices that consist of an extended metal structure attached to the x-ray tube head.
- **Variable-aperture collimator:** A device that consists of two or more pairs of lead shutters that are independently adjustable. Square or rectangular fields are possible, and the x-ray field can be illuminated by a coincidence light field. **Positive-beam–limiting (PBL)** devices automatically collimate to the image receptor size.

EXERCISES

1. Which of the following is *not* a beam-restricting device?
   a. A cone
   b. A PBL device
   c. A variable-aperture collimator
   d. Added filtration

2. An aperture diaphragm should allow x-rays to expose an area:
   a. Equal to the image receptor
   b. Just larger than the image receptor
   c. Just smaller than the image receptor
   d. That varies according to patient size
   e. That varies according to technique

3. When an aperture diaphragm is used:
   a. A PBL device is required.
   b. Added filtration should be increased.
   c. Grid cutoff can occur if the diaphragm is not properly positioned.
   d. Technique should be enhanced.
   e. X-ray field cutoff can occur if the diaphragm is not properly positioned.

4. In a light-localizing, variable-aperture collimator:
   a. Added filtration is required.
   b. Equipped with a PBL device, light field illumination is unnecessary.
   c. If the light bulb burns out, the graduated scale on the adjusting mechanism can be used.
   d. It is not necessary that the crosshairs in the light beam be centered.
   e. Periodic checks of x-ray beam and light field coincidence are necessary.

5. Which of the following is the simplest of all beam-restricting devices?
   a. A fluoroscopic collimator
   b. A radiographic cone
   c. An aluminum filter
   d. An aperture diaphragm
   e. PBL

6. Which of the following devices is normally designed to limit off-focus radiation?
   a. Added filtration
   b. First-stage shutters of a variable-aperture collimator

c. Fixed-aperture circular diaphragms
d. Fixed-aperture rectangular diaphragms
e. Second-stage shutters of a variable-aperture collimator

7. Off-focus radiation:
   a. Consists of scattered electrons
   b. Consists of scattered electrons and x-rays
   c. Improves image quality
   d. Increases patient dose
   e. Results when projectile electrons do not strike the focal spot

8. Which of the following is a beam-restricting device?
   a. 2.5 mm Al added filtration
   b. A cone without an integral diaphragm
   c. A rectangular film mask on a viewbox
   d. A fluoroscopic spot-film device
   e. PBL

9. Cone cutting:
   a. Is useful in high-kVp examinations
   b. Is useful in low-kVp examinations
   c. Occurs when the axis of the cone, tube, and image receptor are not aligned
   d. Occurs when the edge of the cone intercepts the scattered x-ray beam
   e. Occurs when the tip of the cone is too close to the patient

10. If a fixed-aperture, rectangular, beam-restricting device is used:
    a. Added filtration is unnecessary.
    b. An unexposed border should be visible on all four sides of the radiograph.
    c. An unexposed border should be visible on at least two sides of the radiograph.
    d. PBL must be used.
    e. The central axis of the aperture diaphragm must be centered somewhere on the image receptor.

11. A properly designed, light-localizing, variable-aperture collimator:
    a. Concentrates off-focus radiation onto the image receptor
    b. Is designed to enhance off-focus radiation
    c. Needs no added filtration
    d. Requires light field/x-ray beam coincidence
    e. Will have field-defining shutters of aluminum

12. Radiographic cones and cylinders are used principally to reduce which of the following?
    a. Beam quality
    b. Off-focus radiation
    c. Scatter radiation
    d. The need for added filtration
    e. The required radiographic technique

13. Which of the following are the two general types of devices designed to control scatter radiation?
    a. Filtration and beam restrictors
    b. Filtration and image masks
    c. Grids and beam restrictors
    d. Grids and filtration
    e. Image masks and beam restrictors

14. When a diaphragm is used:
    a. A 1 cm unexposed border should be visible on all sides.
    b. A 1 cm unexposed border should be visible on two sides.
    c. A 3 cm unexposed border should be visible on at least three sides.
    d. Added filtration must be increased.
    e. An unexposed border is not necessary.

15. PBL stands for which of the following?
    a. Photon beam level
    b. Photon beam limitation
    c. Photon border level
    d. Positive beam level
    e. Positive beam limitation

16. A diaphragm is machined to just match image receptor size. If an unexposed border is required on the radiograph, the diaphragm opening will:
    a. Have to be enlarged
    b. Have to be reduced
    c. More information is required before a change can be determined
    d. Remain the same
    e. Require additional filtration

17. An aperture diaphragm is designed for 25 cm × 30 cm film. If the SID is 100 cm and the source-to-diaphragm distance is 10 cm, what size should the opening of the diaphragm be?
    a. 2.0 cm × 2.5 cm
    b. 2.0 cm × 3.0 cm
    c. 2.5 cm × 3.0 cm
    d. 2.5 cm × 3.5 cm
    e. 3.0 cm × 3.5 cm

X-rays that leave a patient and are incident on the image receptor are called image-forming radiation. There are two basic components of image-forming radiation: (1) those x-rays that have passed directly through the patient without interaction, and (2) those x-rays that have been scattered within the patient. Only the x-rays that are not significantly scattered carry useful diagnostic information to the image receptor.

Scattered x-rays are the result of Compton interaction. Because the image receptor is not capable of distinguishing primary x-rays from scattered x-rays, it will image a scattered x-ray as having come directly from the x-ray source, when in fact, its direction was from the tissue from which it was scattered. This scattered radiation reduces image contrast.

The main device used to intercept scattered radiation is the grid. There are two principal characteristics of grid construction: (1) **grid ratio** is the thickness of the grid (the height of the grid strip) divided by the width of the interspace material; and (2) **grid frequency** is the number of grid strips per inch or per centimeter.

EXERCISES

1. The principal reason for using a grid is to:
   a. Enhance differential absorption
   b. Improve image contrast
   c. Improve spatial resolution
   d. Reduce patient dose
   e. Remove remnant radiation

2. Which of the following materials would be *most* radiolucent?
   a. Aluminum
   b. Carbon fiber
   c. Copper
   d. Iodine
   e. Lead

3. Which of the following is the most important grid characteristic?
   a. Grid frequency
   b. Grid height
   c. Grid mass
   d. Grid ratio
   e. Grid weight

4. In a grid that has lead strips 0.5 mm apart and 4 mm high, the grid ratio is:
   a. 4:1
   b. 6:1
   c. 8:1
   d. 12:1
   e. 16:1

5. A grid has the following characteristics: grid ratio = 10:1; grid height = 4.5 mm; grid strip width = 40 μm; and interspace width = 450 μm. What is the grid frequency?
   a. 20 lines/cm
   b. 22 lines/cm
   c. 40 lines/cm
   d. 45 lines/cm
   e. 60 lines/cm

6. If only scatter radiation reached the image receptor:
   a. Image contrast would be very high.
   b. Image contrast would be very low.
   c. Image receptor speed would be very high.
   d. Image receptor speed would be very low.
   e. Spatial resolution would be improved.

7. In the design of a radiographic grid, which of the following must be *true*?
   a. The added filtration must be aluminum.
   b. The grid strips are radiolucent.
   c. The grid strips are radiotransparent.
   d. The interspace material is radiolucent.
   e. The interspace material is radiopaque.

8. Grids are principally effective in attenuating which of the following?
   a. All remnant radiation
   b. Photoelectrons
   c. Transmitted x-rays
   d. X-rays after Compton interaction
   e. X-rays after photoelectric interaction

9. If the interspace dimension is constant, increasing the grid ratio will:
   a. Make the grid lighter
   b. Make the grid thicker
   c. Reduce grid mass
   d. Require less grid strip material
   e. Require less interspace material

10. As grid frequency increases:
    a. Grid mass is usually decreased.
    b. The grid ratio is reduced if the thickness of the grid remains constant.
    c. The interspace width becomes thinner if the width of the grid strip remains constant.
    d. The number of grid strips per centimeter increases.
    e. The patient dose is reduced.

11. Which of the following would be the *most* acceptable grid strip material from the standpoint of x-ray attenuation?
    a. Barium
    b. Copper
    c. Iodine
    d. Tungsten
    e. Uranium

12. Which of the following will *not* improve image contrast?
    a. A decrease in kVp
    b. Collimating the x-ray beam

c. The use of a grid
d. The use of added filtration
e. The use of positive-beam limitation (PBL)

13. Grids with a high ratio are:
    a. Easier to manufacture than those with a low ratio
    b. More effective than those with a low ratio
    c. Most effective at low kVp
    d. Produced by increasing grid strip width
    e. Produced by increasing interspace width

14. The efficiency of a grid for reducing scatter radiation is related principally to which of the following?
    a. Grid frequency
    b. Grid interspace
    c. Grid mass
    d. Grid radius
    e. Grid ratio

15. Radiographic grids:
    a. Can be placed anywhere between the source and the image receptor
    b. Can be placed between the patient and the image receptor
    c. Can be placed between the source and the patient
    d. Must be placed between the patient and the image receptor
    e. Must be placed between the source and the patient

16. The construct of a radiographic grid:
    a. Has an aluminum cover for filtration.
    b. Has an aluminum cover to reduce scatter radiation.
    c. Incorporates aluminum or copper as the grid strip material.
    d. Incorporates high-Z interspace material.
    e. Is easier to achieve with an aluminum interspace than with plastic fiber.

17. Use of which of the following will reduce radiographic contrast?
    a. Collimators
    b. Filtration
    c. Grids
    d. Intensifying screens
    e. PBL

14-4

Measuring Grid Performance

The principal function of a radiographic grid is to absorb scattered radiation from the image-forming x-ray beam before it reaches the image receptor. If scattered radiation does reach the image receptor, image contrast is reduced. The function of radiographic grids is to increase image contrast.

The higher the grid ratio and the higher the grid frequency, the greater will be the image contrast. The principal measure of grid performance is the **contrast improvement factor, k:**

$$K = \frac{\text{Radiographic contrast with a grid}}{\text{Radiographic contrast without a grid}}$$

Another measure of grid performance is **selectivity:**

$$\text{Selectivity} = \frac{\text{Transmitted primary x-rays}}{\text{Transmitted scattered x-rays}}$$

Both the contrast improvement factor and selectivity depend on the characteristics of the x-ray beam and the characteristics of the grid. However, the contrast improvement factor depends more on the characteristics of the x-ray beam, whereas selectivity depends more on the construction of the grid.

EXERCISES

1. Which of the following is the *least* important indicator of grid performance?
   a. Contrast improvement factor
   b. Grid frequency
   c. Grid mass
   d. Grid strip height
   e. Grid ratio

2. The contrast improvement factor is defined as the radiographic contrast obtained:
   a. At a density of 1
   b. At a density of 1.0 above base plus fog
   c. With a grid compared with that obtained without a grid
   d. With a collimator compared with that obtained without a collimator
   e. With a screen compared with that obtained without a screen

3. As the grid ratio increases, there is also an increase in which of the following?
   a. Contrast improvement factor
   b. Intensification factor
   c. Spatial resolution
   d. System speed
   e. Width of interspace material

4. In general, the selectivity of a grid depends principally on which of the following?
   a. Contrast improvement factor
   b. Focal length
   c. Grid frequency
   d. Grid mass
   e. Grid radius

5. Radiographic grids with high contrast improvement usually:
   a. Are low-ratio grids
   b. Improve contrast resolution
   c. Improve spatial resolution
   d. Reduce patient dose
   e. Transmit more scatter radiation

6. A radiograph is made at 76 kVp and 25 mAs without a grid. If an 8:1 ratio grid is added, the mAs required then would be approximately:
   a. 25 mAs
   b. 50 mAs
   c. 100 mAs
   d. 150 mAs
   e. 300 mAs

7. Which of the following is the simplest type of grid?
   a. Crossed grid
   b. Focused grid
   c. High-ratio grid
   d. Linear grid
   e. Zero frequency grid

8. The undesirable absorption of image-forming x-rays by a grid is called:
   a. Anode heel effect
   b. Grid cutoff
   c. Malpositioned grid
   d. Primary beam scatter
   e. Upside-down grid

9. Which of the following would be included in the three major classifications of moving grids?
   a. Crossed grid
   b. Focused grid
   c. Linear grid
   d. Reciprocating grid
   e. Zero frequency grid

10. If one had two grids whose characteristics were unknown but grid B weighed twice as much as grid A, one might conclude that grid B would have:
    a. A higher contrast improvement factor
    b. A greater mass effect
    c. A lower grid frequency
    d. A lower grid ratio
    e. A lower selectivity

11. Focused grids:
    a. Cut off the four edges of an image if placed too close to the source
    b. Cut off two edges of an image if placed too far from the tube
    c. Do not move
    d. Reduce the amount of scatter radiation that reaches the image receptor
    e. Reduce the radiation exposure to the patient compared with no grid

12. One factor that does *not* affect the percentage of scatter radiation that reaches the image receptor is:
    a. Grid mass
    b. Grid ratio
    c. kVp
    d. mAs
    e. Patient thickness

13. The value of the Bucky factor increases with which of the following?
    a. Decreasing contrast improvement factor
    b. Decreasing grid ratio
    c. Increasing interspace width
    d. Increasing x-ray quality
    e. Increasing x-ray quantity

14. Which of the following would principally reduce the *production* of scatter radiation?
    a. A decrease in field size
    b. A decrease in SID
    c. An increase in SSD
    d. Use of a filter
    e. Use of a grid

15. Radiographic grids:
    a. Have reduced selectivity as the mass is increased
    b. May have aluminum step wedges incorporated into them
    c. Must include a filter
    d. Usually have contrast improvement factors from 0 to 1.0
    e. Usually have grid ratios between 5:1 and 16:1

16. A crossed radiographic grid:
    a. Allows considerable positioning latitude compared with linear grids
    b. Has a contrast improvement factor equal to a linear grid of equal ratio
    c. Is said to have a grid ratio of 10:1; therefore, it consists of two 5:1 linear grids
    d. Must be used for tomography
    e. Reduces scatter radiation along two axes

17. Which of the following is a disadvantage of moving grids?
    a. They may produce motion blur.
    b. They may result in decreased magnification.
    c. They require higher grid frequency.
    d. They require higher grid ratio.
    e. They require thinner strips.

If the construction and performance characteristics of a grid are known and understood, grid selection and use will be more accurate. Selection of a grid usually requires that one specify the type of grid (parallel, crossed, focused, or moving), the ratio of the grid, and the grid frequency.

Such selection is made on the basis of the types of radiographic examination to be performed. If grid lines are objectionable, moving grids should be used.

Cerebral angiography often requires crossed grids, so that contrast is maximized for imaging small-vessel details. Low-kVp techniques usually demand low-ratio grids, and high-kVp techniques usually require high-ratio grids. For general purpose radiographic rooms, focused grids with ratios of approximately 8:1 to 12:1 usually are used.

Focused grids normally are preferred to parallel grids because with parallel grids, grid cutoff can occur.

$$\text{Distance to grid cutoff} = \frac{\text{Source-to-image-receptor distance}}{\text{Grid ratio}}$$

EXERCISES

1. Which of the following is *not* a grid positioning error?
   a. Air-gap grid
   b. Lateral decentering
   c. Off-center grid
   d. Off-focus grid
   e. Off-level grid

2. In the design of radiographic techniques, the *most* common practice is to use which of the following?
   a. A crossed grid
   b. A focused moving grid
   c. A focused stationary grid
   d. A parallel moving grid
   e. A parallel stationary grid

3. Which of the following techniques will result in the highest patient dose if mAs is changed to maintain optical density?
   a. 5:1 crossed grid; 70 kVp
   b. 5:1 crossed grid; 90 kVp
   c. 10:1 focused grid; 70 kVp
   d. 10:1 focused grid; 90 kVp
   e. 12:1 parallel grid; 70 kVp

4. Grids generally:
   a. Must be cleaned on schedule
   b. Require faster image receptors
   c. Require less mAs
   d. Require periodic replacement because of radiation fatigue
   e. Result in increased patient dose

5. When comparable radiographs are produced, which of the following combinations will result in the lowest patient dose?
   a. High kVp and high-ratio grids
   b. High kVp and low-ratio grids
   c. High kVp and no grid
   d. Low kVp and high-ratio grids
   e. Low kVp and low-ratio grids

6. Grid cutoff:
   a. Is measured by the Bucky factor
   b. Is more pronounced with high-ratio grids
   c. Is more pronounced with low-ratio grids
   d. Never occurs with focused grids
   e. Occurs only with focused grids

7. Air-gap technique:
   a. Increases the Bucky factor
   b. Reduces contrast by absorption of scattered radiation in the air
   c. Requires that the grid and the film must be separated by at least 30 cm
   d. Results in approximately the same patient dose as nongrid techniques
   e. Results in image magnification

8. If radiographic grids are used and the technique is compensated, patient exposure:
   a. Increases with increasing grid ratio
   b. Increases with increasing kVp
   c. Is independent of grid frequency
   d. Is independent of grid mass
   e. Remains unchanged from that with nongrid techniques

9. Bedside examinations require a wide range of SIDs. Which of the following parallel grids would be *most* likely to produce grid cutoff?
   a. 5:1
   b. 6:1
   c. 8:1
   d. 12:1
   e. 16:1

10. In general, which of the following has the greatest contrast improvement factor?
   a. Crossed grids
   b. Focused grids
   c. Moving grids
   d. Parallel grids
   e. Zero grids

11. Which of the following is an undesirable characteristic of linear grids compared with focused grids?
   a. Higher Bucky factor
   b. Increased patient dose
   c. Lower grid frequencies
   d. Lower grid ratios
   e. More grid cutoff

12. What is the result of replacing an 8:1 grid with a 12:1 grid?
   a. Greater positioning latitude
   b. Higher patient dose
   c. Less contrast
   d. Less spatial resolution
   e. Lower patient dose

13. When air-gap radiography is performed:
   a. A high-ratio grid must be used.
   b. A low-ratio grid must be used.
   c. Contrast resolution is improved.
   d. Patient dose is increased.
   e. The heel effect is accentuated.

15-1

Fifteen Percent Rule

The mathematical problems that each radiologic technologist faces in daily practice include (1) mentally applying the 15% rule for kVp to adjust radiographic technique, (2) having a desired total mAs in mind and trying mentally to determine an mA/time combination that will yield that total, and (3) mentally applying the inverse square law for distance changes.

The following exercises will give you an idea of how well you are able to solve applications of the 15% rule in your head.

To obtain the greatest benefit from the following problems, solve them mentally, without a calculator or pencil and paper. If you have trouble with any of these, turn to Part II of the Math Tutor section of this workbook for review. Remember that application of the 15% rule must be done in "steps" for accuracy. For example, to quadruple the optical density starting at 80 kVp, do not simply increase kVp by 30%. Rather, think of the change as two doublings of the optical density (OD), or two steps of 15%. The first doubling is accomplished with an increase of 12 kVp (15% of 80), but the second doubling must be obtained with an increase of 14 kVp (15% of 92), for a total of 106 kVp.

EXERCISES

1. What is 5% of 70?
   a. 0.5
   b. 1.5
   c. 2.5
   d. 3.5
   e. 4.5

2. What is 5% of 90?
   a. 0.5
   b. 1.5
   c. 2.5
   d. 3.5
   c. 4.5

3. What is 15% of 80?
   a. 8
   b. 12
   c. 16
   d. 20
   e. 22

4. What is 15% of 100?
   a. 10
   b. 15
   c. 20
   d. 25
   e. 30

5. What is one half of 15% of 60?
   a. 4.5
   b. 10.5
   c. 12.5
   d. 15
   e. 17

6. What is one half of 15% of 80?
   a. 4
   b. 5
   c. 6
   d. 10
   e. 14

7. Starting at 60 kVp, what new kVp would result in an optical density that is one-half that of the original?
   a. 48 kVp
   b. 51 kVp
   c. 54 kVp
   d. 66 kVp
   e. 69 kVp

8. Original technique: 100 mA, 500 ms, 60 kVp; new technique: 200 mA, 125 ms, _____.
   a. 69 kVp
   b. 70 kVp
   c. 74 kVp
   d. 78 kVp
   e. 80 kVp

9. Original technique: 300 mA, 20 ms, 120 kVp; new technique: 400 mA, 120 kVp, _____.
   a. 5 ms
   b. 10 ms
   c. 15 ms
   d. 25 ms
   e. 30 ms

10. Original technique: 400 mA, 8 ms, 40 kVp; new technique: 50 mA, 90 ms, _____.
    a. 37 kVp
    b. 44 kVp
    c. 46 kVp
    d. 48 kVp
    e. 52 kVp

11. Original technique: 400 mA, 33 ms, 80 kVp; new technique: 300 mA, 33 ms, _____.
    a. 83 kVp
    b. 86 kVp
    c. 90 kVp
    d. 92 kVp
    e. 98 kVp

12. Original technique: 300 mA, 23 ms, 70 kVp; new technique: 150 mA, 100 ms, _____.
    a. 60 kVp
    b. 64 kVp
    c. 77 kVp
    d. 80 kVp
    e. 84 kVp

$$mAs = mA \times s$$

$$\text{Therefore, exposure time (s)} = \frac{mAs}{mA}$$

To get the greatest benefit from this worksheet, try to solve the problems mentally, without writing them down or using a calculator. If you need additional help with technique math, turn to the Math Tutor section of this workbook.

EXERCISES

1. If the required technique is 2.5 mAs and the mA station selected is 100 mA, what is the required exposure time?
   a. 10 ms
   b. 15 ms
   c. 25 ms
   d. 75 ms
   e. 125 ms

2. If the required technique is 7.5 mAs and the mA station selected is 150 mA, what is the required exposure time?
   a. 10 ms
   b. 20 ms
   c. 30 ms
   d. 40 ms
   e. 50 ms

3. If the required technique is 20 mAs and the mA station selected is 300 mA, what is the required exposure time?
   a. 15 ms
   b. 67 ms
   c. 87 ms

   d. 133 ms
   e. 140 ms

4. If the required technique is 80 mAs and the mA station selected is 400 mA, what is the required exposure time?
   a. 15 ms
   b. 50 ms
   c. 150 ms
   d. 200 ms
   e. 350 ms

5. If the required technique is 33 mAs and the mA station selected is 100 mA, what is the required exposure time?
   a. 17 ms
   b. 33 ms
   c. 170 ms
   d. 330 ms
   e. 670 ms

6. If the required technique is 20 mAs and the mA station selected is 400 mA, what is the required exposure time?
   a. 5 ms
   b. 10 ms
   c. 20 ms
   d. 33 ms
   e. 50 ms

7. If the required technique is 25 mAs and the mA station selected is 200 mA, what is the required exposure time?
   a. 125 ms
   b. 150 ms
   c. 225 ms

d. 275 ms

e. 325 ms

8. If the required technique is 60 mAs and the mA station selected is 300 mA, what is the required exposure time?
   a. 100 ms
   b. 200 ms
   c. 300 ms
   d. 400 ms
   e. 600 ms

9. If the required technique is 240 mAs and the mA station selected is 400 mA, what is the required exposure time?
   a. 600 ms
   b. 900 ms
   c. 1200 ms
   d. 1500 ms
   e. 1800 ms

10. If the required technique is 5 mAs and the mA station selected is 100 mA, what is the required exposure time?
    a. 5 ms
    b. 15 ms
    c. 25 ms
    d. 50 ms
    e. 100 ms

11. If the required technique is 40 mAs and the mA station selected is 200 mA, what is the required exposure time?
    a. 25 ms
    b. 50 ms
    c. 100 ms
    d. 150 ms
    e. 200 ms

12. If the required technique is 5 mAs and the mA station selected is 300 mA, what is the required exposure time?
    a. 10 ms
    b. 17 ms
    c. 34 ms
    d. 50 ms
    e. 67 ms

13. If the required technique is 1.6 mAs and the mA station selected is 100 mA, what is the required exposure time?
    a. 16 ms
    b. 17 ms
    c. 34 ms
    d. 40 ms
    e. 50 ms

14. If the required technique is 1.25 mAs and the mA station selected is 50 mA, what is the required exposure time?
    a. 10 ms
    b. 25 ms
    c. 75 ms
    d. 125 ms
    e. 250 ms

15. If the required technique is 15 mAs and the mA station selected is 100 mA, what is the required exposure time?
    a. 15 ms
    b. 25 ms
    c. 50 ms
    d. 150 ms
    e. 250 ms

16. If the required technique is 120 mAs and the mA station selected is 300 mA, what is the required exposure time?
    a. 100 ms
    b. 200 ms
    c. 300 ms
    d. 400 ms
    e. 500 ms

17. If the required technique is 1.25 mAs and the mA station selected is 100 mA, what is the required exposure time?
    a. 1.25 ms
    b. 12.5 ms
    c. 25 ms
    d. 40 ms
    e. 50 ms

18. If the required technique is 4 mAs and the mA station selected is 200 mA, what is the required exposure time?
    a. 2 ms
    b. 4 ms
    c. 10 ms
    d. 20 ms
    e. 40 ms

19. If the required technique is 12.5 mAs and the mA station selected is 100 mA, what is the required exposure time?
    a. 1.25 ms
    b. 5 ms
    c. 12.5 ms
    d. 25 ms
    e. 125 ms

Use the "square law" to find a new mAs that will compensate for a change in distance. Whereas the **inverse square law** is used to predict radiation intensity and therefore optical density, the **square law** is used to compensate radiographic technique so that optical density is maintained constant when SID changes.

The square law:

$$\frac{mAs_2}{mAs_1} = \frac{(SID_2)^2}{(SID_1)^2}$$

where mAs_1 is the original mAs used at SID_1 (the original SID), and mAs_2 is the new mAs needed to maintain equal optical density (OD) if the SID is changed to SID_2.

EXERCISES

1. When radiographic technique is changed from 30 mAs, 100 cm SID to 75 cm SID, what should be the new mAs?
   a. 17 mAs
   b. 20 mAs
   c. 24 mAs
   d. 30 mAs
   e. 32 mAs

2. When radiographic technique is changed from 12.5 mAs, 100 cm SID to 150 cm SID, what should be the new mAs?
   a. 18 mAs
   b. 20 mAs
   c. 22 mAs
   d. 28 mAs
   e. 32 mAs

3. When radiographic technique is changed from 10 mAs, 100 cm SID to 180 cm SID, what should be the new mAs?
   a. 20 mAs
   b. 26 mAs
   c. 30 mAs
   d. 32 mAs
   e. 36 mAs

4. When radiographic technique is changed from 5 mAs, 100 cm SID to 240 cm SID, what should be the new mAs?
   a. 14 mAs
   b. 19 mAs
   c. 24 mAs
   d. 29 mAs
   e. 36 mAs

5. When radiographic technique is changed from 48 mAs, 80 cm SID to 90 cm SID, what should be the new mAs?
   a. 51 mAs
   b. 55 mAs
   c. 59 mAs
   d. 61 mAs
   e. 71 mAs

6. When radiographic technique is changed from 22.5 mAs, 100 cm SID to 200 cm SID, what should be the new mAs?
   a. 50 mAs
   b. 70 mAs
   c. 78 mAs
   d. 84 mAs
   e. 90 mAs

7. When radiographic technique is changed from 36 mAs, 150 cm SID to 113 cm SID, what should be the new mAs?
   a. 20 mAs
   b. 26 mAs
   c. 30 mAs
   d. 38 mAs
   e. 48 mAs

8. When radiographic technique is changed from 10 mAs, 150 cm SID to 225 cm SID, what should be the new mAs?
   a. 17 mAs
   b. 22.5 mAs
   c. 27.5 mAs
   d. 32.5 mAs
   e. 36 mAs

9. When radiographic technique is changed from 60 mAs, 70 kVp, 150 cm SID to 113 cm SID, what should be the new mAs?
   a. 34 mAs
   b. 86 mAs
   c. 96 mAs
   d. 102 mAs
   e. 116 mAs

10. A PA chest examination done at 100 cm SID tabletop technique requires 1.5 mAs. What is the required mAs when testing is conducted with a dedicated chest imaging system with a fixed 180 cm SID?
    a. 1 mAs
    b. 2 mAs
    c. 3 mAs
    d. 5 mAs
    e. 10 mAs

11. If the dedicated chest room in Question 10 was designed for a fixed SID of 300 cm, what would be the required mAs?
    a. 1 mAs
    b. 3 mAs
    c. 5 mAs
    d. 13.5 mAs
    e. 20 mAs

12. A dedicated mammography imaging system has a fixed SID of 55 cm and normal technique calls for 200 mAs. If this system is replaced by a 75 cm mammography imaging system, what will be the approximate new mAs?
    a. 200 mAs
    b. 275 mAs
    c. 325 mAs
    d. 375 mAs
    e. 500 mAs

Characteristics of the Imaging System

Proper radiographic exposure must take into account several variable characteristics of the x-ray imaging system. Perhaps the most important characteristic is the type of high-voltage generator incorporated into the imaging system. In general, compared with single-phase generators, full-wave–rectified and more complex waveform generators require a lower kVp and less mAs to produce acceptable radiographs. The radiologic technologist has no control over this characteristic.

Essentially all x-ray imaging systems now have selectable added filtration. The choices of added filtration available to the radiologic technologist usually range from 0 to 4 mm Al, resulting in total filtration of 1.5 to 5.5 mm Al. In general, when one increases added filtration, a reduction in kVp and an increase in mAs are required to maintain constant optical density.

EXERCISES

1. Which of the following is a popular focal-spot combination (small/large) for a dedicated mammography imaging system?
   a. 0.05 mm/0.2 mm
   b. 0.1 mm/0.3 mm
   c. 0.1 mm/3 mm
   d. 0.3 mm/1.0 mm
   e. 0.3 m/1.2 mm

2. The approximate filtration of the x-ray beam contributed by the light-localizing collimator is:
   a. 0.1 mm Al
   b. 0.5 mm Al
   c. 1.0 mm Al
   d. 2.0 mm Al
   e. 3.0 mm Al

3. The radiologic technologist cannot change the type of high-voltage generator used because:
   a. A change can be made only by the medical physicist.
   b. It is fixed at the time of purchase.
   c. Only the radiologic engineer can make that change.
   d. Only the radiologist can make that change.
   e. The service engineer determines this at installation.

4. Compared with half-wave rectification for a fixed exposure time:
   a. Full-wave rectification will have four times the number of pulses.
   b. High-frequency will have six times the number of pulses.
   c. Three-phase will have at least six times the number of pulses.
   d. Three-phase will have at least 12 times the number of pulses.
   e. Three-phase will have four times the number of pulses.

5. The principal advantage of a large focal spot compared with a small focal spot is:
   a. Spatial resolution is enhanced.
   b. Contrast resolution is improved.
   c. Faster image receptors can be used.
   d. Voltage ripple is reduced.
   e. A greater number of x-rays can be produced.

6. An acceptable radiograph is made with the large focal spot. If the examination were repeated with the small focal spot using the same technique:
   a. Patient dose would be lower.
   b. The image would be darker.
   c. The image would be lighter.
   d. The image would be sharper.
   e. The image would have better contrast.

7. General purpose x-ray tubes usually have inherent filtration of:
   a. 0.1 mm Al
   b. 0.5 mm Al
   c. 1.0 mm Al
   d. 2.0 mm Al
   e. 3.0 mm Al

8. Which of the following has the *least* voltage ripple?
   a. High-frequency
   b. Single-phase, full-wave
   c. Single-phase, half-wave
   d. Three-phase, six-pulse
   e. Three-phase, 12-pulse

9. Three-phase rectified power has which of the following?
   a. Three pulses per cycle
   b. Six pulses per cycle
   c. Nine pulses per cycle
   d. Fifteen pulses per cycle
   e. Eighteen pulses per cycle

10. An acceptable radiograph is made with the large focal spot. If the examination were repeated with the small focal spot:
    a. kVp should be reduced.
    b. mAs and kVp should be increased.
    c. mAs and kVp should be reduced.
    d. mAs should be reduced.
    e. No technique change is required.

11. The principal advantage of a small focal spot compared with a large focal spot is:
    a. Better detail
    b. Use of faster image receptors
    c. Higher heat capacity
    d. Reduced voltage ripple
    e. Production of a greater number of x-rays

12. An acceptable radiograph is made with 1.0 mm Al added filtration and the small focal spot. If the examination were repeated with 3.0 mm Al added filtration, what would be the *most* likely technique change?
    a. Increase kVp
    b. Increase kVp and mAs
    c. Increase mAs
    d. Increase SID
    e. Use the larger focal spot size

13. An acceptable radiograph is produced with a half-wave–rectified x-ray imaging system. If the examination is repeated on a full-wave imaging system, what should be changed?
    a. Exposure time
    b. kVp
    c. mAs
    d. Object-to-image receptor distance (OID)
    e. SID

14. An acceptable radiograph is made with 1.0 mm Al added filtration. If the examination were repeated with 3.0 mm Al added filtration and appropriate technique changes made:
    a. Image blur would be reduced.
    b. Image contrast would improve.
    c. Patient dose would be reduced.
    d. Spatial resolution would improve.
    e. Such an exposure would not be possible.

15. An acceptable radiograph is made with a single-phase generator. If a repeat examination is performed with a three-phase generator, what technique change should be made?
    a. Increase kVp and mAs
    b. Increase mAs
    c. No change is required
    d. Reduce kVp
    e. Reduce kVp and mAs

16. What is the principal advantage of high-frequency generators?
    a. Better spatial resolution
    b. Enhanced radiation quality
    c. Increased radiation quantity and quality
    d. Reduced radiation quantity
    e. Reduced radiation quantity and quality

In general radiography, overlying and underlying tissues are superimposed. In tomography, these tissues are blurred. Tomography requires deliberate and controlled motion unsharpness. The principal purpose of tomography is to improve image contrast; however, this improvement occurs at the expense of increased patient dose.

Magnification radiography requires an increase in OID to produce a magnified image. The degree of magnification is given by the magnification factor (MF).

$$MF = \frac{Image\ size}{Object\ size} = \frac{SID}{SOD}$$

Magnification radiography works best with a small x-ray tube focal spot. It usually can be performed without radiographic grids, yet it still results in a somewhat higher patient dose.

EXERCISES

1. During conventional tomography, the image receptor:
   a. Is focused by the angle of movement.
   b. Is focused to the automatic plane of interest.
   c. Moves opposite the x-ray tube in a seesaw motion.
   d. Moves with the x-ray tube similarly to the x-ray tube tower assembly in fluoroscopy.
   e. Remains fixed.

2. During conventional tomography, structures that lie outside the object plane are blurred because of which of the following?
   a. Absorption blur
   b. Geometric blur
   c. Image receptor blur
   d. Motion blur
   e. Subject blur

3. With linear tomography, which of the following is *true?*
   a. The source and the image receptor are the same distance from the focal plane.
   b. The source and the image receptor cover different tomographic angles.
   c. The source and the image receptor move at the same speed.
   d. The source and the image receptor move in opposite directions.
   e. The source and the image receptor move the same distance.

4. Which of the following combinations determines the thickness of the cut in a tomograph?
   a. Collimation and filtration
   b. SID and length of tube travel
   c. OID and speed of tube travel
   d. SID and speed of tube travel
   e. SOD and length of tube travel

5. Conventional tomography uses which of the following principles?
   a. Tridimensional image
   b. Optical illusion
   c. Motion blur
   d. Random movement
   e. Stereoscopy

6. During conventional tomography, the fulcrum is in the:
   a. Film plane
   b. Focal plane
   c. Image receptor plane
   d. Object plane
   e. Tomographic layer

7. When the tomographic angle is 0 degrees, the tomographic layer is:
   a. Indefinable
   b. Infinity
   c. Thin
   d. Very thick
   e. Zero

8. To obtain a tomographic layer of approximately 1 mm, the tomographic angle should be approximately:
   a. 10 degrees
   b. 20 degrees
   c. 40 degrees
   d. 50 degrees
   e. 60 degrees

9. Which of the following is the *major* disadvantage of conventional tomography?
   a. Cost
   b. Enhanced contrast
   c. Image blur
   d. Lost spatial resolution
   e. Patient dose

10. The *major* advantage of conventional tomography is better:
    a. Contrast resolution.
    b. Cost
    c. Image blur
    d. Patient dose
    e. Spatial resolution

11. Conventional tomography has been called which of the following?
    a. Cisternography
    b. Heel effect
    c. Laminography
    d. Myelography
    e. The line-focus principle

12. Which of the following tomographic angles would be considered for use in zonography?
    a. 5 degrees
    b. 15 degrees
    c. 25 degrees

d. 35 degrees
e. 60 degrees

13. The tomographic angle is the angle of x-ray tube movement during which of the following?
    a. Anode preparation
    b. Cathode boost
    c. Fulcrum adjustment
    d. Fulcrum motion
    e. X-ray exposure

14. Adequate magnification radiography requires that which of the following must have a large value?
    a. Focal spot
    b. OID
    c. SID
    d. SOD
    e. SSD

15. Magnification radiography normally is used to image what type of structure?
    a. High-contrast
    b. Large
    c. Low-contrast
    d. Moving
    e. Small

16. The magnification factor is equal to which of the following?
    a. SID + OID
    b. SID ÷ SOD
    c. SOD + OID
    d. SOD ÷ SID
    e. SSD × SID

17. For magnification cerebral angiography, which of the following focal-spot sizes would be *best*?
    a. 0.3 mm
    b. 0.6 mm
    c. 1.0 mm
    d. 2.0 mm
    e. 10 mm

18. The major disadvantage of magnification radiography is increased:
    a. Artifacts
    b. Blur
    c. Cost
    d. Noise
    e. Patient dose

19. If the MF is 1.5 and the image size is 9 cm, what is the object size?
    a. 3 cm
    b. 6 cm
    c. 12 cm
    d. 13.5 cm
    e. 15 cm

20. The tomographic angle is:
    a. Determined by the tabletop angle
    b. Equal to the anode angle
    c. That found between the anatomic part and the image receptor
    d. That found between the vertical and the image plane
    e. That of tube movement during x-ray exposure

16-1

Film Factors

The characteristic curve, sometimes called an **H & D curve,** describes the relationship between **optical density** and **radiation intensity.** The characteristic curve is helpful in predicting a number of image receptor factors, such as optical density (OD), contrast, speed, and latitude. OD describes the degree of blackening on a film. It is related to the fraction of light transmitted through the exposed and processed film.

Image contrast is the difference between light and dark areas on a radiograph. High-contrast radiographs are nearly white-on-black, whereas low-contrast radiographs are very gray. Latitude is the reciprocal of contrast and describes the range of exposure techniques that will result in an acceptable image.

EXERCISES

1. Which of the following is *not* necessary for constructing a characteristic curve?
   a. Densitometer
   b. Processor
   c. Sensitometer
   d. Slit camera
   e. Step wedge

2. The diagnostically useful portion of a characteristic curve most often includes which of the following?
   a. The base density
   b. The base density plus fog
   c. The shoulder
   d. The straight-line portion
   e. The toe

3. If the OD of a radiograph is such that only 1% of incident light is transmitted, the OD has a value of:
   a. 0.01
   b. 0.1
   c. 1.0
   d. 2.0
   e. 3.0

4. The generally accepted range of useful ODs on a radiograph is:
   a. 0.1 to 0.25
   b. 0.25 to 2.5
   c. 1.0 to 3.0
   d. 1.5 to 4.0
   e. 3.0 to 5.0

5. Which of the following radiographic techniques should result in the widest exposure latitude?
   a. High kVp, contrast film, high grid ratio
   b. High kVp, direct exposure, high grid ratio
   c. High kVp, latitude film, low grid ratio
   d. Low kVp, direct exposure, high grid ratio
   e. Low kVp, screen-film, low grid ratio

6. As the time of film development is increased beyond the manufacturer's recommendations:
   a. Contrast increases.
   b. Fog increases.
   c. Latitude narrows.
   d. Spatial resolution is reduced.
   e. Speed decreases.

7. An exposure of 100 mR is equal to a log
   relative exposure of:
   a. 0.2
   b. 0.3
   c. 2.0
   d. 3.0
   e. 4.0

8. When one increases the exposure by four times,
   that is an increase in log relative exposure of:
   a. 0.1
   b. 0.3
   c. 0.6
   d. 2.0
   e. 4.0

9. Base density refers to which of the following?
   a. A log relative exposure of 0.25
   b. A log relative exposure of 0.5
   c. The fog of the base
   d. The optical density of the base
   e. The physical density of the film

10. Which of the following is the main component
    of radiographic noise?
    a. Graininess
    b. Quantum mottle

    c. Random mottle
    d. Structure mottle
    e. Uniform mottle

11. An optical density of 3.0 on a radiograph:
    a. Indicates good technique
    b. Indicates higher radiopacity than a
       density of 4
    c. Indicates underexposure
    d. Is usually on the toe of the characteristic
       curve
    e. Must be viewed with a hot light

12. Unexposed but processed film may appear
    cloudy and dull because of which of the
    following?
    a. Average gradient
    b. Base density
    c. Contrast
    d. Latitude
    e. Scatter radiation

Exercises 13 through 17 refer to the following
illustration.

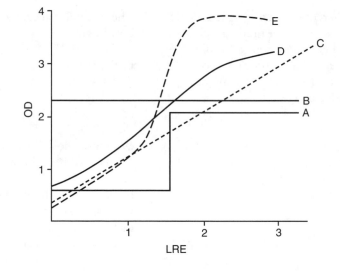

13. Which characteristic curve best represents a
    screen-film combination?
    a. A
    b. B
    c. C
    d. D
    e. E

14. Which characteristic curve *best* represents
    digital x-ray imaging?
    a. A
    b. B
    c. C
    d. D
    e. E

15. Which characteristic curve represents the fastest image receptor?
    a. A
    b. B
    c. C
    d. D
    e. E

16. Which characteristic curve shows highest base plus fog density?
    a. A
    b. B
    c. C
    d. D
    e. E

17. Which characteristic curve exhibits greatest contrast?
    a. A
    b. B
    c. C
    d. D
    e. E

To obtain a high-quality radiograph, an understanding of geometry is necessary. The x-ray source, the anatomic object, and the image receptor all lie in different planes; therefore, the image will always be larger than the object—a condition called **magnification**. Under some circumstances (e.g., cerebral angiography, mammography), magnification is desired and planned. Normally, however, it is preferable to have as little magnification as possible.

The degree of magnification is identified by the magnification factor (MF).

$$MF = \frac{Image\ size}{Object\ size} = \frac{SID}{SOD}$$

The size of the object is rarely accessible for measurement; consequently, the MF usually is determined by the ratio of SID to SOD. SOD usually can be estimated accurately.

Image **distortion** occurs when the object is not positioned in a plane that is parallel to the plane of the image receptor. This situation occurs frequently in clinical practice and is one of the principal reasons why precise patient positioning is necessary.

EXERCISES

1. Image magnification increases with increasing:
   a. Image size
   b. Object size
   c. OID
   d. SID
   e. SOD

2. Distortion primarily occurs:
   a. Because subject anatomy is inclined
   b. Because subject anatomy is thick rather than thin
   c. When improper kVp was selected
   d. When subject anatomy is flat
   e. When subject anatomy lies parallel to the image receptor

3. Distortion:
   a. Can be corrected by proper patient positioning
   b. Is controlled by focal-spot size
   c. Never accompanies magnification
   d. Occurs only lateral to the central axis of the x-ray beam
   e. Occurs only when the image is inclined

4. To reduce magnification, one should do which of the following?
   a. Reduce OID
   b. Reduce SID
   c. Reduce SSD
   d. Use the small focal spot
   e. Use tighter collimation

5. If the SID is 100 cm and an object is placed 20 cm from the image receptor, what is the magnification factor (MF)?
   a. 0.8
   b. 1.0
   c. 1.25
   d. 1.4
   e. 1.6

6. In a particular radiographic examination, the SID is 100 cm and the SOD is 86 cm. The image size-to-object size ratio is approximately:
   a. 0.86:1
   b. 1.12:1
   c. 1.16:1
   d. 2.14:1
   e. 3:1

7. Distortion of an x-ray image results from unequal:
   a. Exposure of the object
   b. Focal spot
   c. Heel effect
   d. Magnification
   e. SID

8. In magnification radiography, when the object is placed equidistant between the source and the image receptor, the size of the image will be:
   a. 1.33 times object size
   b. 2.0 times object size
   c. Four times object size
   d. One-half the object size
   e. The same size as the object

9. A 20 cm object is radiographed at 40 cm from the focal spot, and the SID is 60 cm. The size of the image will be:
   a. 30 cm
   b. 40 cm
   c. 50 cm
   d. 60 cm
   e. 70 cm

10. When an object is present to one side of the central axis of the x-ray beam:
    a. Distortion will disappear.
    b. Subject contrast will remain unchanged.
    c. The magnification factor will be larger.
    d. The magnification factor will be smaller.
    e. The magnification factor will remain unchanged.

11. To obtain minimum magnification, one should do which of the following?
    a. Make sure the object is positioned on the central axis.
    b. Position the anatomy close to the image receptor.
    c. Select a short SID.
    d. Select a short SSD.
    e. Use maximum collimation.

12. Which of the following conditions contributes *least* to image distortion?
    a. A thick object at a short SID
    b. A thin object at a long SID
    c. Angling of the central ray
    d. Object position
    e. Off-axis imaging

13. To minimize magnification, one should do which of the following?
    a. Position the object as close to the image receptor as is practical.
    b. Position the x-ray tube as close to the patient as is practical.
    c. Use high kVp, low mAs.
    d. Use the large focal spot.
    e. Use the small focal spot.

14. A foreshortened image:
    a. Can be corrected by increasing kVp and reducing mAs
    b. Can be corrected by reducing kVp and increasing mAs
    c. Can be corrected by reducing SID
    d. Can never be smaller than the object
    e. Results from an inclined object

15. Image magnification can be reduced with the use of which of the following?
    a. A cone
    b. Increased filtration
    c. Shorter OID
    d. Shorter SID
    e. Shorter SSD

16. Which of the following is *not* one of the geometric factors that affect radiographic quality?
    a. Collimation
    b. Distortion
    c. Focal-spot size
    d. Magnification
    e. SID

17. The magnification factor is *not* dependent on:
    a. Focal spot size
    b. OID
    d. SOD
    e. SSD
    c. SID

18. The magnification factor increases with increasing:
    a. Focal-spot size
    b. OID
    c. SID
    d. SOD
    e. SSD

The smaller the focal-spot size is, the sharper is the image. Conversely, the larger the focal-spot size is, the greater are the image blur and the loss of image detail. This blur is called **focal-spot blur** (**FSB**) because the focal spot is more of an area than a point.

Focal-spot size is the principal parameter that controls spatial resolution.

The extent of FSB is also affected by the spatial relationships among source, object, and image receptor in a way similar to the relationships that influence magnification and distortion.

Mathematically, the FSB can be calculated as follows:

$$\text{FSB} = \text{Effective focal spot} \times \frac{\text{OID}}{\text{SOD}}$$

Although measurements of FSB usually are made on the central axis, it should be apparent that FSB off of the central axis varies. FSB on the cathode side is larger than that on the anode side. This phenomenon is a consequence of the line-focus principle.

EXERCISES

1. In mammography, which of the following conditions would be *most* effective in improving the sharpness of detail of microcalcifications near the chest wall?
   a. Positioning the anode on the same side as the chest wall
   b. Positioning the cathode on the same side as the chest wall
   c. Using a long OID
   d. Using a short SID
   e. Using a short SSD

2. Which of the following is *most* responsible for radiographic spatial resolution?
   a. Film graininess
   b. Focal-spot size
   c. Screen mottle
   d. SID
   e. Use of a grid

3. The sharpness of detail in a radiograph is *best* increased by the use of which of the following?
   a. High-speed screens
   b. Large focal spot
   c. Long SID
   d. Medium-speed screens
   e. Small focal spot

4. A radiograph that shows a relative lack of FSB would be:
   a. High in contrast
   b. Low in distortion
   c. Low in optical density
   d. Magnified
   e. Sharp in detail

5. An intravenous pyelogram (IVP) is routinely conducted with an anteroposterior projection to:
   a. Improve contrast resolution.
   b. Maximize the effect of the contrast medium.
   c. Minimize the FSB of the kidneys.
   d. Reduce the dose.
   e. Use the lowest kVp possible.

6. Geometric blur is controlled principally by which imaging system characteristic?
   a. Contrast resolution
   b. Focal-spot size
   c. Noise
   d. Sensitivity
   e. Spatial resolution

7. The best way to minimize FSB without affecting optical density is to use a very:
   a. High-contrast image receptor
   b. Long OID
   c. Long SSD
   d. Short SID
   e. Small focal spot

8. Another term for FSB is:
   a. Actual focal spot
   b. Disumbra
   c. Effective focal spot
   d. Penumbra
   e. Umbra

9. A radiograph of the abdomen is taken at 100 cm SID with a 2.0 mm effective focal spot. If the OID is 10 cm, what is the FSB?
   a. 0.1 mm
   b. 0.2 mm
   c. 0.3 mm
   d. 0.1 cm
   e. 0.2 cm

10. When one images an object lateral to the central axis of the x-ray beam, the FSB will be:
    a. Larger on the anode side
    b. Larger on the cathode side
    c. Magnified
    d. Reduced
    e. The same as on the central axis

11. Increasing which of the following is effective in reducing FSB?
    a. Focal-spot size
    b. kVp
    c. Object size
    d. OID
    e. SID

12. When the focal spot is switched from large to small:
    a. FSB will be greater on the anode side.
    b. kVp must be increased for the same optical density.
    c. mAs must be increased for the same optical density.
    d. Motion blur will be enhanced.
    e. Penumbra will be reduced.

13. FSB can be reduced by:
    a. Increasing focal-spot size
    b. Increasing processing time or temperature
    c. Reducing OID
    d. Reducing SID
    e. Reducing SSD

14. Image contrast is the product of image receptor contrast and:
    a. Focal-spot contrast
    b. Grid contrast
    c. Resolution
    d. Screen contrast
    e. Subject contrast

15. Spatial resolution is *principally* affected by which of the following?
    a. Film speed
    b. Focal-spot size
    c. kVp
    d. mAs
    e. Screen speed

16. When proper radiographic detail cannot be obtained because of a large OID, what change in technique may be used to improve the detail?
    a. Increase image receptor speed
    b. Increase SID
    c. Increase time
    d. kVp
    e. Reduce mAs

17. For a radiograph with magnification of 2, which of the following focal-spot sizes will limit the FSB to 0.4 mm or less?
    a. 0.2 mm
    b. 0.3 mm
    c. 0.4 mm
    d. 0.5 mm
    e. 0.6 mm

WORKSHEET
16-4 Subject Factors

Maximizing radiographic contrast and image detail within the limitations of the examination is a principal objective of the radiologic technologist. Radiographic contrast is the product of the film contrast and the subject contrast.

Subject contrast varies with tissue thickness, mass, density, and atomic number. The greater the difference in each of these factors for various tissues, the greater will be the subject contrast. Subject shape also affects subject contrast.

Two factors controlled by the radiologic technologist are kVp and motion. In general, as kVp increases, subject contrast decreases. Blur caused by motion of the patient, tube, or image receptor is called **motion blur** and results in a loss of contrast resolution and spatial resolution.

EXERCISES

1. Which of the following radiographic techniques is likely to produce the *best* visualization of low subject contrast structures?
   a. 72 kVp, 100 mA, 100 ms
   b. 84 kVp, 200 mA, 100 ms
   c. 93 kVp, 400 mA, 50 ms
   d. 100 kVp, 200 mA, 100 ms
   e. 107 kVp, 800 mA, 25 ms

2. Short exposure times are recommended for radiography of the stomach to do which of the following?
   a. Enhance contrast
   b. Improve spatial resolution
   c. Minimize geometric blur
   d. Reduce magnification
   e. Reduce motion blur

3. An upper gastrointestinal image demonstrates motion blur. To increase image detail, the radiologic technologist could do which of the following?
   a. Increase grid ratio
   b. Increase kVp and reduce exposure time
   c. Increase mA and exposure time
   d. Reduce OID
   e. Reduce SID

4. Certain areas in a radiograph appear blurred while others are sharp. The radiologic technologist probably can adjust for this by doing which of the following?
   a. Increasing SID
   b. Reducing mAs and increasing kVp
   c. Reducing OID
   d. Using a different cassette
   e. Using a smaller focal spot

5. Absorption blur can be reduced by which of the following?
   a. Increasing OID
   b. Increasing kVp
   c. Patient compression
   d. Decreasing SID
   e. Use of contrast media

6. Motion blur gets worse with increasing:
   a. Field size
   b. Grid ratio
   c. Image receptor speed
   d. kVp
   e. Patient movement

7. Subject contrast is:
   a. Film contrast minus radiographic contrast
   b. Radiographic contrast divided by film contrast
   c. Radiographic contrast minus film contrast
   d. Radiographic contrast times film contrast
   e. The sum of radiographic contrast and film contrast

8. Which of the following does *not* affect subject contrast?
   a. Grid ratio
   b. kVp
   c. mAs
   d. Object shape
   e. Object size

9. Which of the following factors *most* often affects subject contrast with imaging microcalcifications during mammography?
   a. Atomic number of the microcalcification
   b. Breast mass density
   c. Breast shape
   d. Breast thickness
   e. Mass density of the microcalcification

10. Which of the following anatomic structures should exhibit the *greatest* subject contrast with muscle?
    a. Bladder
    b. Heart
    c. Kidney
    d. Liver
    e. Lung

11. Absorption blur is *most* closely related to which of the following?
    a. Film blur
    b. Focal-spot blur
    c. Geometric blur
    d. Object shape
    e. Screen blur

12. Extremity x-ray examination results in which of the following?
    a. High distortion
    b. High noise
    c. High patient dose
    d. Long-scale contrast
    e. Short-scale contrast

13. Subject contrast is enhanced with the use of contrast media because:
    a. Absorption blur is reduced.
    b. Compton effect is increased.

c. Focal-spot blur is reduced.
d. Mass density is increased.
e. Photoelectric interaction is increased.

14. The principal cause of motion blur is movement of which of the following?
    a. The Bucky mechanism
    b. The image receptor
    c. The patient
    d. The table
    e. The x-ray tube

15. Which of the following will reduce motion blur?
    a. Long exposure time
    b. Short SID
    c. Increased kVp
    d. Increased mAs
    e. Proper patient instructions

16. To improve bony detail in a radiograph, the radiologic technologist could do which of the following?
    a. Decrease kVp and mAs
    b. Decrease kVp and SID
    c. Decrease SID and mAs
    d. Use a faster screen
    e. Use a smaller focal spot

17. Which factor *most* often reduces the visualization of low-contrast structures on a properly exposed radiograph?
    a. Focal-spot size
    b. Grid ratio
    c. Patient motion
    d. Type of film
    e. Type of screens

18. Sharpness of detail on a radiograph is *principally* improved by which of the following?
    a. Increasing kVp
    b. Increasing scatter radiation
    c. Reducing image noise
    d. Reducing patient motion
    e. Reducing radiation dose

19. Radiographic spatial resolution is improved by the use of which of the following?
    a. A grid
    b. A larger focal spot
    c. Reduced kVp
    d. Reduced mAs
    e. Slower radiographic intensifying screens

The radiologic technologist has many decisions to make before performing a patient examination, each of which will influence the quality of the resultant radiographic image. These decisions relate to choice of equipment, patient preparation and positioning, and selection of radiographic factors from the operating console. In general, a change in the selection of one factor will influence the selection of other factors; however, this is not always the case.

EXERCISES

1. Magnification is reduced by which of the following?
   a. Increasing kVp
   b. Increasing screen speed
   c. Increasing SID and OID
   d. Increasing SID and reducing OID
   e. Reducing focal-spot size

2. Focal spot blur can be reduced by which of the following?
   a. Increasing kVp
   b. Increasing mAs
   c. Increasing the OID
   d. Reducing SOD
   e. Using the small focal spot

3. When radiographic technique factors are adjusted to provide an acceptable image and then filtration is added to the x-ray tube, which of the following will increase?
   a. Average energy of the x-ray beam
   b. Optical density
   c. Patient dose
   d. Radiographic contrast
   e. Spatial resolution

4. Ensuring good screen-film contact also ensures reduced:
   a. Blur
   b. Contrast resolution
   c. Magnification
   d. Patient dose
   e. Radiographic noise

5. Use of contrast media principally affects which of the following?
   a. Blur
   b. Contrast resolution
   c. Mass density
   d. Optical density
   e. Speed

6. Reducing field size through proper collimation usually results in improved:
   a. Blur
   b. Contrast resolution
   c. Magnification
   d. Patient dose
   e. Spatial resolution

7. Which of the following is *most* often influenced by focal-spot size?
   a. Absorption blur
   b. Contrast resolution
   c. Geometric blur
   d. Motion blur
   e. Patient dose

8. In a radiographic examination of the lumbar spine, which of the following techniques would result in greatest exposure to the patient?
   a. 70 kVp/200 mAs
   b. 80 kVp/100 mAs
   c. 95 kVp/50 mAs
   d. 110 kVp/25 mAs
   e. 120 kVp/25 mAs

9. Which of the following does *not* affect image blur?
   a. Focal-spot size
   b. kVp
   c. OID
   d. SID
   e. SOD

10. Which of the following is the *principal* reason for using direct-exposure radiography?
    a. Better resolution of low-contrast tissues
    b. Better spatial resolution
    c. Higher contrast
    d. Less motion blur
    e. Lower patient dose

11. If other factors remain constant, which of the following would result in the *highest* optical density?
    a. 100 mA, 750 ms, 90 cm SID
    b. 200 mA, 500 ms, 90 cm SID
    c. 300 mA, 300 ms, 100 cm SID
    d. 400 mA, 200 ms, 100 cm SID
    e. 500 mA, 100 ms, 100 cm SID

12. An anteroposterior examination of the abdomen is taken at 80 kVp, 50 mAs, and 100 cm SID. If the scale of contrast is to be shortened, the radiologic technologist must do which of the following?
    a. Increase both mAs and kVp
    b. Reduce both mAs and kVp
    c. Reduce kVp and increase mAs
    d. Reduce mAs and increase kVp
    e. Shorten the SID

13. Assume that the usual exposure time for a lateral cervical spine radiograph at 100 cm SID is 100 ms. At an SID of 90 cm, all other factors remaining the same, the *correct* exposure time would be:
    a. 10 ms
    b. 25 ms
    c. 50 ms
    d. 80 ms
    e. 180 ms

14. When radiographic technique factors are adjusted to obtain an acceptable image, patient dose will increase as which of the following increases?
    a. Film speed
    b. Grid ratio
    c. SID
    d. SOD
    e. SSD

15. Geometric blur can be reduced by which of the following?
    a. Improving film-screen contact
    b. Increasing processing time or temperature
    c. Increasing SID and OID
    d. Increasing SSD and OID
    e. Reducing focal-spot size

16. When technique factors are adjusted to obtain an acceptable image, motion blur will increase with which of the following?
    a. Increase in focal-spot size
    b. Increased field size
    c. Low-ratio grid (compared with high-ratio grid)
    d. Reduced total filtration
    e. Slow radiographic intensifying screens (compared with fast screens)

17. With other factors constant, optical density will increase with increasing:
    a. Focal-spot size
    b. Grid ratio
    c. mAs
    d. SID
    e. SSD

18. Radiographic contrast is increased by which of the following?
    a. Increasing grid ratio
    b. Raising kVp
    c. Reducing the air gap
    d. Reducing the heel effect
    e. Using a slower film

19. When the mAs is adjusted to provide constant optical density after an increase in kVp:
    a. Absorption blur is reduced.
    b. Geometric blur is reduced.
    c. Latitude is reduced.
    d. Motion blur is reduced if the same mA is used.
    e. Spatial resolution will improve.

16-6 Patient Factors

The radiologic technologist has control over the following: exposure technique factors, patient factors, and image quality factors.

Radiographic technique is the selection of the proper x-ray exposure factors with the x-ray imaging system necessary to produce a high-quality radiograph.

The two principal patient factors are the thickness of the body part that is being examined and its composition. In general, the thicker and more dense the part is, the higher the voltage and milliampere-seconds settings should be.

EXERCISES

1. The chest represents high-contrast anatomy (high subject contrast). Therefore, which of the following is *most* appropriate?
   a. High kVp
   b. High mAs
   c. Long SID
   d. Low kVp
   e. Low mAs

2. The anatomic part to be examined must be measured because:
   a. A change of focal spots may be required.
   b. A different image receptor may be required.
   c. The mass density of the part is determined by thickness.
   d. The selected radiographic technique depends on anatomy thickness.
   e. The SSD changes with anatomy thickness.

3. When fixed kVp technique is used for various anatomic thicknesses, a change will be required in which of the following?
   a. Added filtration
   b. kVp
   c. mAs
   d. SID
   e. SSD

4. The anatomic part must be measured for variable kVp technique because a change will be required in which of the following?
   a. Added filtration
   b. kVp
   c. mAs
   d. SID
   e. SSD

5. In the diagnostic x-ray range, the smallest change in kVp that can be perceived on the radiographic image is approximately:
   a. 2 kVp
   b. 4 kVp
   c. 6 kVp
   d. 8 kVp
   e. 12 kVp

6. In general, a chest radiograph should be taken with:
   a. A generalization about this is not possible; decisions are thickness dependent.
   b. High kVp and high mAs
   c. High kVp and low mAs
   d. Low kVp and high mAs
   e. Low kVp and low mAs

7. What is the approximate mass density of lung tissue?
   a. .32 g/cm^3
   b. 0.85 g/cm^3
   c. 1.0 g/cm^3
   d. 1.85 g/cm^3
   e. 4.0 g/cm^3

8. In general, a mammogram should be taken with:
   a. A generalization about this is not possible; decisions are thickness dependent.
   b. High kVp and high mAs
   c. High kVp and low mAs
   d. Low kVp and high mAs
   e. Low kVp and low mAs

9. What is the effective atomic number of fat?
   a. 6.3
   b. 7.4
   c. 7.6
   d. 10.5
   e. 13.8

10. What is the approximate mass density of bone?
    a. 0.001 g/cm^3
    b. 0.85 g/cm^3
    c. 1.0 g/cm^3
    d. 1.85 g/cm^3
    e. 4.0 g/cm^3

11. What is the effective atomic number of lung tissue?
    a. 6.3
    b. 7.4
    c. 7.6
    d. 10.5
    e. 13.8

12. What is the effective atomic number of soft tissue?
    a. 6.3
    b. 7.4
    c. 7.6
    d. 10.5
    e. 13.8

13. What is the approximate mass density of fat?
    a. 0.001 g/cm^3
    b. 0.91 g/cm^3
    c. 1.0 g/cm^3
    d. 1.85 g/cm^3
    e. 4.0 g/cm^3

14. What is the effective atomic number of bone?
    a. 6.3
    b. 7.4
    c. 7.6
    d. 10.5
    e. 13.8

15. For a given anatomic part, the smallest change in mAs that can be perceived on the radiographic image is approximately:
    a. 5%
    b. 15%
    c. 30%
    d. 50%
    e. 70%

16. What is the mass density of soft tissue?
    a. 0.001 g/cm^3
    b. 0.85 g/cm^3
    c. 1.0 g/cm^3
    d. 1.85 g/cm^3
    e. 4.0 g/cm^3

17. Which of the following tissue characteristics is most important when photoelectric interaction prevails, as in mammography?
    a. Effective atomic number
    b. Electron density
    c. Mass density
    d. Optical density
    e. Tissue shape

18. Which of the following tissue characteristics is most important when Compton interaction prevails, as in computed tomography?
    a. Effective atomic number
    b. Electron density
    c. Mass density
    d. Optical density
    e. Tissue shape

Radiographic technique factors set by the radiologic technologist consist of current, exposure time (ms), voltage, and SID (cm). These factors influence the radiographic exposure to the patient. The selected combination of these factors determines the quality of the radiograph. *Image quality factors* refer to terms used to evaluate the characteristics of a radiographic image.

The principal terms are *optical density, contrast, definition,* and *distortion.*

The radiologic technologist selects a combination of exposure technique factors to produce a radiograph with an acceptable scale of contrast, the correct optical density and spatial and contrast resolution, and a minimum of distortion of the image.

EXERCISES

1. If a radiographic technique calling for 100 mA at 100 ms is changed to 50 mA at 2000 ms:
   a. Grayscale contrast will become longer.
   b. Grayscale contrast will become shorter.
   c. There will be no change in grayscale contrast.
   d. There will be no change in exposed time.
   e. There will be no change in x-ray tube capacity.

2. A longer grayscale on a radiograph can be obtained by doing which of the following?
   a. Increasing kVp
   b. Increasing mAs
   c. Reducing kVp
   d. Reducing mAs
   e. Using a larger focal spot

3. For a mobile abdominal radiographic examination, radiographic contrast can be increased by doing which of the following?
   a. Increasing the kVp and decreasing the mAs
   b. Increasing the OID
   c. Increasing the SID
   d. Using a faster image receptor
   e. Using a high-ratio grid

4. A radiograph that exhibits a long grayscale contrast is one with which of the following?
   a. Few shades of gray that have great differences
   b. Few shades of gray that have minimal differences
   c. Good spatial resolution
   d. Many shades of gray that have great differences
   e. Many shades of gray that have minimal differences

5. From the following set of exposure technique factors, select the set that is *most* likely to produce a radiograph with the best spatial resolution:
   a. A
   b. B
   c. C
   d. D
   e. E

	mAs	kVp	OID	SID	FOCAL SPOT	IMAGE RECEPTOR
A	10	60	8 cm	90 cm	2.0 mm	High speed
B	20	68	10 cm	90 cm	2.0 mm	High speed
C	25	72	5 cm	180 cm	1.0 mm	Medium speed
D	30	86	5 cm	90 cm	1.0 mm	Medium speed
E	50	94	4 cm	100 cm	100 cm	Medium speed

6. Which of the preceding exposure technique factors would result in the worst spatial resolution?
   a. A
   b. B
   c. C
   d. D
   e. E

7. If a radiographic technique designed for an 8:1 grid is changed to accommodate a 10:1 grid:
   a. Grayscale contrast will become longer.
   b. Grayscale contrast will become shorter.
   c. There will be no change in contrast resolution.
   d. There will be no change in grayscale contrast.
   e. There will be no change in x-ray tube capacity.

8. Which of the following is the function of optimizing contrast?
   a. To control detail sharpness
   b. To control quantum mottle
   c. To determine optical density
   d. To improve spatial resolution
   e. To make detail visible

9. A radiographic technique that would ensure visibility of detail for a cervical spine is:
   a. Increasing the OID
   b. Reducing the SID
   c. Reducing the SSD
   d. Selecting the large focal spot
   e. Using a beam restriction device

10. A radiograph was made using these factors: 200 mA, 300 ms, 70 kVp, 100 cm SID. A mobile radiograph is then conducted at 80 cm. To maintain the same optical density, approximately what mAs should be selected?
    a. 15 mAs
    b. 20 mAs
    c. 28 mAs
    d. 38 mAs
    e. 48 mAs

Exercises 11 through 14 refer to the following exposure technique factors:
    A. 100 mA, 500 ms, 60 kVp, no grid
    B. 200 mA, 750 ms, 50 kVp, 16:1 grid
    C. 400 mA, 100 ms, 60 kVp, no grid
    D. 600 mA, 700 ms, 70 kVp, 8:1 grid
    E. 800 mA, 200 ms, 80 kVp, 8:1 grid

11. Which technique factors should result in greatest latitude?
    a. A
    b. B
    c. C
    d. D
    e. E

12. Which technique factors should result in highest contrast?
    a. A
    b. B
    c. C
    d. D
    e. E

13. Which technique factors should result in highest optical density?
    a. A
    b. B
    c. C
    d. D
    e. E

14. Which technique factors should result in highest patient dose?
    a. A
    b. B
    c. C
    d. D
    e. E

15. When an examination is changed from an 8:1 grid technique to a nongrid technique, and compensating changes are made in other technique factors:
    a. Contrast resolution will improve.
    b. Optical density will decrease.
    c. Optical density will increase.
    d. Patient dose will increase.
    e. There will be no change in optical density.

16. If a technique of 100 mA, 1000 ms is changed to 200 mA, 500 ms:
    a. Optical density will be reduced.
    b. Optical density will increase.
    c. Patient dose will increase.
    d. There will be no change in contrast resolution.
    e. There will be no change in optical density.

16-8

Radiographic Technique Charts

Radiographic technique charts are guides that are prepared for specific x-ray imaging systems for the purpose of assisting radiologic technologists in selecting exposure factors for each radiographic procedure.

There are four types of radiographic technique charts: variable kilovoltage, fixed kilovoltage, high kilovoltage, and automatic exposure.

For the variable-kilovoltage chart, voltage is adjusted for different tissue thickness. The fixed-kilovoltage chart uses an optimum voltage selection for each body part, and the milliampere-seconds setting is the variable used to accommodate for differences in tissue thickness.

High kilovoltage means that the voltage selection is in excess of 100 kVp. Radiographic technique charts of this type are used primarily for barium studies and chest radiography. The automatic exposure chart serves as a guide for control panel selections when automatic exposure control systems are used.

EXERCISES

1. Which of the following technique charts provides the *least* amount of patient radiation exposure?
   a. Anatomically programmed radiography (APR)
   b. Automatic exposure
   c. Fixed kilovoltage
   d. High kilovoltage
   e. Variable kilovoltage

2. Accuracy in positioning the patient is *most* critical with which of the following?
   a. APR
   b. Automatic exposure
   c. Fixed-kilovoltage technique chart
   d. High-kilovoltage technique chart
   e. Variable-kilovoltage technique chart

3. Before a radiographic technique chart is prepared, which of the following would be *most* important?
   a. Calculating the mAs distance rule
   b. Calibrating the x-ray imaging system
   c. Marking all kVp stations on the control panel
   d. Marking each image receptor
   e. Measuring the part size with calipers

4. Which of the following is a basic characteristic of the variable-kilovoltage chart?
   a. Large focal spot
   b. Long scale of contrast
   c. Low mAs selection
   d. Short exposure time
   e. Short scale of contrast

5. Which of the following is the procedure for selection of the kVp for a body part when the variable-kilovoltage chart is used?
   a. Measure the part, multiply by 2, and then add 30.
   b. Measure the part, multiply by 5, and then add 30.

c. Preselect the kVp, and multiply the mAs by 2.

d. Preselect the kVp, multiply by 2, and then add 20.

e. Preselect the kVp, multiply by 2, and then add 30.

6. Which of the following will increase exposure latitude?
   a. Automatic exposure
   b. Faster image receptor
   c. Fixed-kilovoltage chart
   d. High-kilovoltage chart
   e. Variable-kilovoltage chart

7. The optical density present on the radiograph can best be controlled by which of the following?
   a. Collimation
   b. Focal-spot size
   c. kVp
   d. mAs
   e. Measurement of the part

8. Penetration of the anatomic part by the x-ray beam can best be controlled by which of the following?
   a. Calibration of the equipment
   b. kVp
   c. mAs
   d. Measurement of the part
   e. Tissue thickness

9. Which of the following procedures would make best use of a high-kilovoltage chart?
   a. Barium enema
   b. Chest
   c. Knee
   d. Mammography
   e. Pelvis

10. Which of the following technique charts requires accurate measurement?
    a. Automatic exposure control
    b. Combination fixed and variable
    c. Fixed kilovoltage
    d. High kilovoltage
    e. Variable kilovoltage

11. Which of the following technique charts requires higher patient radiation dose?
    a. Automatic exposure control
    b. Combination fixed and variable kilovoltage
    c. Fixed kilovoltage

d. High kilovoltage
e. Variable kilovoltage

12. Which of the following technique charts has the shortest scale of contrast?
    a. Automatic exposure control
    b. Combination fixed and variable kilovoltage
    c. Fixed kilovoltage
    d. High kilovoltage
    e. Variable kilovoltage

13. Which of the following technique charts has the *least* exposure latitude?
    a. Automatic exposure control
    b. Combination fixed and variable kilovoltage
    c. Fixed kilovoltage
    d. High kilovoltage
    e. Variable kilovoltage

14. Which of the following technique charts requires accurate patient positioning?
    a. Automatic exposure control
    b. Combination fixed and variable kilovoltage
    c. Fixed kilovoltage
    d. High kilovoltage
    e. Variable kilovoltage

15. Which of the following technique charts recommends a 2 kVp change for each centimeter of thickness?
    a. Automatic exposure control
    b. Combination fixed and variable kilovoltage
    c. Fixed kilovoltage
    d. High kilovoltage
    e. Variable kilovoltage

16. Which of the following technique charts requires no specific mAs selection?
    a. Automatic exposure control
    b. Combination fixed and variable kilovoltage
    c. Fixed kilovoltage
    d. High kilovoltage
    e. Variable kilovoltage

17. Which of the following technique charts results in higher contrast?
    a. Automatic exposure control
    b. Combination fixed and variable kilovoltage
    c. Fixed kilovoltage
    d. High kilovoltage
    e. Variable kilovoltage

WORKSHEET

17-1

Image Artifacts

Perhaps the most important quality control program is that associated with the automatic processor. Daily attention to the automatic processor is essential, and this attention should be properly recorded.

An artifact is any irregular optical density on a radiograph that is not caused by the proper shadowing of the object by the primary x-ray beam. Processing, exposure, and handling and storage are the three types of artifacts a radiologic technologist is likely to encounter.

EXERCISES

1. Patient motion during exposure will result in which of the following?
   a. A handling artifact
   b. A processing artifact
   c. A storage artifact
   d. An exposure artifact
   e. An imaging system artifact

2. A guide shoe is a component of which of the following?
   a. A cassette
   b. A darkroom countertop
   c. A film bin
   d. An automatic processor
   e. An image receptor

3. A chemical fog artifact:
   a. Appears as streaks
   b. Is an exposure artifact
   c. Is removed by extended washing
   d. Results in lower image contrast
   e. Results in lower optical density

4. The yellow appearance of a radiograph after a long time:
   a. Indicates that the developer was overreplenished
   b. Indicates that the developer was underreplenished
   c. Is a processing artifact
   d. Is a storage artifact
   e. Results from extended processing

5. Which of the following tasks should be performed daily?
   a. Analyze fixer retention
   b. Assess darkroom fog
   c. Clean screens
   d. Monitor automatic processor
   e. Obtain phantom images

6. Corrective action should be triggered whenever automatic processor monitoring shows a change in mid-density of:
   a. ±0.1
   b. ±0.2
   c. ±0.3
   d. ±0.5
   e. ±1.0

7. The repeat rate:
   a. Is the number of repeated images
   b. Should be determined monthly
   c. Should be determined annually
   d. Should not exceed 2%
   e. Should not exceed 4%

8. Which of the following is a part of processor quality control?
   a. Analyze fixer replenishment rate
   b. Assess image reproducibility
   c. Assess x-ray reproducibility
   d. Clean screens
   e. Determine x-ray beam quality

9. For most hospitals and busy imaging centers, the recommended frequency of automatic processor cleaning is:
   a. Daily
   b. Weekly
   c. Monthly
   d. Semiannually
   e. Annually

10. The operation of the automatic processor should be observed and the developer temperature recorded at least once each:
    a. Day
    b. Week
    c. Month
    d. Quarter
    e. Year

11. Wet pressure sensitization would be classified as which of the following?
    a. A handling artifact
    b. A processing artifact
    c. A storage artifact
    d. An exposure artifact
    e. An imaging system artifact

12. Pi lines are so called because they:
    a. Are visible on the latent image
    b. Look like a section of pie
    c. Look like a whole sliced pie
    d. Occur at regular intervals
    e. Occur on the finished radiograph

13. Static artifacts appear *most often* during what conditions of temperature and humidity, respectively?
    a. High, high
    b. High, low
    c. This varies
    d. Low, high
    e. Low, low

14. If residual thiosulfate is *not* properly removed during washing, the radiograph will:
    a. Be overdeveloped
    b. Be underdeveloped
    c. Have to be repeated
    d. Turn blue
    e. Turn yellow

15. Which of the following is a source of fog?
    a. Excess fixing
    b. Excess hypo retention
    c. Improper safelight
    d. Improper screen cleaning
    e. Poor screen-film contact

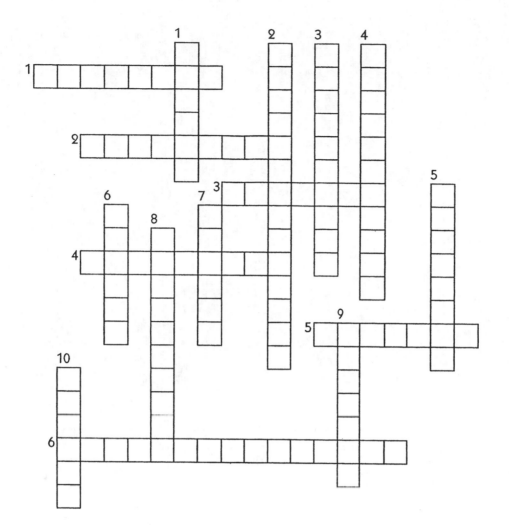

ACROSS

1. _____ fog looks like light or radiation fog and is usually a uniform, dull gray.
2. Warped cassettes cause _____ artifacts.
3. Dirt or chemical stain on a roller can cause

   _____ _____.
4. _____ fog and light fog look alike.
5. Chemistry not properly squeezed from the film creates a _____ effect.
6. When radiographers mix up cassettes, _____ _____ can occur.

DOWN

1. Dirty or _____ rollers can cause emulsion pickoff.
2. An artifact is any _____ on a radiograph that is not caused by superimposition of anatomy in the primary x-ray beam.
3. Cassettes that have not been checked for proper screen-film contact cause a _____ in the area of poor contact on the radiographic image.

4. _____-_____ sensitization is caused when irregular rollers cause pressure during development and produce small circular patterns.
5. Inadequate processing chemistry can result in a chemical fog called a _____ stain.
6. Crown, tree, and smudge are three distinct patterns of _____.
7. If a patient is placed under the tube when the tube is not centered to the table or Bucky tray, _____-_____ artifacts will occur.
8. Kinking or abrupt bending before processing can cause scratches that look like _____ marks.
9. A radiograph with patient motion appears blurred or _____.
10. Gelatin buildup can result in _____ deposits on the film.

X-ray imaging systems are increasingly more sophisticated and complicated. Although the operation of such imaging systems often is made easier by continuing developments in design, the assurance that the equipment is functioning properly becomes more difficult to monitor. Such monitoring is called a **quality control program.**

A quality control program designed for an x-ray imaging system involves a number of observations and measurements of the various parts and subsystems of the system.

EXERCISES

1. Compared with a quality control program, a quality assurance program:
   a. Deals with equipment
   b. Deals with people
   c. Is normally performed weekly
   d. Is normally performed monthly
   e. Is normally performed annually

2. Which of the following is an essential element of a quality control program?
   a. Equipment performance evaluation
   b. Error correction
   c. Image interpretation
   d. Personnel performance evaluation
   e. Repair procedures

3. Radiographic kVp should be evaluated:
   a. Weekly
   b. Monthly
   c. Semiannually
   d. Annually
   e. Not required

4. The variable-aperture, light-localizing collimator must confine the x-ray beam to:
   a. ±2% of the SID
   b. ±5% of the SID
   c. Inside the light field
   d. Outside the light field
   e. Within the light field

5. The actual radiographic kVp should be within what value of the indicated kVp?
   a. ±1 kVp
   b. ±2 kVp
   c. ±4 kVp
   d. ±6 kVp
   e. ±10 kVp

6. Which of the following devices may be used to assess the accuracy of the exposure timer?
   a. Densitometer
   b. Penetrameter
   c. Ramp filter
   d. Sensitometer
   e. Solid-state detector

7. If the automatic exposure timer fails, a backup timer should terminate the exposure at:
   a. 3 s or 300 mAs
   b. 6 s or 600 mAs
   c. 9 s or 900 mAs
   d. 12 s or 1200 mAs
   e. 15 s or 1500 mAs

8. Output radiation intensity should be reproducible to within:
   a. 1%
   b. 3%

c. 5%
d. 10%
e. 20%

9. During normal fluoroscopy, the radiation intensity at the tabletop will result in dose rates of approximately:
   a. 0 to 2 mrad/min
   b. 2 to 10 mrad/min
   c. 0 to 2 rad/min
   d. 2 to 6 rad/min
   e. 6 to 15 rad/min

10. When cassette spot films are used instead of photofluorospot films:
    a. A grid must be used.
    b. Compression must be applied.
    c. Patient dose is higher.
    d. Patient dose is lower.
    e. X-ray beam collimation is required.

11. All fluoroscopic automatic exposure systems should be evaluated:
    a. Weekly
    b. Monthly
    c. Semiannually
    d. Annually
    e. Not required

12. Conventional tomography images should lie within what distance of the indicated tomographic plane?
    a. ±1 mm
    b. ±5 mm
    c. ±10 mm
    d. ±15 mm
    e. A range of values (depending on tube motion)

13. Mammography kVp must be accurate to within:
    a. ±1 kVp
    b. ±3 kVp
    c. ±5 kVp
    d. ±10 kVp
    e. It depends on the imaging system.

14. The patient couch of a CT imaging system must move automatically with an accuracy of:
    a. 1 mm
    b. 2 mm
    c. 3 mm
    d. 5 mm
    e. 10 mm

15. Which of the following organizations accredits hospitals?
    a. ACMP
    b. ACPM
    c. ACR
    d. CRCPD
    e. The Joint Commission

16. The minimum filtration required for general purpose radiography and fluoroscopy is:
    a. 2.0 mm Al
    b. 2.1 mm Al
    c. 2.3 mm Al
    d. 2.5 mm Al
    e. 3.0 mm Al

17. Which of the following can be used to measure effective focal-spot size?
    a. Densitometer
    b. Ion chamber
    c. Sensitometer
    d. Slit camera
    e. Solid-state detector

18. The ability of an x-ray imaging system to produce constant radiation output at various combinations of mA and exposure time, resulting in the same mAs, is called:
    a. Accuracy
    b. Linearity
    c. Precision
    d. Reproducibility
    e. Uniformity

19. A photometer is an instrument that is used to measure
    a. Artifacts
    b. Contrast resolution
    c. Illumination
    d. Optical density
    e. Spatial resolution

ACROSS

1. _____ is particularly helpful in locating foreign bodies.
2. Tomography achieves radiographic contrast by _____ structures above and below the object plane.
3. Tomography may be ordered for diagnosis when conventional radiography cannot be used because of _____.
4. The larger a tomographic angle is, the _____ the imaged section will be.

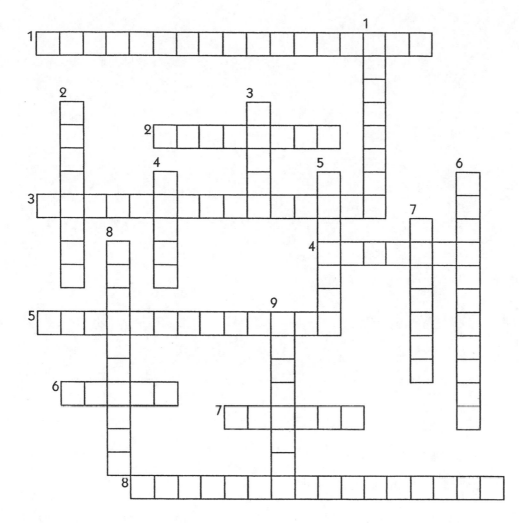

5. One of the two multidirectional movements that produce the sharpest tomographic images is the _____ movement.
6. In magnification radiography, _____ is preferred.
7. In _____ tomography, the grid lines should be parallel to the length of the table.
8. Despite the fact that CT and MRI have replaced most plain-film tomographic examinations, _____ still is frequently performed, even in modern departments.

DOWN
1. The most important requirement for viewing stereoradiographs is to be sure that radiographs are viewed in the same _____ in which the images were taken.
2. Magnification radiography is used principally by _____ radiologists.

3. _____ are not needed in magnified radiography.
4. In multidirectional tomography, the image receptor should remain _____.
5. When CT and MRI images can be viewed from any direction, this phenomenon can be called _____.
6. Many radiologists are proficient at crossing their eyes to perform _____.
7. During exposure in linear tomography, changes in the distance from x-ray tube to patient and in the angulation of the x-ray beam can result in a lack of _____ optical density.
8. The section of tissue between two select parallel planes is the only area that is in focus with _____.
9. In making stereoradiographs, make sure the tube shift is across any _____ linear structures.

19-1

Basis for Mammography
X-Ray Imaging System
Magnification Mammography

Mammography is an examination of the breast with the use of low-energy x-rays. General purpose x-ray imaging systems cannot be used successfully for mammography; a dedicated mammography x-ray imaging system is required.

Breast compression reduces motion blur, absorption blur, and patient dose and improves spatial and contrast resolution.

The mammographic imaging system must be able to accurately produce x-rays in the range of 23 to 30 kVp. The system should have a molybdenum/rhodium-targeted x-ray tube. Such a tube emits radiation with K-characteristic x-rays at 19 and 23 keV, respectively. Because of the low filtration of mammography, the radiation exposure of the patient can be considerably higher than in general radiography.

EXERCISES

1. Low kVp is required for mammography because of which of the following?
   a. High mAs
   b. Patient positioning and compression
   c. Composition of breast tissue
   d. Type of image receptor used
   e. Varying thickness of breast tissue

2. When molybdenum is used for the x-ray tube target:
   a. kVp can be higher.
   b. mAs can be lower.
   c. No added filtration is required.
   d. No bremsstrahlung x-rays are produced.
   e. Useful characteristic x-rays are used.

3. If the cathode of the x-ray tube is positioned toward the chest wall during a cranial-caudad view:
   a. Absorption blur will be reduced.
   b. Exposure time will be reduced.
   c. Geometric blur will be greater toward the chest wall.
   d. The central ray will miss the breast.
   e. Optical density on the nipple side will be greater.

4. In mammography, low kVp is selected to do which of the following?
   a. Improve spatial resolution.
   b. Increase Compton absorption.
   c. Increase photoelectric absorption.
   d. Reduce patient dose.
   e. Reduce skin reaction.

5. When a mammogram taken at 23 kVp is compared with one taken at 28 kVp:
   a. For the same exit dose, the 28 kVp examination will require a higher entrance dose.
   b. If the mAs is constant, exposure time will be less, at 23 kVp.
   c. If the mAs is constant, the number of x-rays reaching the image receptor will be the same.
   d. Radiographic contrast will be enhanced, at 28 kVp.
   e. The ratio of entrance dose to exit dose will be higher, at 23 kVp.

6. The principal reason why molybdenum-targeted x-ray tubes are used in mammography is that molybdenum produces which of the following?
   a. A high atomic number
   b. A high melting point
   c. A higher heat capacity
   d. Useful bremsstrahlung x-rays
   e. Useful characteristic x-rays

7. Successful mammography cannot be done at 90 kVp because:
   a. Compton interactions are too few.
   b. Differential absorption is too low.
   c. Exposure time is too long.
   d. Patient dose is too high.
   e. X-ray tube heat is too great.

8. During mammography:
   a. More filtration is required.
   b. Radiographic contrast is low.
   c. The half-value layer is relatively low.
   d. Radiation quality is relatively high.
   e. X-ray transmission predominates.

9. Regarding the incidence of breast cancer in women, which of the following is *true*?
   a. Each year, about 10,000 new cases appear in the United States.
   b. It is on the decline.
   c. More than 80% of breast cancer results in death.
   d. The most critical decade is that of 30 to 40 years.
   e. The odds of developing breast cancer are 1 in 8.

10. In screen-film mammography, which of the following is *most* often responsible for image contrast?
    a. mAs
    b. kVp
    c. Tissue atomic number
    d. Tissue mass
    e. Tissue mass number

11. X-ray tube potential below 20 kVp is *not* used because:
    a. Characteristic x-rays are not produced.
    b. Compton interaction predominates.
    c. Generators are not available for such low voltage.
    d. There are no x-rays below 20 keV.
    e. X-ray penetration is not sufficient.

12. X-ray imaging systems specially designed for mammography:
    a. Create high anode heat
    b. Have devices to reduce motion and absorption blur
    c. Have SIDs that are greater than 100 cm
    d. Have x-ray tube target angles that are less than 10 degrees
    e. Use extra large focal-spot x-ray tubes

13. If an x-ray tube is positioned so that the anode is toward the chest wall during a cranial-caudad view:
    a. Image-forming x-rays will have more uniform intensity at the image receptor.
    b. Patient dose will be lower.
    c. Spatial resolution will be higher toward the nipple.
    d. Exposure time will be about one half.
    e. Radiation exposure will be greater at the nipple than at the chest wall.

14. The principal reason why mammography is widely used is that:
    a. It is easy.
    b. It is inexpensive.
    c. It is reimbursable.
    d. The incidence of breast cancer is high.
    e. The radiation dose is low.

15. Which of the following target/filter combinations is *most* appropriate for screening mammography?
    a. Mo/Al
    b. Mo/Mo
    c. Rh/Mo
    d. W/Al
    e. W/Mo

16. Compression during mammography is necessary to do which of the following?
    a. Comfort the patient
    b. Increase OID
    c. Increase SID
    d. Reduce geometric blur
    e. Use the small focal spot

17. Mammography grids are designed to do which of the following?
    a. Improve optical density
    b. Improve resolution contrast
    c. Improve spatial resolution
    d. Reduce geometric blur
    e. Reduce patient dose

The mammography image receptor of choice is the single-emulsion film/detail screen. The recently introduced solid-state digital detector shows great promise.

EXERCISES

1. During mammography, it is important:
   a. To use 2.5 mm Al filtration
   b. To select a kVp greater than 30
   c. To use at least 0.5 mm Al equivalent filtration
   d. To use grids
   e. To keep the SID as short as is practicable

2. An advantage to the use of a molybdenum-targeted x-ray tube for mammography is that:
   a. Bremsstrahlung radiation predominates over characteristic radiation.
   b. The tube can handle more heat.
   c. The tube is recommended for all types of image receptors.
   d. The tube's emission spectrum is better for differential absorption in breast tissue.
   e. The radiation dose is less than one-half that of a tungsten-targeted tube.

3. When film is loaded for mammography:
   a. The base should be in contact with the screen.
   b. The emulsion should be in contact with the cover.
   c. The film should be on the x-ray tube side of the radiographic intensifying screen.
   d. The radiographic intensifying screen should be on the x-ray tube side of the film.

e. The spatial resolution is the same as for routine radiography.

4. Which of the following techniques is *most* appropriate for screen-film mammography?
   a. Molybdenum target, 60 cm SID, 25 kVp
   b. Molybdenum target, 100 cm SID, 25 kVp
   c. Molybdenum target, long SID, 50 kVp
   d. Tungsten target, long SID, 20 kVp
   e. Tungsten target, long SID, 50 kVp

5. Poor mammographic screen-film contact results in which of the following?
   a. Higher patient dose
   b. Large region blurring
   c. Lower patient dose
   d. Patient discomfort
   e. Small region blurring

6. MQSA requires what spatial resolution expressed as a minimum spatial frequency?
   a. 5 lp/mm
   b. 6 to 10 lp/mm
   c. 11 to 15 lp/mm
   d. 16 to 20 lp/mm
   e. 21 to 25 lp/mm

7. Why is SID reduced in mammography compared with conventional radiography?
   a. To decrease exposure time
   b. To decrease geometric unsharpness
   c. To improve differential absorption
   d. To improve spatial resolution
   e. To reduce patient dose

8. What is the ideal technique for 4.5 cm compressed breast, 50-50 glandular/fat tissue?
    a. 22 kVp/60 mAs
    b. 22 kVp/150 mAs
    c. 26 kVp/60 mAs
    d. 26 kVp/150 mAs
    e. 28 kVp/150 mAs

9. Which of the following is *true* about the mammographic screen-film image receptor?
    a. A single screen is between the source and the film.
    b. Fixed grids are used.
    c. The receptor is nonscreen.
    d. The speed is approximately 200.
    e. Two screens with double-emulsion film are used.

10. Aggressive breast compression improves all *except:*
    a. Examination speed
    b. Exposure time
    c. Image contrast
    d. Patient dose
    e. Quantum mottle

11. When a change is made from film "A" to film "B," film "B" has twice the speed, and the same radiographic intensifying screen is used:
    a. Exposure time is half.
    b. Geometric blur is accentuated.
    c. Image noise is increased.
    d. Motion blur is reduced.
    e. Patient dose is increased.

12. When the radiographic intensifying screen is changed from screen "X" to screen "Y," which has twice the x-ray-to-light conversion efficiency, and the same film is used:
    a. Exposure time is doubled.
    b. Geometric blur is accentuated.
    c. Image noise is increased.
    d. Motion blur is reduced.
    e. Patient dose is increased.

Quality Control Team
Quality Control Program

The purposes of a mammography quality control (QC) program are to produce the best possible diagnostic image through good equipment performance and to ensure that the patient receives the best available care with the least radiation exposure. QC falls under the larger umbrella of quality assurance (QA), which is an administrative program that ensures that all tasks of the QC team are carried out at the highest level. Continuous quality improvement is an extension of any QC/QA program and includes administrative protocols for the continuous improvement of mammographic quality.

The mammography QC team includes a radiologist, a medical physicist, and a mammographer. Radiologists oversee the QA program and track diagnostic results. Medical physicists examine and monitor the performance of imaging equipment, and they chart and record data to ensure compliance with the latest recommendations and standards. Mammographers perform many tests and evaluations that involve equipment, processing, and mammographic images.

EXERCISES

1. Which of the following describes the difference between QC and QA?
   a. QC deals with the performance of imaging apparatus.
   b. QC defines the quality of the QA team.
   c. QC is focused on patient scheduling, examination, and reporting.
   d. QA is concerned principally with image processing.
   e. QA is the responsibility of the mammographer.

2. Which mammography staff member is principally responsible for the QC/QA program?
   a. Administrator
   b. Mammographer
   c. Medical physicist
   d. QC technologist
   e. Radiologist

3. CQI stands for which of the following?
   a. Cautious quality improvement
   b. Competent quality imaging
   c. Continuous quality improvement
   d. Controlled quality insistence
   e. None of the above

4. The assessment of glandular dose in mammography is principally the responsibility of which of the following staff members?
   a. Administrator
   b. Mammographer
   c. Medical physicist
   d. QC technologist
   e. Radiologist

5. The responsibilities of the medical physicist must be carried out at *least:*
   a. Daily
   b. Weekly
   c. Monthly

d. Quarterly
e. Annually

6. Which member of the mammography QC/QA team is principally responsible for daily QC/QA?
   a. Administrator
   b. Mammographer
   c. Medical physicist
   d. QC mammographer
   e. Radiologist

7. The duties of the QC mammographer include tasks that should be performed:
   a. Daily
   b. Daily and weekly
   c. Daily, weekly, and quarterly
   d. Daily, weekly, quarterly, and annually
   e. Daily, quarterly, and annually

8. Which of the following is a QC responsibility of the medical physicist?
   a. Collimation assessment
   b. Daily processor QC
   c. Fixer retention analysis
   d. Repeat analysis
   e. Screen-film contact assay

9. Which of the following tasks must the QC mammographer perform daily?
   a. Compression evaluation
   b. Darkroom cleanliness assessment
   c. Fixer retention assay
   d. Phantom image analysis
   e. Screen-film contact evaluation

10. Which of the following tasks must the QC mammographer perform daily?
    a. Compression evaluation
    b. Fixer retention assay
    c. Phantom image analysis
    d. Processor QC
    e. Screen-film contact evaluation

11. Which of the following tasks should the QC mammographer perform weekly?
    a. Compression evaluation
    b. Darkroom cleanliness
    c. Fixer retention assay
    d. Phantom image analysis
    e. Screen-film contact evaluation

12. Which of the following tasks should the QC mammographer perform monthly?
    a. Darkroom cleanliness
    b. Fixer retention assay

c. Formal conference with the radiologist
d. Screen-film contact evaluation
e. Visual checklist

13. Which of the following tasks should the QC mammographer perform quarterly?
    a. Darkroom cleanliness
    b. Darkroom fog analysis
    c. Fixer retention assay
    d. Formal conference with the radiologist
    e. Production of phantom images

14. Which of the following tasks should the QC mammographer perform semiannually?
    a. Darkroom cleanliness
    b. Darkroom fog analysis
    c. Fixer retention assay
    d. Formal conference with the radiologist
    e. Production of phantom images

15. What is the principal reason to routinely require darkroom cleanliness?
    a. Ensure constant spatial resolution.
    b. Improve image contrast.
    c. Reduce chemical fog.
    d. Reduce image artifacts.
    e. Reduce light fog.

16. Materials used for the construction of a mammography darkroom should be chosen with regard to which of the following properties?
    a. Ensuring abrasive surfaces
    b. Maximizing light absorption
    c. Minimizing dust collection
    d. Providing ease of chemical absorption
    e. Reducing light reflection

17. The film used to conduct a processor program should:
    a. Be that special film provided by the manufacturer
    b. Be the first sheets of each new box
    c. Be unprocessed discarded film
    d. Be used randomly throughout the clinical supply
    e. Come from a dedicated supply

18. Which of the following is *not* critical to the proper start of a processor QC program?
    a. Calibrated ion chamber
    b. Clean processor tanks and racks
    c. Dedicated box of film
    d. Proper chemistry, as specified by the manufacturer
    e. Proper temperature and replenishment rates

19. When processor QC is performed, the sensito-
    metric strip of film should be processed:
    a. In alternation with the guide rail
    b. While the least exposed end is fed first
    c. While the most exposed end is fed first
    d. With the long edge against the guide rail
    e. With the short edge against the guide rail

20. Mammography film should be processed:
    a. With the chest wall side fed first
    b. With the emulsion side fed down
    c. With the emulsion side fed up
    d. With the nipple side fed first
    e. With the use of film from the middle of
       the box

21. The densitometer is used in mammography QC
    to do which of the following?
    a. Ensure constant spatial resolution.
    b. Evaluate exposure reproducibility.
    c. Improve contrast resolution.
    d. Measure average gradient.
    e. Measure optical density.

22. In the start-up phase of processor QC, a
    sensitometric strip should be evaluated:
    a. Each day for 5 consecutive days
    b. Each day for 1 month
    c. Twice daily for 3 consecutive days
    d. Twice daily for 5 consecutive days
    e. Twice daily for 1 month

23. The step on the sensitivity strip called the *speed
    index* is also the:
    a. Base step
    b. Contrast step
    c. Gamma point
    d. Mid-density step
    e. Resolution step

24. The mid-density step on the sensitometric strip
    is that with optical density closest to:
    a. 1.2 but not less than 1.2
    b. 1.2 but not more than 1.2
    c. 1.2 but not less than 1.3
    d. 1.3 but not more than 1.3
    e. 1.4

25. The contrast index of a sensitivity strip is also
    known as the:
    a. Average gradient
    b. Base plus fog index
    c. Contrast difference
    d. Density difference
    e. Resolution index

26. Steps on the sensitometric strip assigned for
    density difference are those associated with the
    following optical densities:
    a. 0.5 and 2.2
    b. 0.5 and 2.5
    c. 1.0 and 2.2
    d. 1.2 and 2.2
    e. 1.2 and 2.5

27. The value for base plus fog on the sensitometric
    strip is determined from:
    a. An unexposed area of the strip
    b. The response with no film in the
       densitometer
    c. The step closest to OD equal to 1.2
    d. The step with the highest OD
    e. The step with the lowest OD

28. During evaluation of screens for cleanliness, if
    dust or dirt artifacts are observed:
    a. The density difference reading should be
       repeated.
    b. The mid-density reading should be repeated.
    c. Phantom images should be repeated.
    d. The screen must be cleaned immediately.
    e. The screen should be cleaned as soon as
       possible.

29. What is the principal reason to measure
    mid-density?
    a. Ensure clinical contrast.
    b. Ensure constant spatial resolution.
    c. Evaluate the constancy of image receptor
       speed.
    d. Verify processor chemical replenishment
       rates.
    e. Verify processor chemical temperature.

30. What is the principal reason to evaluate density
    difference on a sensitivity strip?
    a. Detect light chemical fog.
    b. Ensure constancy of image contrast.
    c. Ensure proper processor chemistry.
    d. Provide best spatial resolution.
    e. Reduce base plus fog.

31. During routine processor QC, mid-density may
    vary by how much before corrective action is
    necessary?
    a. 0.05 OD
    b. 0.1 OD
    c. 0.15 OD
    d. 0.2 OD
    e. 0.3 OD

32. During a routine processor QC, density difference may vary by how much before corrective action is necessary (clinical images)?
    a. 0.05 OD
    b. 0.1 OD
    c. 0.15 OD
    d. 0.2 OD
    e. 0.3 OD

33. During processor QC, what is the reason for measuring the optical density of an unexposed portion of the sensitometric film?
    a. Ensure constant contrast.
    b. Evaluate the level of fog in the processing chain.
    c. Improve contrast resolution.
    d. Maintain spatial resolution.
    e. Monitor the chemical temperature and replenishment rate.

34. The mid-density assay of the sensitometric strip should be repeated if the value falls outside of the identified range by how much?
    a. 0.05 OD
    b. 0.1 OD
    c. 0.15 OD
    d. 0.2 OD
    e. 0.3 OD

35. The density difference assay of the sensitometric strip should be repeated if the value falls outside of the identified range by how much?
    a. 0.05 OD
    b. 0.1 OD
    c. 0.15 OD
    d. 0.2 OD
    e. 0.3 OD

36. The established base plus fog optical density value is allowed to vary by:
    a. +0.03
    b. ±0.03
    c. ±0.05
    d. ±0.05
    e. ±0.1

37. Screen cleanliness is a QC task that must be evaluated:
    a. Daily
    b. Weekly
    c. Monthly
    d. Quarterly
    e. Semiannually

21-1

Illumination
Human Vision

The fluoroscopic examination has improved continually since its first demonstration in 1896 by Thomas A. Edison. Fluoroscopy used to require dark adaptation for scotopic vision (rod vision). Now, all fluoroscopic images are viewed under photopic vision (cone vision) with the use of a cathode ray tube or a flat panel display device for image viewing.

Image brightness is assured through an automatic feedback loop called *automatic brightness control (ABC)*.

EXERCISES

1. In a modern fluoroscope, the fluoroscopic x-ray tube:
   a. Can be under or over the table
   b. Is always over the table
   c. Is always the same as the radiographic tube
   d. Is always under the table
   e. Must have very high capacity

2. The fluoroscope was invented by:
   a. Alexander Bell
   b. Hollis Potter
   c. Jan Marconi
   d. Thomas Edison
   e. Wilhelm Roentgen

3. Compared with a radiographic examination, the primary purpose of a fluoroscopic examination is to visualize:
   a. Cross-sectional images
   b. Dynamic images
   c. Longitudinal images
   d. Static images
   e. Transverse images

4. Fluoroscopy normally requires a tube current of:
   a. 0.1 to 1.0 mA
   b. 1 to 5 mA
   c. 5 to 10 mA
   d. 10 to 100 mA
   e. 10 to 1000 mA

5. Compared with radiography, the x-ray technique required for fluoroscopy calls for which of the following?
   a. Higher kVp
   b. Higher mA
   c. Lower kVp
   d. Lower mA
   e. Shorter exposure

6. Automatic brightness stabilization (ABS) is designed to compensate for changes in which of the following?
   a. Examination time
   b. Patient composition
   c. Patient dose
   d. Patient positioning
   e. Technique selection

7. The Bucky slot cover of a fluoroscope is a:
   a. Cassette holder
   b. Film changer
   c. Film support device
   d. Film transport device
   e. Protective device

8. Which of the following units of measurement is used to express fluoroscopic image brightness?
   a. cd/m²
   b. Coulomb
   c. Coulomb/kilogram
   d. Lambert
   e. Roentgen

9. Which of the following structures is *most* sensitive to color?
   a. Cones
   b. Fovea centralis
   c. Rods
   d. Cornea
   e. Iris

10. What is the function of the iris?
    a. Control the light level
    b. Distinguish colors
    c. Focus the light onto the retina
    d. Protect the eye
    e. Sense visible-light photons

11. The cones are:
    a. Essentially color blind
    b. Located at the fovea centralis
    c. Located on the periphery of the retina
    d. Used for photopic vision
    e. Very sensitive to light

12. The fovea centralis is:
    a. Essential to focusing
    b. Next to the lens
    c. Part of the retina
    d. The blind spot
    e. The disc-like structure

13. Visual acuity is the ability to do which of the following?
    a. Control the amount of light entering the eye
    b. Detect differences in brightness
    c. Distinguish colors
    d. Perceive fine detail
    e. Vary depth of field

14. The rods are used principally for which of the following?
    a. Bright vision
    b. Color perception
    c. Dim vision
    d. Focusing
    e. Visual acuity

15. In general, during fluoroscopy as compared with radiography:
    a. A smaller focal spot is used.
    b. Patient dose is lower.
    c. Spatial resolution is better.
    d. The mA is lower.
    e. The SID is longer.

16. Which of the following describes the fluoroscopic system designed to maintain constant image intensity?
    a. Automatic brightness stabilization (ABS)
    b. Automatic channel selector (ACS)
    c. Automatic programmed radiography (APR)
    d. Charge-coupled device (CCD)
    e. Positive-beam limitation (PBL)

17. Which of the following structures is responsible for the vision of dim objects?
    a. Cornea
    b. Fovea centralis
    c. Iris
    d. Pupil
    e. Rod

18. Which of the following ocular structures immediately precedes the vitreous humor along the path of incident light?
    a. Cone
    b. Cornea
    c. Fovea centralis
    d. Iris
    e. Lens

19. Which of the following properties is associated with rods but *not* with cones?
    a. Color detection
    b. Contrast perception
    c. Ray focusing
    d. Scotopic vision
    e. Visual acuity

The image-intensifier tube was introduced to radiology in the 1950s for the principal purpose of reducing patient dose. The image-intensifier tube improves image quality and diagnostic accuracy.

The dose reduction produced by the image intensifier, called **brightness gain,** is the product of the geometric gain, or **minification,** and the **flux gain.**

Direct digital and solid-state flat-panel image receptors have recently been offered as a replacement for the image-intensifier tube.

EXERCISES

1. Photoelectric emission:
   a. Is the emission of electrons from a heated wire
   b. Is the emission of electrons from an illuminated surface
   c. Is the emission of photons
   d. Occurs at the input phosphor of an image-intensifier tube
   e. Occurs at the output phosphor of an image-intensifier tube

2. At what stage of image-intensified fluoroscopy is the number of image-forming photons lowest?
   a. Entering the input phosphor
   b. Entering the photocathode
   c. Leaving the input phosphor
   d. Leaving the output phosphor
   e. Leaving the photocathode

3. Image-intensifier brightness gain increases with increasing:
   a. Flux gain
   b. kVp
   c. mA
   d. Output phosphor size
   e. Radiation exposure

4. When an image intensifier receives x-rays at the input phosphor, what is emitted at the output phosphor?
   a. Electrons
   b. Infrared light
   c. Ultraviolet light
   d. Visible light
   e. X-rays

5. Which of the following is the input phosphor of image intensifiers?
   a. Cadmium tungstate
   b. Calcium tungstate
   c. Cesium iodide
   d. Sodium iodide
   e. Zinc cadmium sulfide

6. Which of the following is the output phosphor of image intensifiers?
   a. Cadmium tungstate
   b. Calcium tungstate
   c. Cesium iodide
   d. Sodium iodide
   e. Zinc cadmium sulfide

7. The photocathode converts:
   a. Electrons into visible light
   b. Visible light into electrons

c. Visible light into x-rays
d. X-rays into electrons
e. X-rays into visible light

8. Which of the following is the component of the image intensifier responsible for focusing the electron beam?
   a. Electrostatic lens
   b. Glass envelope
   c. Input phosphor
   d. Output phosphor
   e. Photocathode

9. The ability of an image intensifier to enhance image illumination is called:
   a. Automatic brightness
   b. Brightness gain
   c. Flux gain
   d. Illumination gain
   e. Minification gain

10. The minification gain of an image intensifier increases with increasing:
    a. Input phosphor size
    b. kVp
    c. mA
    d. Output phosphor size
    e. Tube voltage

11. Which of the following is a representative brightness gain for an image intensifier?
    a. 200
    b. 2000
    c. 20,000
    d. 200,000
    e. 2,000,000

12. If an image intensifier is described as a $^{25}/_{12}$ tube, $^{25}/_{12}$ refers to which of the following?
    a. Area of the input phosphor in square inches
    b. Diameter of the input phosphor in cm
    c. Diameter of the output phosphor in centimeters
    d. Radius of the input phosphor in inches
    e. Radius of the output phosphor in centimeters

13. When a multifocus image intensifier is operated in the magnification mode:
    a. A larger area of input phosphor is used.
    b. Contrast resolution is reduced.
    c. Patient dose is lower.
    d. Spatial resolution is reduced.
    e. The electron focal point is closer to the input phosphor.

14. An image that displays vignetting:
    a. Is dim around the periphery
    b. Is dim in the center
    c. Has higher contrast resolution
    d. Has higher spatial resolution
    e. Shows the barrel stay artifact

15. With a multifocus image intensifier in the magnification mode:
    a. Contrast resolution is reduced.
    b. Noise is increased.
    c. Patient dose is reduced.
    d. Spatial resolution is improved.
    e. Field of view is increased.

16. In a 10/7/5 image intensifier:
    a. Contrast resolution is best in the 10 mode.
    b. Spatial resolution is best in the 10 mode.
    c. The field of view is largest in the 10 mode.
    d. There are three different input phosphors.
    e. There are three different output phosphors.

17. An image intensifier has a 5 cm output phosphor and a 45 cm input phosphor. The brightness gain is 10,000. The flux gain is approximately:
    a. 10
    b. 80
    c. 120
    d. 1000
    e. 5000

18. Place the following in proper sequence for image-intensified fluoroscopy:
    1. Electric signal to light
    2. Electrons to light
    3. Light to electric signal
    4. Light to electrons
    5. X-ray to light
    a. 1, 2, 3, 4, 5
    b. 2, 3, 4, 5, 1
    c. 3, 5, 2, 1, 4
    d. 4, 3, 2, 1, 5
    e. 5, 4, 2, 3, 1

19. Which of the following applies to the output phosphor?
    a. Electrons emitted
    b. Light absorbed
    c. Light emitted
    d. X-rays absorbed
    e. X-rays emitted

21-3

Image Monitoring

The fluoroscopic image produced at the output phosphor of an image-intensifier tube is the size of a postage stamp and cannot be viewed directly. This image is manipulated for viewing, or **monitoring,** with a closed-circuit television system. The output image of the image-intensifying tube is detected by a television camera tube, usually a **vidicon,** or a CCD and then is displayed on a television or a flat-panel monitor.

Such images can be monitored with an optically coupled cine camera that usually is restricted to use during specialized examinations, such as cardiac catheterization. If static images are required during the examination, they are made with an optically coupled spot-film camera. Both spot-film and cine cameras use single-emulsion photographic film that has dimensional sizes of 16 to 105 mm.

EXERCISES

1. Vertical television resolution is limited principally by which of the following?
   a. Bandpass
   b. Field rate
   c. Frame rate
   d. Lines per frame
   e. Modulation

2. The electron beam in a television camera tube is produced by which of the following means?
   a. Electroemission
   b. Photoconduction
   c. Photoemission
   d. Thermionic emission
   e. Thermoluminescence

3. What is the cinefluorography component of image-intensifier fluoroscopy?
   a. Cesium iodide
   b. Electrons from light
   c. Minification
   d. Synchronized
   e. Vidicon

4. What is the photoemissive component of image-intensified fluoroscopy?
   a. Cesium iodide
   b. Electrons from light
   c. Minification
   d. Synchronized
   e. Vidicon

5. Which of the following is photoconductive?
   a. Electron gun
   b. Electrostatic grid
   c. Signal plate
   d. Target
   e. Window

6. What is the principal disadvantage of coupling the television camera to the image intensifier with the use of fiber optics?
   a. Cassette-loaded spot film cannot be used.
   b. Fragility is increased.
   c. Image noise is increased.
   d. Photospot camera cannot be used.
   e. Spatial resolution is reduced.

7. Which of the following refers to the image-intensifier input phosphor?
   a. Cesium iodide
   b. Electrons from light

c. Minification
d. Synchronized
e. Vidicon

8. Which is a critical component in optically coupling an image intensifier with a photospot camera?
a. Electrostatic lens
b. Face plate
c. Objective lens
d. Signal plate
e. Subjective lens

9. What is the *most* important component of a television monitor?
a. Cathode ray tube
b. Charge-coupled device
c. Coupling device
d. Electromagnetic coils
e. Television camera tube

10. In an optical coupling arrangement, which is nearest the television camera?
a. Beam splitter
b. Camera lens
c. Deflection coil
d. Mirror
e. Objective lens

11. What is the component of the television monitor in which the video signal is transformed into an image?
a. Electron beam
b. Electron gun
c. Electrostatic grid
d. Phosphor screen
e. Target assembly

12. What is the electron beam of the television camera tube?
a. A fan beam
b. An area beam
c. Blanked
d. Collimated
e. Modulated

13. One television frame is equivalent to which of the following?
a. 17 ms
b. 262½ lines
c. 1024 lines
d. One television field
e. Two television fields

14. Fluoroscopic television operates at a frame rate of:
a. 30 f/s
b. 60 f/s
c. 262½ f/s
d. 525 f/s
e. 1024 f/s

15. Horizontal television resolution is limited principally by which of the following?
a. Bandpass
b. Field rate
c. Frame rate
d. Lines per frame
e. Modulation

16. What is normally the weakest imaging link in television fluoroscopy?
a. Image-intensifier tube
b. Optical coupling device
c. Spot-film device
d. Television camera
e. Television monitor

17. Common frame rates during cinefluorography are 15, 30, and 60 f/s because:
a. Flicker is not observed at these rates.
b. It is linked to patient dose.
c. Of the frame rate requirement of the television camera tube
d. Of the frequency of the power supply
e. The film format requires it.

18. When the electron beam of the CRT is blanked, it is:
a. Demodulated
b. In a vertical retrace
c. In an active trace
d. Modulated
e. Turned on

19. Which of the following is *true* about cineradiography?
a. Frame rate is unimportant.
b. Patient exposure rates are lower than those used for fluoroscopy.
c. The x-ray beam is off when the shutter is closed, as a patient protection measure.
d. The x-ray beam is off when the shutter is closed, to prevent damage to the film transport system.
e. The x-ray beam is on during film transport.

20. What is the television camera tube component of image-intensified fluoroscopy?
    a. Cesium iodide
    b. Electrons from light
    c. Minification
    d. Synchronized
    e. Vidicon

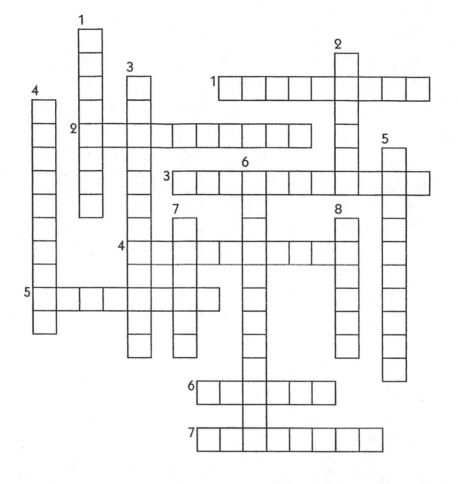

ACROSS

1. Type of television camera tube used in television fluoroscopy.
2. Daylight vision, involving the cones.
3. Produced studies on illumination that resulted in the development of the image intensifier in the 1950s.
4. Type of electron emission that occurs after heat stimulation.
5. Night vision, involving the rods.
6. Invented the fluoroscope in 1896.
7. Ability to detect differences in brightness.

DOWN

1. Property that describes the number of times per second that an electron beam can be modulated or changed; used to determine horizontal resolution.

2. Ability to perceive fine detail.
3. Photoemissive surface composed of cesium and antimony compounds that emit electrons when stimulated by light.
4. Ability of the image-intensifier tube to enhance the illumination level of an image.
5. Reduction in brightness at the periphery.
6. Ratio of the square of the diameter of the input phosphor to the square of the diameter of the output phosphor.
7. Input phosphor with which x-rays interact after exiting the patient and the glass envelope.
8. Line of varying intensity of light.

22-1

Types of Procedures
Basic Principles
IR Suite

IR stands for *interventional radiography*. Radiographers who have passed the American Registry of Radiologic Technologists (ARRT) examination for cardiovascular and interventional radiography have the letters (CV) in their credentials.

Angiography refers to methods of imaging contrast-filled vessels. Vascular imaging and therapeutic intervention through vessels require a special suite equipped with advanced radiographic and fluoroscopic imaging systems. Special guidewires and catheters are used in interventional radiology to access the vascular network without surgery. Different catheter tips are designed to access specific arteries.

Charge-coupled devices (CCDs) are rapidly replacing the television camera tube as the image recorder. CCDs are photosensitive silicon chips that can be used anywhere that light will be converted to a digital video image. The advantages of CCDs for IR are many and include high spatial resolution, lack of spatial distortion, a linear response, lower patient dose, and the lack of warm-up and maintenance requirements.

EXERCISES

1. Which of following suffixes is proper for a radiologic technologist certified by the ARRT as a vascular technologist?
   a. RT (ARRT) (CVIR)
   b. RT (CV)
   c. RT (CV) (ARRT)
   d. RT (CVIR)
   e. RT (CVIR) (ARRT)

2. The spatial resolution of the CCD can be as high as:
   a. 1 lp/mm
   b. 2 lp/mm
   c. 5 lp/mm
   d. 10 lp/mm
   e. 15 lp/mm

3. A CCD:
   a. Has a life span of approximately 100,000 exposures
   b. Is associated with low DQE
   c. Requires regular maintenance
   d. Results in higher patient dose but better contrast resolution than a television camera
   e. Has a sensitive element composed of a layer of crystalline silicon

4. The term *angiography* refers to which of the following?
   a. Contrast examinations of arteries
   b. Contrast examinations of veins
   c. Contrast examinations of vessels
   d. Examination of brain vessels
   e. Examination of leg vessels

5. Transbrachial select coronary angiography refers to examination of which of the following?
   a. Angiointerventional radiography
   b. Angioplasty
   c. Coronary arteries through an artery of the arm
   d. Coronary arteries through an artery of the leg
   e. The brachial artery

6. Who pioneered transfemoral neuroangiography?
   a. Charles Dotter
   b. Mason Jones
   c. Melvin Judkins
   d. Nick Brian
   e. Vincent Hinck

7. Who pioneered the femoral approach to coronary angiography?
   a. Charles Dotter
   b. Mason Jones
   c. Melvin Judkins
   d. Nick Brian
   e. Vincent Hinck

8. Who developed a method of arterial access that uses a needle and catheter and makes cutdown of the vessel unnecessary?
   a. Charles Dotter
   b. Mason Jones
   c. Melvin Judkins
   d. Sven-Ivar Seldinger
   e. Vincent Hinck

9. Which of the following statements about cut-film changers is **not** true?
   a. An 8:1 or 10:1 carbon fiber focused grid is normally used.
   b. The supply and receiving magazines of cut-film changers are lined with lead.
   c. Cut-film changers normally produce 12 images per second.
   d. Cut-film changers replaced roll-film changers.
   e. Normally, an 800-speed screen-film combination is used.

10. Transbrachial selective coronary angiography was introduced in the early:
    a. 1950s
    b. 1960s
    c. 1970s
    d. 1980s
    e. 1990s

11. What is the principal reason to use guidewires in cardiovascular angiography and interventional radiology?
    a. Better visualization under fluoroscopy
    b. Ease of entry at the puncture site
    c. Safe introduction of the catheter into the vessel
    d. Visualization of arteries
    e. Visualization of veins

12. What is the approximate length of a conventional guidewire?
    a. 50 cm
    b. 100 cm
    c. 145 cm
    d. 200 cm
    e. 300 cm

13. Selective catheterization of specific arteries is promoted by which of the following?
    a. Curve of the catheter
    b. Degree of difficulty
    c. Degree of disease
    d. Gauge of the catheter
    e. Shape of the tip of the catheter

14. A fenestrated catheter is:
    a. A large-volume catheter
    b. A small-volume catheter
    c. One with a sharp curve at the tip
    d. One with a straight tip
    e. One with side holes at the tip

15. A catheter is fenestrated to:
    a. Accommodate more contrast material
    b. Improve image contrast
    c. Improve spatial resolution
    d. Reduce possible whiplash
    e. Simplify vessel puncture

16. To prevent clotting of blood within the catheter, what is the normal procedure?
    a. Saline flush
    b. Water flush
    c. Aspirin administration
    d. Heparinized saline flush
    e. Catheter occlusion

17. For vascular studies, choice of radiopaque contrast medium is based on which of the following?
    a. Air
    b. Barium
    c. Calcium
    d. Iodine
    e. Mylithem

18. After angiography:
    a. A physical examination is necessary to assess the patient's medical history for allergies and other conditions.
    b. Manual compression on the femoral site is not necessary once the catheter is removed.

c. The patient usually can be released immediately.

d. The patient is instructed to remain immobile for several hours.

e. The patient is visited by the radiologist to establish rapport.

19. When applied to contrast media, what does *osmolality* refer to?
    a. Atomic number of the media
    b. Concentration of ions in the media
    c. Mass density of the media
    d. Risk of the media
    e. Viscosity of the media

20. What is a principal complication of transfemoral angiography?
    a. Blood loss
    b. Hemorrhage of the puncture site
    c. Oxygen deprivation
    d. Patient anxiety
    e. Vessel collapse

21. Which of the following is an imaging procedure that would be conducted in an IR suite?
    a. Angioplasty
    b. Arthrectomy
    c. Embolization
    d. Myelography
    e. Thrombolysis

22. Which of the following is an interventional procedure that would be conducted in an IR suite?
    a. Arteriography
    b. Arthrography
    c. Cardiac catheterization
    d. Myelography
    e. Stent placement

23. In an IR suite, a door between the operating console and the examination room:
    a. Is a protective barrier
    b. Is not required
    c. Must be double-hinged
    d. Must be double-wide
    e. Should accommodate a stretcher

24. Which of the following is a minimum requirement for an IR x-ray tube?
    a. 0.3 mm small focal spot
    b. 5 cm diameter anode
    c. 80 kW power rating
    d. 300,000 kHU anode heat capacity
    e. Molybdenum-targeted anode

25. For the spatial resolution requirements of the magnification of small vessels, the focal spot must be:
    a. No smaller than 0.3 mm
    b. No larger than 0.3 mm
    c. No smaller than 0.5 mm
    d. No larger than 0.5 mm
    e. None of the above

26. What is a characteristic of an IR x-ray tube?
    a. Large target angle
    b. Small-diameter anode disc
    c. Small target angle
    d. 50 kW power rating
    e. 300,000 kHU anode heat capacity

27. If an aortogram is performed with a 0.3 mm focal spot and an SID of 100 cm and the artery is 15 cm from the image receptor, what is the magnification factor?
    a. 0.85
    b. 1.08
    c. 1.10
    d. 1.18
    e. 1.25

28. If a carotid arteriogram is performed with a 0.3 mm focal spot at 100 cm SID and the artery is 10 cm from the image receptor, what is the focal-spot blur?
    a. 0.033
    b. 0.33
    c. 0.27
    d. 2.7
    e. 3.3

29. Cardiac catheterization is performed with a 0.3 mm focal spot and an SID of 100 cm. The coronary artery is 15 cm from the image receptor. What is the approximate spatial resolution for this procedure?
    a. 0.05 mm
    b. 0.11 mm
    c. 0.16 mm
    d. 0.53 mm
    e. 1.1 mm

30. Which of the following high-voltage generators is **most** desirable for the IR suite?
    a. High-frequency
    b. Single-phase
    c. Single-phase full-wave rectified
    d. Three-phase six-pulse
    e. Three-phase twelve-pulse

31. Which of the following IR image receptors is used during cardiac catheterization?
    a. 105 mm photofluorographic camera
    b. Cassette-loaded spot film
    c. Cinefluorographic camera
    d. Digital fluoroscopy spot film
    e. Serialographic changer

32. Which of the following has been the principal IR image receptor since the 1950s?
    a. 105 mm photofluorographic camera
    b. Cassette-loaded spot film
    c. Cinefluorographic camera
    d. Digital fluoroscopy spot film
    e. Serialographic changer

Computed tomography (CT) represents one of the most important developments in medical imaging of the 20th century. The development of slip-ring technology and high-frequency generators promoted the introduction of spiral computed tomography. This was followed by multislice computed tomography for faster imaging of a larger tissue volume.

The CT imaging system has three principal sections: the gantry, the operating console, and the computer. The gantry assembly includes a high-voltage generator, an x-ray tube, a detector array, and the patient couch.

EXERCISES

1. A CT imaging system produces which type of image?
   a. Axial
   b. Biaxial
   c. Fulcrum plane
   d. Longitudinal
   e. Transverse

2. In its simplest configuration, the CT imaging system consists of an x-ray source and which of the following?
   a. A detector
   b. A selenium plate
   c. A video display terminal
   d. An image intensifier
   e. An x-ray beam collimator

3. Which of the following is characteristic of first-generation CT imaging systems?
   a. A pencil x-ray beam
   b. A selenium or film image receptor
   c. Multiple sources and multiple detectors
   d. Rotate-only geometry
   e. Slip rings

4. CT imaging systems incorporate:
   a. Charged electrostatic plates
   b. High-frequency radiographic grids
   c. Light-localizing, variable-aperture collimators
   d. Multiple reconstruction algorithms
   e. Single-focus x-ray tubes

5. Sensitivity profile in CT is determined principally by the:
   a. Bow-tie filter
   b. Predetector collimator
   c. Prepatient collimator
   d. Reconstruction algorithm
   e. Ramp function

6. Spatial resolution for CT imaging systems is approximately:
   a. 1 cm
   b. 10 cm
   c. 100 mm
   d. 1 mm
   e. 10 mm

7. Second-generation CT imaging systems:
   a. Have a multiple detector array
   b. Have rotate-rotate geometry

    c. Require imaging speeds from 1 to 5 minutes
    d. Require special patient preparation
    e. Use increments of 1 degree per view

8. Third-generation CT imaging systems have which of the following?
    a. Multiple-detector, area-beam geometry
    b. Rotate-rotate geometry
    c. Rotate-translate geometry
    d. Single-detector, fan-beam geometry
    e. Translate-translate geometry

9. Fourth-generation CT imaging systems:
    a. Are faster than third-generation CT imaging systems
    b. Have rotate-rotate geometry
    c. Incorporate area-beam geometry
    d. May use selenium or film as the image receptor
    e. Require prepatient collimation

10. Which of the following subsystems would normally be associated with the gantry assembly?
    a. Image postprocessing
    b. The algorithms
    c. The detector array
    d. The physician's viewing console
    e. The software

11. Which of the following has been used as a detector in a CT imaging system?
    a. Bismuth germanate
    b. $CaWO_4$
    c. High-pressure air
    d. Selenium
    e. Silver halide

12. A comparison of scintillation and gas-filled detectors shows that:
    a. Both have approximately the same total detection efficiency.
    b. Both rely heavily on Compton interaction.
    c. Only scintillation detectors require prepatient collimation.
    d. The gas-filled detectors have higher intrinsic efficiency.
    e. The scintillation detectors have higher geometric efficiency.

13. Noise on a CT image can be reduced by:
    a. Increasing kVp
    b. Increasing mAs
    c. Increasing matrix size
    d. Reducing image time
    e. Reducing pixel size

14. In a CT imaging system, prepatient collimation:
    a. Controls pixel size
    b. Controls scatter radiation that reaches the detector
    c. Determines image noise
    d. Determines patient dose
    e. Determines slice thickness

15. The translate-rotate mode:
    a. Collects data only during the rotate portion
    b. Describes both first- and second-generation CT imaging systems
    c. Requires higher heat capacity x-ray tubes
    d. Requires only solid-state detectors
    e. Results in imaging times as short as 1 s

16. Each translation of a source detector assembly produces which of the following?
    a. A matrix
    b. A pixel
    c. A projection
    d. A voxel
    e. An image

17. Slice thickness can also be expressed as which of the following?
    a. Dose profile
    b. Low-contrast profile
    c. Resolution profile
    d. Sensitivity profile
    e. Spatial profile

18. The thickness of section in CT depends primarily on:
    a. kVp
    b. mAs
    c. Matrix size
    d. Predetector collimation
    e. Prepatient collimation

19. CT is performed at high kVp principally to:
    a. Improve image contrast.
    b. Minimize beam hardening.
    c. Reduce patient dose.
    d. Reduce scatter radiation.
    e. Reduce x-ray tube loading.

20. Streak artifacts on a CT image are usually due to:
    a. Beam hardening
    b. Bone/soft tissue interface
    c. Bowel gas
    d. Detector imbalance
    e. Metal clips

Every medical image has two principal characteristics: spatial resolution and contrast resolution.

Spatial resolution refers to the ability of an imaging system to image small, high-contrast objects such as calcifications in soft tissue. Spatial resolution is best measured by **spatial frequency** and **modulation transfer function (MTF).**

Contrast resolution refers to the ability of the imaging system to reproduce objects such as cysts and tumors that do not vary much from surrounding tissue in their x-ray absorption properties.

EXERCISES

1. A 120 × 120 matrix will consist of how many pixels?
   a. 120
   b. 240
   c. 625
   d. 14,400
   e. 65,536

2. What is the pixel size of an image reconstructed from a 24 cm diameter region of interest (ROI) in a 320 × 320 matrix?
   a. 0.25 mm
   b. 0.5 mm
   c. 0.75 mm
   d. 1.3 mm
   e. 1.5 mm

3. A CT image is made with a 5 mm slice thickness and a 0.5 mm pixel size. What is the size of the voxel?
   a. 0.75 mm^3
   b. 1.00 mm^3
   c. 1.25 mm^3
   d. 1.5 mm^3
   e. 25 mm^3

4. Which of the following Hounsfield unit (HU) values **most** closely represents the value for blood?
   a. −80 HU
   b. −40 HU
   c. −2 HU
   d. 20 HU
   e. 100 HU

5. A CT imaging system has a limiting resolution of 7 lp/cm. An object of what size can be resolved?
   a. 0.35 mm
   b. 0.5 mm
   c. 0.7 mm
   d. 1.4 mm
   e. 3.5 mm

6. Which of the following is characteristic of a CT image but **not** of a conventional radiograph?
   a. Anatomic structures are superimposed.
   b. Better contrast resolution is obtained.
   c. Better spatial resolution is obtained.
   d. More scatter radiation reaches the image receptor.
   e. Overlying and underlying tissues are blurred.

7. An image matrix contains which of the following?
   a. Algorithms
   b. Equations of information
   c. Picture elements
   d. Silver halide information units
   e. Slice sensitivity 1.00

8. A Hounsfield unit:
   a. Has a value from −100 to +100
   b. Has a value from −500 to +500
   c. Is the numeral value of a pixel
   d. Is the numeral value of anode heat generated
   e. Is the volume of a voxel expressed in mm^3

9. The precise pixel value in HU depends on which of the following?
   a. 32 shades of gray
   b. Light field, x-ray beam coincidence
   c. Pixel size
   d. The x-ray attenuation coefficient
   e. X-ray beam size

10. Spatial resolution refers to which of the following?
    a. The ability to classify large low-contrast objects
    b. The ability to identify small high-contrast objects
    c. The ability to identify tissues of varying composition
    d. The binary number system
    e. The constancy of the imaging system over time

11. When a CT image is described, contrast resolution:
    a. Is limited by the MTF of the system
    b. Is limited by the noise of the system
    c. Is not as good as in conventional radiography
    d. Is the same as spatial resolution
    e. Means that contrast material was injected

12. Partial volume artifacts are more likely with:
    a. Higher kVp
    b. Higher mA
    c. Larger pixel size
    d. Thicker slices
    e. Thinner slices

Exercises 13 through 15 refer to the figure below.

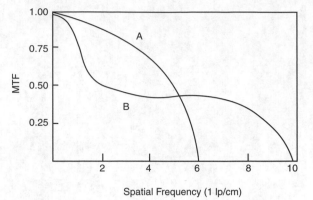

13. The MTF curves describe two imaging systems. Which of the following statements is **true**?
    a. System A detects smaller objects than system B.
    b. System A has better spatial resolution than system B.
    c. System A has more image noise than system B.
    d. System B has better contrast for coarse details than system A.
    e. System B has better spatial resolution than system A.

14. A device has the MTF characteristics represented by B. Which of the following statements is **true** for that device?
    a. At 2 lp/cm, only one half of an object can be imaged.
    b. At 10 lp/cm, the response is excellent.
    c. It can image a 0.5 mm object.
    d. Its imaging ability increases with increasing spatial frequency.
    e. Longer imaging time than in A will be required.

15. The MTF characteristics of system A suggest that it:
    a. Can image down to approximately 0.8 mm
    b. Can image down to approximately 6 cm
    c. Images large objects better than small objects
    d. Images small objects better than large objects
    e. Is a better system than B

16. Noise on a CT image increases with an
    increase in:
    a. kVp
    b. mA
    c. Matrix size
    d. Pixel size
    e. Slice thickness

17. During CT imaging, beam hardening artifacts:
    a. Are due to the polyenergetic beam
    b. Can be corrected by preprocessing
    c. Produce CT numbers higher in the periphery
    d. Result in brighter pixels in the center of the
       patient
    e. Result in higher attenuation in the center of
       the patient

18. Spatial resolution in CT imaging depends
    principally on:
    a. Focal spot size
    b. kVp
    c. Pixel size
    d. Postpatient collimation
    e. Slice thickness

Spiral computed tomography (CT) reduces motion blur, imaging time, and partial volume artifact. It is made possible by slip-ring technology that allows the gantry to rotate continuously without interruption. Interpolation allows collected data to be reconstructed at any position along the z-axis, which is the long axis of the body. The volume of the tissue image is determined by examination time, couch travel, pitch, and collimation.

The spiral CT pitch is the relationship between patient couch movement and x-ray beam collimation. Increasing the pitch ratio to above 1.0 increases the volume of tissue that can be imaged and reduces patient dose.

Multislice spiral CT uses several parallel detector arrays, each of which contains thousands of individual detectors, to produce four or more spiral slices at the same time. The signal from each radiation detector is connected to a computer-controlled electronic amplifier and switching device called a *data acquisition system (DAS)*.

The DAS selects detector combinations for signal summation and sends the signals to a computer for reconstruction of the image. Multislice spiral CT can image larger tissue volume faster than single-slice spiral CT.

EXERCISES

1. Which of the following terms is equivalent to *spiral?*
   a. Elliptical
   b. Helical
   c. Interpolation
   d. Paraboloid
   e. Trispiral

2. Which of the following molecules takes on the structure of a spiral?
   a. Carbohydrate
   b. Deoxyribonucleic acid
   c. Free radical
   d. Lipid
   e. Protein

3. Which of the following is specifically characteristic of spiral CT?
   a. Continuous bidirectional rotation of the x-ray tube
   b. Continuous x-ray tube rotation in one direction
   c. Rotating detector array
   d. Stationary patient couch
   e. Step-like motion of the patient couch

4. During spiral CT examination of a supine patient, the z-axis:
   a. Is the anterior-posterior axis
   b. Is the lateral axis, left to right
   c. Is the lateral axis, right to left
   d. Is the long axis of the body
   e. Varies with the examination

5. The ability to reconstruct an image at any z-axis position is due to:
   a. Extrapolation
   b. Filtered back projection
   c. Fourier transformation
   d. Interpolation
   e. Linear estimation

6. A principal advantage of reconstruction in any z-axis position is:
   a. Image acquisition during a single breath-hold
   b. Improved contrast resolution
   c. Improved spatial resolution
   d. Larger volume of tissue imaged
   e. Reduction of partial volume

7. The simplest form of three-dimensional imaging is:
   a. Isometric
   b. Maximum-intensity projection
   c. Shaded surface display
   d. Shaded volume display
   e. Slip-ring technology

8. Which of the following reconstruction techniques exhibits the **most** image noise?
   a. 180-degree interpolation
   b. 360-degree interpolation
   c. Back-projected conventional CT
   d. Filtered back projection conventional CT
   e. High-dose CT

9. During a 360-degree x-ray rotation, the patient couch moves 15 mm during each revolution. Slice thickness is 10 mm. What is the slice pitch?
   a. 0.66
   b. 1.25
   c. 1.5
   d. 1.66
   e. 2.0

10. Which of the following is one advantage of spiral CT over conventional CT?
    a. Better patient dose utilization
    b. Improved contrast resolution
    c. Improved spatial resolution
    d. Lack of motion artifact
    e. Large matrix reconstruction

11. Which of the following is another advantage of spiral CT over conventional CT?
    a. Better patient dose utilization
    b. Improved contrast resolution
    c. Improved spatial resolution
    d. Large matrix reconstruction
    e. Reduced scanning time

12. If a 20-second spiral CT examination is acquired at a pitch of 1.5 with collimation of 10 mm, what volume of tissue was imaged?
    a. 3 cm
    b. 30 cm
    c. 300 cm
    d. 3 mm
    e. 30 mm

13. Thirty centimeters of tissue along the z-axis is to be imaged with a 5 mm slice thickness at a pitch of 2.0. What imaging time is required?
    a. 20 s
    b. 25 s
    c. 30 s
    d. 35 s
    e. 40 s

14. How much z-axis tissue will be imaged during a 20 s procedure if the slice width is 5 mm at a pitch of 1 and the gantry rotation time is 2 s?
    a. 5 cm
    b. 10 cm
    c. 100 cm
    d. 5 mm
    e. 10 mm

15. Why is it recommended that beam pitch should **not** exceed 2.0?
    a. Increased noise
    b. Poor contrast resolution
    c. Poor patient dose utilization
    d. Poor spatial resolution
    e. Poor z-axis resolution

16. Which of the following is another term for slice thickness?
    a. Dose profile
    b. Interpolation profile
    c. Reconstruction index
    d. Section sensitivity profile
    e. Z-axis profile

17. With increasing slice pitch:
    a. Image noise is reduced.
    b. Patient dose is increased.
    c. Sagittal/coronal reconstruction is improved.
    d. The section sensitivity profile decreases.
    e. The section sensitivity profile increases.

18. When a shaded surface display reformation is implemented, the image will appear:
    a. As CT angiography
    b. As z-axis reformation
    c. Isometric
    d. Surface-rendered
    e. Volume-rendered

19. Which of the following technique developments made spiral CT possible?
    a. Dose-efficiency detectors
    b. High-frequency generators
    c. Interpolation algorithms
    d. Slip rings
    e. Volume imaging

20. CT angiography relies on a reconstruction process that is called:
    a. Longitudinal reformation
    b. Maximum intensity projection
    c. Shaded surface display
    d. Surface-rendered
    e. Volume rendered

21. Which of the following characteristics is specific to a spiral CT x-ray tube?
    a. High anode heat capacity
    b. High rotation speed
    c. Large effective focal spots
    d. Large target angle
    e. Small effective focal spots

22. Approximately what is the minimum power requirement for the high-voltage generator and x-ray tube for spiral CT?
    a. 10 kW
    b. 20 kW
    c. 30 kW
    d. 40 kW
    e. 50 kW

23. The single **most** important advantage of spiral CT is which of the following?
    a. Imaging of a large volume of anatomy at low patient dose
    b. Imaging of a large volume of anatomy in one breath-hold
    c. Improved contrast resolution
    d. Improved spatial resolution
    e. Improved z-axis resolution

24. What range of beam pitch is recommended for multislice spiral CT?
    a. 0.5 to 1
    b. 0.5 to 2
    c. 0.5 to 4
    d. 1
    e. 1 to 2

25. DAS stands for which of the following?
    a. Data acquisition system
    b. Digital acquired space
    c. Digital activation signal
    d. Digital analog server
    e. Digital analog system

26. The largest number of individual detectors in a multislice CT imager is approximately:
    a. Two
    b. Four
    c. Ten
    d. Hundreds
    e. Thousands

27. Which of the following statements about multislice CT is **true**?
    a. Higher-resolution multislice spiral CT results in low patient radiation dose.
    b. Larger detector size results in better spatial resolution.
    c. Narrower slice scanning results in better contrast resolution at the same mA.
    d. The simplest approach to multislice scanning is the use of eight detector arrays, each of equal width.
    e. Wider multislices allow imaging of a greater tissue volume.

28. A principal advantage of multislice spiral CT compared with step-and-shoot CT is all of the following **except**:
    a. Better spatial resolution
    b. Faster imaging
    c. Larger tissue volume
    d. Lower patient dose
    e. Three-dimensional image reconstruction

24-1 History of Computers Anatomy of a Computer

 The hardware of a computer is the nuts, bolts, and chips of the system.

Hardware essentially exists in three stages: input devices, the central processing unit (CPU), and output devices.

Everything visible and material about a computer is hardware.

The input and output devices, called I/O devices, are the most visible of the computer parts. Some serve only as input or output devices, but most perform a dual function.

Primary memory is provided by the least visible of all the hardware: small memory modules made up of very large-scale integrated circuits on very small silicon chips. The CPU also is located on such a chip.

EXERCISES

1. Which of the following best represents an analog device?
   a. A gasoline pump register
   b. A meter rule
   c. A photograph
   d. A point-of-sale register
   e. A raffle ticket

2. Which of the following is a difference between random access memory (RAM) and read-only memory (ROM)?
   a. One cannot write to ROM.
   b. RAM is faster than ROM.
   c. RAM is on the hard drive and ROM is on a floppy disk.
   d. RAM is solid state and ROM is tape.
   e. ROM is not found in primary memory.

3. Many milestones stand out in the development of the modern computer, but perhaps the **most** important is the:
   a. CPU
   b. Discovery of x-rays
   c. ENIAC
   d. Flip-flop
   e. Transistor

4. The arithmetic unit in a computer:
   a. Can be primary or secondary memory
   b. Contains the control unit
   c. Is an analog device
   d. Is an I/O device
   e. Is synchronized by an internal clock

5. Primary memory usually is found:
   a. In a modem
   b. In the CPU
   c. On diskettes
   d. On magnetic tape
   e. On the hard drive

6. Which of the following has the largest memory capacity?
   a. A floppy disk
   b. A Winchester disk
   c. An optical disc
   d. An optical tape
   e. The CPU

7. A logic terminal is one that:
   a. Can be programmed
   b. Does not contain a microprocessor
   c. Logically fits with the rest of the system

d. Performs logic functions
e. Requires a microprocessor

8. In which of the following is RAM located?
   a. A floppy disk
   b. A magnetic tape
   c. A modem
   d. An optical disc
   e. The CPU

9. The term *stored program* means which of the following?
   a. Digital instead of analog must be used.
   b. Instructions can be placed in memory.
   c. Memory can be expanded.
   d. Only binary data can be manipulated.
   e. The binary number system must be used.

10. The control unit:
    a. Can contain primary or secondary memory
    b. Contains the arithmetic unit
    c. Contains the LUT
    d. Is an I/O device
    e. Is synchronized by an internal clock

11. Which of the following is normally associated with the first generation of computers?
    a. An abacus
    b. Diodes
    c. Peg wheels
    d. Transistors
    e. Vacuum tubes

12. Most primary memory devices consist of which of the following?
    a. A disk
    b. A magnetic ferrite core
    c. A semiconductor
    d. A tape
    e. Transistors

13. Which of the following is an I/O device?
    a. CPU
    b. LUT
    c. Memory module
    d. Modem
    e. Winchester disk

14. Most computer-assisted radiologic imaging devices incorporate which of the following?
    a. A calculator
    b. A mainframe computer
    c. A microcomputer
    d. A minicomputer
    e. An I/O device

15. Optical character recognition (OCR) is:
    a. A hardware device
    b. A software system
    c. A visual counter
    d. Part of the CPU
    e. Part of the cathode-ray tube (CRT)

16. Secondary memory is available as a:
    a. CPU
    b. Keypad
    c. Magnetic tape
    d. Modem
    e. Video display terminal (VDT)

17. Which of the following would be found in the CPU?
    a. A modem
    b. A Winchester disk
    c. An arithmetic unit
    d. LUT
    e. Secondary storage

18. Which of the following would **least** likely be a part of a radiologic imaging VDT?
    a. Alphabetic keypad
    b. CRT
    c. Image receptor
    d. Modem
    e. Special function keypad

19. Which of the following is an arithmetic function?
    a. And/or
    b. Multiplication
    c. Product
    d. Session
    e. Transfer file

24-2 Computer Software Processing Methods

The written instructions that guide a computer through its various operations are called *computer programs*. These constitute the software of a computer. System software exists as instructions written in a very low-level computer language and based on the binary number system.

Individual application computer programs are written in various computer languages. High-level computer languages such as FORTRAN, BASIC, and COBOL are written in English-oriented symbols that can be assembled, compiled, or interpreted into a machine-oriented language.

Machine language is the lowest-level language used in computer programs. It consists of a series of binary digits (bits) assembled according to a code to represent instructions for the CPU or numeric and alphabetic characters.

The binary code is based on the binary number system, which contains only two digits—zero and one. Eight bits make a byte, and two bytes make a word. It is the bits, bytes, and words that move through a computer operation from input to output.

EXERCISES

1. Software includes which of the following?
   a. LUT
   b. The CPU
   c. The operating system
   d. The operating terminal
   e. The ROM

2. When a computer is turned on, the first interaction occurs through the:
   a. Applications program
   b. Bootstrap
   c. File manager and scheduler
   d. I/O manager
   e. Memory manager

3. The binary code for the decimal number 18 is:
   a. 10101
   b. 10001
   c. 1001
   d. 1010
   e. 10010

4. The sum of $2^3 + 2^2 + 2^0$ is:
   a. 8
   b. 13
   c. 84
   d. 842
   e. 96

5. The number 47 falls between:
   a. 2^4 and 2^5
   b. 2^5 and 2^6
   c. 2^6 and 2^7
   d. 2^7 and 2^8
   e. 2^8 and 2^9

6. Which of the following is a high-level computer language?
   a. Dbase
   b. Display writer
   c. FORTRAN
   d. LUT
   e. MS Windows

7. Which of the following is an applications program?
   a. Basic
   b. COBOL
   c. Logo
   d. Windows 2000
   e. WordStar

8. Alphabetic characters usually are encoded by how many bits?
   a. 2
   b. 4
   c. 8
   d. 16
   e. 32

9. The operating system:
   a. Competes with the CPU
   b. Is found in the modem
   c. Is usually in decimal form
   d. Is usually programmed in the highest-level language
   e. Organizes data flow through the computer

10. Which of the following terms does **not** fit with the others?
    a. Assembler
    b. Compiler
    c. Computer language
    d. Interpreter
    e. Operating system

11. Which of the following is a high-level language?
    a. Assembly
    b. Bootstrap
    c. FORTRAN
    d. Machine-oriented
    e. Windows 2000

12. Which of the following is the oldest of currently used computer languages?
    a. ADA
    b. BASIC
    c. COBOL
    d. FORTRAN
    e. PASCAL

13. An algorithm is:
    a. A computer language
    b. An equation in a computer language
    c. An I/O device
    d. An operating system
    e. Rarely used in diagnostic imaging

14. The computer language that is particularly suited to business is which of the following?
    a. ADA
    b. BASIC
    c. COBOL
    d. FORTRAN
    e. PASCAL

15. Which type of computer processing is used in radiologic imaging?
    a. Batch processing
    b. Off-line processing
    c. On-line processing
    d. Real-time processing
    e. Time share processing

16. Which of the following equalities is **correct?**
    a. $2^8 = 512$
    b. $2^{10} = 1024$
    c. $3^4 = 27$
    d. $10^4 = 1000$
    e. $12^3 = 1654$

17. Which of the following is the programming language that is easiest to learn?
    a. COBOL
    b. BASIC
    c. FORTRAN
    d. PASCAL

18. The type of program that a user might write to classify radiologic images would be:
    a. A bootstrap program
    b. An applications program
    c. An assembler program
    d. An iterative program
    e. An operating system

19. The zero or one in the binary system is called a:
    a. Bit
    b. Byte
    c. Chomp
    d. CPU
    e. Word

20. To encode is to change from:
    a. Alphabetic characters to decimal characters
    b. Bits to bytes
    c. Bytes to bits
    d. Numbers to words
    e. Ordinary characters to binary digits

21. Which of the following number systems uses the **greatest number of** digits?
    a. Binary
    b. Decimal
    c. Duodecimal
    d. Exponential
    e. Hexadecimal

22. Which of the following computer measures is the largest?
    a. Bit
    b. Byte
    c. Chomp
    d. Smack
    e. Word

ACROSS

1. Type of memory that is retained even if power to the computer is lost
2. Designed a system to record census data in 1890; started a company that eventually evolved into IBM
3. System of many transistors and other electronic elements fused onto a chip
4. One of two individuals who designed and built the first electronic digital computer
5. I/O device consisting of a keyboard and a cathode ray tube display
6. Tiny piece of semiconductor material, usually silicon
7. Computer programs that tell the computer what to do and how to store data
8. One of two mathematicians who built mechanical calculators using pegged wheels to perform automatically the four arithmetic functions
9. Type of data processing in which a computer performs operations on defined data without human input or intervention

10. One of the individuals involved in developing UNIVAC, the first commercially successful, general purpose, stored-program electronic digital computer
11. Primary control center unit built around a microprocessor
12. Term indicating that a computer is powered by electrical devices rather than by a mechanical device

DOWN

1. Leader of a team of scientists at Bell Laboratories who, in 1948, developed the transistor
2. Type of memory used for storing computational instructions or data that might change from time to time; sometimes called *read-write memory*
3. Computer on a chip
4. Device that identifies the route of entry and directs data from an input device to destinations; transfers computed results to the output device selected
5. Operation in which information is transferred into primary memory
6. Type of memory module that consists of groups of silicon chips etched with extremely small storage circuits
7. Operation in which results of a computation are transferred from primary memory to storage or to the user
8. Secondary memory device that stores digital data on a mirrored surface by modulating the reflective properties of that surface
9. In 1842, designed an analytic engine to perform general calculations automatically
10. Visible components of a computer
11. Secondary memory device that stores data in a series of concentric magnetic tracks

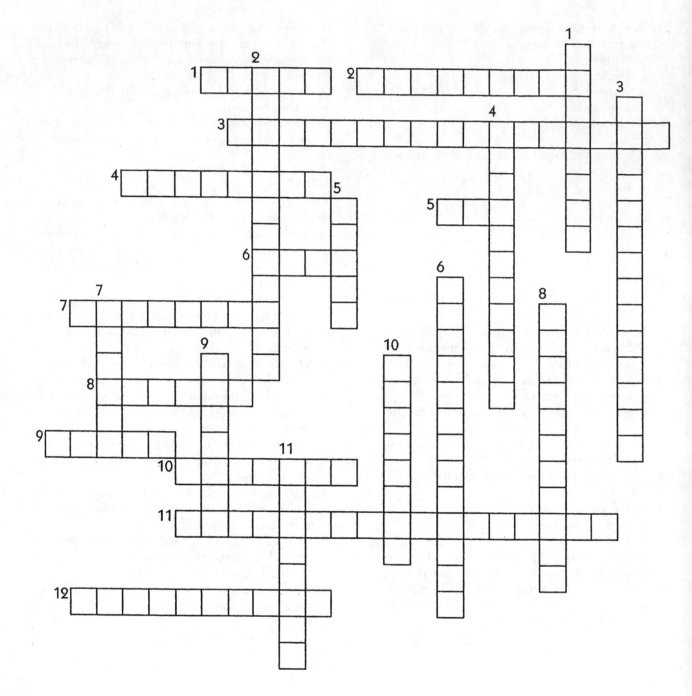

25-1 Computed Radiography Image Receptor

Computed radiography (CR) first appeared in 1984, but it took a decade for CR to become clinically acceptable. CR was the first example of digital radiography. Wet chemistry processing of a latent image is replaced with laser stimulation of metastable electrons that serve as the latent image.

The image receptor in CR is a photostimulable phosphor (PSP) made of barium fluorohalide such as barium fluorobromide (BaFlBr). It appears physically much as a radiographic intensifying screen. With a PSP, however, no light is emitted in response to x-ray exposure. Rather, electrons are energized into a metastable state by the interaction of x-rays.

When an intense laser light is incident on the PSP, light is emitted as the metastable electrons return to their ground state. The intensity of this laser-stimulated light is proportional to the x-ray intensity at the image receptor.

EXERCISES

1. What is the principal difference between screen-film radiography and computed radiography?
   a. Analog vs digital
   b. Involves light
   c. Requires processing
   d. The cassette
   e. Uses an imaging plate

2. The laser light used in CR:
   a. Is in the ultraviolet light region
   b. Is more energetic than the stimulated light
   c. Is pulsed across the photostimulable phosphor
   d. Has longer wavelength than the stimulated light
   e. Produces light of intense fluorescence

3. Which of the following steps can be eliminated during switching from screen-film radiography to CR?
   a. Hang images
   b. Perform examination
   c. Process image
   d. Reload cassette
   e. Repeat examination

4. An electron that is described as being metastable:
   a. Is outside of the atom
   b. Is present in positive and negative form
   c. Is the transformation of an x-ray
   d. Has been captured by the nucleus
   e. Has higher energy than it should have

5. Doping of a photostimulable phosphor with Europium results in:
   a. Better contrast resolution
   b. Better spatial resolution
   c. Higher x-ray absorption
   d. Lower patient dose
   e. More stimulable light emission

6. The activator in a photostimulable phosphor is there to:
   a. Define laser wavelength.
   b. Enhance electron metastability.
   c. Increase x-ray absorption.
   d. Select the proper wavelength.
   e. Shape the wavelength of stimulable emission.

7. Which of the following is most intense?
   a. Laser light
   b. Normal visual light

c. Optical lens support
d. Stimulable emission
e. X-ray beam

8. Which of the following is monochromatic?
   a. Infrared light
   b. Laser light
   c. Stimulated emission
   d. Visible light
   e. X-ray beam

9. Photostimulable phosphor image receptors are effective because:
   a. Metastable states are produced.
   b. Optical density is proportional to dose.
   c. Spatial resolution is improved.
   d. Their response follows the H & D curve.
   e. They are composed of detector elements (DELs).

10. The electron binding energy of a photostimulable phosphor is closest to:
    a. 10 keV
    b. 20 keV
    c. 35 keV
    d. 50 keV
    e. 75 keV

11. As a descriptor of a photostimulable phosphor, the term *turbid* refers to an appearance of:
    a. Black
    b. Clear
    c. Color
    d. Cloudy
    e. Gray

12. Europium is an activator in the photostimulable phosphor. An activator is responsible for:
    a. Contrast resolution
    b. Emitted light intensity
    c. Reduced patient dose
    d. Spatial resolution
    e. X-ray absorption

13. Photostimulable phosophor image receptors:
    a. Are relatively insensitive to x-rays
    b. Become radiation fatigued with age
    c. Can be fogged by background radiation
    d. Have better spatial resolution than screen-film radiography
    e. Require higher patient dose

14. To remove the image of background radiation or a previous image, one should:
    a. Clear the image receptor with a cleaning solution.
    b. Expose the image receptor to intense light.
    c. Expose the image receptor to intense x-ray exposure.
    d. Store the image receptor for 3 days.
    e. Transfer the image receptor signal to digital storage.

15. Which of the following is the proper sequence for producing a computed radiographic image?
    a. Erase/read/expose
    b. Expose/erase/read
    c. Expose/read/erase
    d. Read/erase/expose
    e. Read/expose/erase

The computed radiography reader (processor) appears much like a film daylight loader system. However, appearance is the only similarity between the two. Inside the computed radiography reader are mechanical drive mechanisms, optical shaping lenses and mirrors, and photosensitive detectors.

The mechanical drive mechanism supports a "slow" scan of the imaging plate by moving the plate slowly through the reader. The optical assembly supports a "fast" scan mode by deflecting the laser beam back and forth across the imaging plate as it is slow scanned.

Interaction of the laser beam with the imaging plate results in photostimulable emission, which is measured by a photodiode and quantified. The intensity of photostimulable emission is proportional to the intensity of the x-ray exposure to that portion of the imaging plate. The diameter of the laser beam and scan motion determine the size of each pixel.

EXERCISES

1. The photostimulable emission in computed radiography:
   a. Has longer wavelength than the laser-stimulating light
   b. Has shorter wavelength than the laser-stimulating light
   c. Is discrete, as is the laser-stimulating light
   d. Is in the far infrared region of the spectrum
   e. Is monochromatic, as is the laser-stimulating light

2. The slow-scan portion of the computed radiography reader:
   a. Has a speed that is determined by the emission rate
   b. Is under mechanical control
   c. Is under optical control
   d. Relies on a photometric response
   e. Requires mirrors and prisms

3. Spatial resolution in computed radiography is principally determined by:
   a. Fast-scan rate
   b. Field of view
   c. Laser beam diameter
   d. Phosphor size
   e. Slow-scan rate

4. The source of the stimulating light is:
   a. Emitted light
   b. The laser
   c. The optical path
   d. The photometer
   e. X-radiation

5. What is the approximate diameter of the laser beam?
   a. <1 μm
   b. 10 μm
   c. 100 μm
   d. 1000 μm
   e. >1000 μm

6. How does the computed radiography reader maintain the laser beam as a circle?
   a. Beam-shaping optics
   b. Fast-scan regulation

c. Intensity control
d. Light-collecting optics
e. Slow-scan regulation

7. Which of the following is NOT a photodetector?
   a. ADC
   b. CCD
   c. CMOS
   d. PD
   e. PMT

8. The x-ray capture element of a computed radiography imaging plate is the:
   a. BaFlBr
   b. Cassette
   c. CCD
   d. Laser beam
   e. Light-collecting optics

9. The characteristic curve of a computed radiography imaging plate is described as:
   a. Detective quantum efficiency
   b. Image buffer
   c. Image receptor response function
   d. Modulation transfer function
   e. Sampling quantization

10. A screen-film image receptor is responsive over how many orders of magnitude?
    a. One
    b. Two
    c. Three
    d. Four
    e. Five

11. An advantage of computed radiography over screen-film radiography, regardless of the type of examination, is the relatively constant:
    a. Image contrast
    b. Image processing
    c. Optical density
    d. Patient positioning
    e. Radiographic technique

12. Patient radiation dose reduction in computed radiography is limited by:
    a. Fast-scan mode
    b. Image contrast
    c. Patient size
    d. Slow-scan mode
    e. System noise

13. Which of the following statements applies when computed radiography is compared with screen-film radiography?
    a. kVp is less important.
    b. Image processing is faster.
    c. mAs is less important.
    d. Optical density is better.
    e. Patient positioning is easier.

14. Which of the following is an advantage of computed radiography over screen-film radiography?
    a. Easier viewing
    b. Fewer repeats
    c. Patient positioning
    d. Patient scheduling
    e. Technique selection

15. A computed radiography image receptor is responsive to an x-ray beam over how many orders of magnitude?
    a. One
    b. Two
    c. Three
    d. Four
    e. Five

Digital radiography produces digital radiographic images with a flat-panel solid-state image receptor. Three designs are in use: photostimulable phosphor charge-coupled device (CCD), amorphous silicon (a-Si), and amorphous selenium (a-Se).

EXERCISES

1. Which of the following is the principal disadvantage of the use of an area beam in digital radiography?
   a. Increased patient dose
   b. Lack of postexamination processing
   c. Reduced spatial resolution
   d. Scatter radiation
   e. Short exposure time

2. Rapid translation of the source-collimator-detector assembly across the patient during scanned projection digital radiography will do which of the following?
   a. Improve contrast resolution
   b. Reduce spatial resolution
   c. Reduce system noise
   d. Require higher kVp
   e. Slow the examination

3. Digital radiography:
   a. Has better spatial resolution
   b. Is faster
   c. Produces an initial image in analog form
   d. Requires computer processing
   e. Uses film as the image receptor

4. A scanned projection radiograph (SPR):
   a. Has better spatial resolution
   b. Has worse contrast than digital fluoroscopy
   c. Is like a tomograph
   d. Is virtually scatter-free
   e. Removes superposition of structures

5. Which of the following is a part of SPR?
   a. Analog-to-digital converter
   b. Area beam
   c. Data acquisition system
   d. Detector array
   e. Video monitor

6. The x-ray tube in digital radiography must have high heat capacity because of which of the following?
   a. High kVp
   b. High mA
   c. Long exposure time
   d. Reduced spatial resolution
   e. The number of images acquired

7. The principal advantage of the use of an area beam in digital radiography is which of the following?
   a. Improved contrast resolution
   b. Low patient dose
   c. Postexamination processing
   d. Scatter radiation rejection
   e. Short exposure time

8. Which of the following is an advantage of an area beam over SPR in digital radiography?
   a. Improved contrast
   b. Improved spatial resolution

c. Less technique required
d. Low noise
e. Reduced motion blur

9. Which of the following is used as an image receptor in digital radiography?
   a. An image intensifier
   b. $CaWO_4$
   c. $CdWO_4$
   d. Se
   e. Rare earth phosphors

10. The principal disadvantage of area-beam digital radiography is which of the following?
    a. Edge enhancement
    b. Longer exposure time
    c. Noise
    d. Poor contrast resolution
    e. Poor spatial resolution

11. A digital image constructed on a 512×512 matrix will have how many pixels?
    a. 512
    b. 1024
    c. 512^2
    d. 1024^2
    e. 1636

12. The minimum matrix size for an acceptable radiographic image is probably:
    a. $2^4 \times 2^4$
    b. $2^6 \times 2^6$
    c. $2^8 \times 2^8$
    d. $2^{10} \times 2^{10}$
    e. $2^{11} \times 2^{11}$

13. Which of the following is normally unique to digital radiography?
    a. A detector array
    b. Area x-ray beam
    c. Fast image access
    d. Remasking
    e. Reregistration

14. The image receptor in computed radiography is:
    a. a-Se
    b. a-Si
    c. BaFlCl
    d. $CaWO_4$
    e. $CdWO_4$

15. Which of the following is used as a radiation detector in digital radiography?
    a. BGO
    b. $CdWO_4$
    c. Ceramic
    d. Selenium
    e. Xenon

16. The principal limitation of the SPR mode of digital radiography is which of the following?
    a. Cost
    b. Examination time
    c. Image noise
    d. Patient dose
    e. Spatial resolution

17. An x-ray system used for digital radiography must have which of the following?
    a. A high heat capacity x-ray tube
    b. A modem
    c. A rapid film changer
    d. Access to the Internet
    e. At least two video monitors

18. Spatial resolution is improved in SPR by:
    a. Speeding up the examination
    b. Tighter collimation
    c. Using a higher heat capacity tube
    d. Using an image-intensifier tube
    e. Using more detectors per degree

19. The principal advantage of a fan-shaped x-ray beam over an area x-ray beam is which of the following?
    a. Examination time
    b. Hybrid images
    c. Less heat generated
    d. Reduced patient dose
    e. Scatter radiation rejection

20. Temporal subtraction in digital fluoroscopy:
    a. Can produce misregistered images
    b. Requires rapid kVp switching
    c. Results in higher dose than energy subtraction
    d. Takes longer than film subtraction
    e. Uses alternating x-ray beam filters

Digital fluoroscopy has been developed as a replacement for some earlier angiographic procedures such as subtraction angiography. With digital fluoroscopy, such subtraction images are relatively easily and quickly produced, and postprocessing and manipulation of the image are possible.

In digital fluoroscopy, a high signal-to-noise ratio, high-resolution video system is coupled with a computer. The video signal is digitized, manipulated in the computer by one of several techniques, and finally displayed on the video monitor. Alternatively, solid-state flat-panel image receptors produce direct digital images.

EXERCISES

1. The principal reason for image integration is to:
   a. Improve contrast resolution.
   b. Improve spatial resolution.
   c. Reduce examination time.
   d. Reduce image noise.
   e. Reduce patient dose.

2. The maximum frame acquisition rate in digital fluoroscopy is about:
   a. 1 frame per second
   b. 4 frames per second
   c. 10 frames per second
   d. 30 frames per second
   e. 60 frames per second

3. The signal-to-noise ratio of a conventional TV camera tube is about:
   a. 100:1
   b. 200:1
   c. 1000:1
   d. 2000:1
   e. 5000:1

4. Compared with conventional fluoroscopy, digital fluoroscopy is conducted:
   a. At much higher x-ray tube current
   b. At much lower x-ray tube current
   c. With a different type of image intensifier
   d. With a different type of video monitor
   e. With higher-capacity x-ray tubes

5. Digital imaging systems can display images on a 1024 × 1024 matrix. How many pixels are present in such a matrix?
   a. 1000
   b. 1024
   c. 2048
   d. 1,048,576
   e. It depends on the gray scale.

6. A conventional radiograph is which of the following?
   a. A digital image
   b. A geometric image
   c. A linear image
   d. An analog image
   e. An exponential image

7. Which of the following components found in digital fluoroscopy is **not** found in conventional fluoroscopy?
   a. A video monitor
   b. An automatic brightness stabilizer (ABS)
   c. An analog-to-digital converter (ADC)
   d. An image intensifier
   e. A source-to-image receptor distance (SID) indicator

8. During digital fluoroscopy, the image receptor is which of the following?
   a. Film
   b. The cassette
   c. The image-intensifier tube
   d. The TV camera tube
   e. The video monitor

9. A principal advantage of digital fluoroscopy over conventional fluoroscopy for subtraction studies is:
   a. Contrast enhancement
   b. Examination speed
   c. Less contrast material
   d. Low patient dose
   e. Noise enhancement

10. The approximate pixel size for a 12-inch image-intensifier tube and a 256 reconstruction matrix is:
    a. 0.4 mm
    b. 0.8 mm
    c. 1.0 mm
    d. 2.5 mm
    e. 4 mm

11. During digital fluoroscopy:
    a. Both cine and spot film modes can be used.
    b. Neither cine nor spot film modes can be used.
    c. The x-ray beam is continuous and at high mA.
    d. The x-ray beam is continuous and at low mA.
    e. The x-ray beam is pulsed.

12. Digital fluoroscopy is conducted:
    a. At relatively low mA
    b. In the progressive TV mode
    c. With direct-exposure film
    d. With low patient dose
    e. With low signal-to-noise ratio

13. How many video monitors are required for digital fluoroscopy?
    a. None
    b. One
    c. Two
    d. Three
    e. Four

14. The time-interval difference mode is best used for which of the following?
    a. Dynamic studies
    b. Extremities

   c. High-dose examinations
   d. Large fields
   e. Long exposure times

15. Reregistration of an image is used to do which of the following?
    a. Correct any error in patient identification
    b. Correct for motion
    c. Increase edge enhancement
    d. Reduce noise
    e. Reduce patient dose

16. The combination of temporal subtraction and energy subtraction techniques is called:
    a. Enhanced subtraction
    b. Hybrid subtraction
    c. No subtraction
    d. Radiographic subtraction
    e. Resonance subtraction

17. The minimum acceptable TV signal-to-noise ratio for digital fluoroscopy is:
    a. 100:1
    b. 200:1
    c. 1000:1
    d. 2000:1
    e. 5000:1

18. Interrogation time:
    a. Is the time spent questioning the patient
    b. Is the time needed to switch off the x-ray tube
    c. Is the time needed to switch on the x-ray tube
    d. Is the total exposure time
    e. Refers to the total examination time

19. A digital imaging system with a dynamic range of 2^{10} will be able to reproduce how many shades of gray?
    a. 32
    b. 256
    c. 512
    d. 1024
    e. 4096

20. The approach to digital radiography used in computed tomography (CT) is called:
    a. Area-beam imaging
    b. Computed radiography
    c. Digital subtraction angiography
    d. Digital vascular imaging
    e. Scanned projection radiography

21. An advantage of digital imaging over conventional imaging is which of the following?
    a. Increased latitude
    b. Increased resolution
    c. Postprocessing
    d. Reduced noise
    e. Reduced speed

22. A pixel is a:
    a. Matrix of numbers
    b. Range of numbers
    c. Three-dimensional digital image cell
    d. Two-dimensional digital image cell
    e. Unit of fluoroscopy dose

23. Between the TV camera and the computer of a digital fluoroscopic system is a/an:
    a. Analog-to-digital converter
    b. Digital-to-analog converter
    c. Image-intensifier tube
    d. Image storage device
    e. Second video monitor

24. The mask image is usually the:
    a. First image
    b. Image at the peak of contrast
    c. Image just preceding contrast
    d. Last contrast image
    e. Last image

25. Energy subtraction is based on which of the following?
    a. Changing mAs
    b. Contrast enhancement
    c. K-edge absorption
    d. Noise reduction
    e. Time differences

26. As one integrates video frames in digital fluoroscopy:
    a. Image noise is lower.
    b. Patient dose increases.
    c. Spatial resolution is improved.
    d. The signal-to-noise ratio increases.
    e. Video noise is louder.

27. Which of the following components is uniquely essential to digital fluoroscopy?
    a. ADC
    b. CRT
    c. High-frequency generator
    d. TV camera pickup tube
    e. TV monitor

28. A misregistration artifact:
    a. Cannot be corrected or compensated
    b. Is not really an artifact
    c. Occurs when a patient moves
    d. Requires more hardware than is usually available
    e. Usually follows a change in kVp

29. Remasking:
    a. Can correct for patient motion
    b. Reduces spatial resolution
    c. Requires a change in kVp
    d. Requires a repeat examination
    e. Will increase patient dose

30. A matrix of what size can be held by 10 bytes of memory?
    a. 256×256
    b. 512×512
    c. 1024×1024
    d. 2084×2084
    e. 4096×4096

31. A 7-bit pixel can display how many shades of gray?
    a. 7
    b. 49
    c. 64
    d. 128
    e. 256

32. How much computer memory is required to store 10 chest images in a 256×256 matrix with 64 shades of gray?
    a. 1 MB
    b. 4 MB
    c. 16 MB
    d. 64 MB
    e. 128 MB

33. How many numbers can be stored in 7 bits?
    a. 64
    b. 128
    c. 256
    d. 512
    e. 1024

34. How many bits are required to display 512 shades of gray?
    a. 5
    b. 6
    c. 7
    d. 8
    e. 9

35. How many shades of gray are possible in a pixel of size 2^{10}?
    a. 64
    b. 128
    c. 256
    d. 512
    e. 1024

36. For computational and storage purposes, a string of bits is arranged in a/an:
    a. Array
    b. Byte
    c. Matrix
    d. Sector
    e. Track

37. For a digital subtraction angiography image, 256 photons are incident on a pixel. What is the signal-to-noise ratio?
    a. 2
    b. 4
    c. 6
    d. 10
    e. 16

Spatial Resolution

The ability of an imaging system to render on the image a faithful reproduction of a small, high-contrast object is termed *spatial resolution*. The smaller the object that can be imaged, the better is the spatial resolution.

It is easy to image smaller and smaller objects and to state spatial resolution in terms of object size—1 cm, 1 mm, or 1 μm. In medical imaging, spatial resolution is expressed in terms of spatial frequency—frequency in space. Spatial frequency is a measure of how quickly, in space, an object changes.

Tissues can be identified by their spatial frequency. Calcified lung nodules or breast microcalcifications are high spatial frequency objects. Abdominal tissue, fat, and soft tissue masses are low spatial frequency objects. It is difficult for any imaging system to image both high-frequency objects and low-frequency objects.

As a generalization, digital imaging systems have better contrast resolution but poorer spatial resolution than screen-film imaging systems.

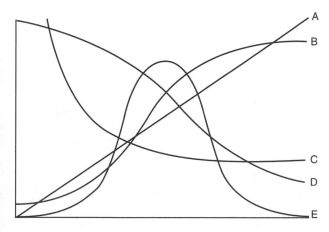

EXERCISES

1. Spatial frequency consists of units of:
   a. Line length
   b. Line pair
   c. Line pair/millimeter
   d. Millimeter
   e. Millimeter/line pair

2. What value of modulation transfer function (MTF) is often used by imaging system vendors to describe their imaging system?
   a. 0%
   b. 10%
   c. 25%
   d. 50%
   e. 100%

3. As an object gets smaller, which of the following gets bigger?
   a. ll
   b. lp
   c. lp/mm
   d. mm
   e. mm/lp

4. Which of the curves above represents a modulation transfer function?
   A
   B
   C
   D
   E

5. A breast microcalcification is spherical and 300 μm in diameter. What is the spatial frequency of this tissue object?
   a. 0.5 lp/mm
   b. 0.6 lp/mm
   c. 1.0 lp/mm
   d. 1.7 lp/mm
   e. 2.7 lp/mm

6. Screen-film radiography can image to 8 lp/mm. This represents an object of approximately what size?
   a. 25 μm
   b. 63 μm
   c. 128 μm
   d. 250 μm
   e. 500 μm

7. Which of the curves above represents a contrast-detail curve?
   A
   B
   C
   D
   E

8. Modulation in imaging is a term that is best described as the:
   a. Ability to image rate of change
   b. Frequency of tissue
   c. Intrinsic contrast of tissue
   d. Repeat rate
   e. Size of an object

9. A calcified lung nodule measures 1 cm. What spatial frequency does this represent?
   a. 0.05 lp/mm
   b. 0.1 lp/mm
   c. 0.5 lp/mm
   d. 1.0 lp/mm
   e. 5.0 lp/mm

10. Which of the curves above represents a characteristic screen-film response?
    A
    B
    C
    D
    E

11. The best a multislice computed tomography imaging system can image is 1.5 lp/mm. This represents an object of what size?
    a. 125 μm
    b. 333 μm
    c. 400 μm
    d. 550 μm
    e. 675 μm

12. The modulation transfer function for a digital imaging system has a cutoff spatial frequency of 5 lp/mm. What is the pixel size?
    a. 10 μm
    b. 25 μm
    c. 50 μm
    d. 100 μm
    e. 200 μm

13. Which of the curves above represents the digital image receptor radiation response?
    A
    B
    C
    D
    E

14. Why does digital radiography have a higher modulation transfer function at low spatial frequencies than does screen-film imaging?
    a. Better contrast resolution
    b. Fewer repeats
    c. Higher detective quantum efficiency (DQE)
    d. Less kVp dependence
    e. Lower patient dose

15. Which of the curves above represents a line spread function?
    A
    B
    C
    D
    E

16. Which of the curves above are related when space is converted to spatial frequency?
    A to D
    B to C
    B to D
    C to A
    E to A

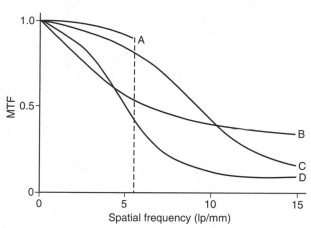

17. Which of the curves above represents best spatial resolution?
    A
    B
    C
    D

18. Which of the curves above represents best contrast resolution?
    A
    B
    C
    D

19. Which of the above curves represents digital radiography?
    A
    B
    C
    D

Contrast Resolution
Contrast Detail

Although it is clear that digital radiography has poorer spatial resolution than screen-film imaging, it is also becoming clearer that the superior contrast resolution of digital imaging is important for image quality and interpretation. Contrast resolution results in the ability to distinguish many shades of gray on an image.

The number of gray levels that an imaging system can produce is called *dynamic range*. The human visual system can see perhaps 30 shades of gray, and that is what we are stuck with when we use screen-film radiography. Today's digital imaging systems are capable of rendering up to 65,536 shades of gray (16 bits), all visible with postprocessing of the image.

One method for evaluating the relative spatial and contrast resolutions of imaging systems is the contrast-detail curve. Use of such a curve shows that spatial resolution is determined by the modulation transfer function (MTF) of the imaging system; contrast resolution is limited by the noise of the system.

EXERCISES

1. Which of the following reduces contrast resolution?
   a. Detective quantum efficiency
   b. kVp
   c. mAs
   d. Modulation transfer function
   e. Noise

2. If the dynamic range of a magnetic resonance imaging system is 12 bits, how many shades of grays are present?
   a. 1024
   b. 2048
   c. 4096
   d. 8192
   e. 16384

3. Patient radiation dose should be lower when digital imaging is used than when screen-film imaging is used, principally because of:
   a. Detective quantum efficiency
   b. kVp
   c. mAs
   d. Modulation transfer function
   e. Noise

4. Contrast resolution in computed tomography is superior because of:
   a. Collimation
   b. Detective quantum efficiency
   c. Image receptor response curve
   d. Modulation transfer function
   e. Spiral motion

5. "Technique creep" is an attempt to reduce patient radiation dose by instituting:
   a. Increased detective quantum efficiency (DQE)
   b. Increased kVp and reduced mAs
   c. Increased mAs and reduced kVp
   d. Increased mAs and reduced noise
   e. No repeats

6. The digital radiographic imaging repeat rate should not exceed:
   a. 0%
   b. 1%
   c. 5%
   d. 10%
   e. 25%

7. Detective quantum efficiency (DQE) is a measure of:
   a. Contrast resolution
   b. Digital data file size
   c. Image noise
   d. Spatial resolution
   e. X-ray absorption

8. The principal advantage of digital radiography over screen-film radiography is:
   a. Contrast resolution
   b. Easier patient positioning
   c. Fewer repeats
   d. Less noise
   e. Reduced radiographic technique

9. How is the x-ray beam incident on the image receptor described?
   a. High kVp
   b. Higher mAs
   c. K-edge absorption
   d. Lower energy
   e. Percent transmission

10. What happens at the K-edge of the phosphor of a receptor?
    a. Higher noise
    b. Higher x-ray absorption
    c. Lower detective quantum efficiency
    d. Lower modulation transfer function
    e. Lower x-ray absorption

11. Which of the following is **not** an image capture element for digital imaging?
    a. BaFBr
    b. CCD
    c. CsI
    d. GdOS
    e. LaOS

12. Which of these contrast-detail curves represents best spatial resolution?
    A
    B
    C
    D
    E

13. Why did you make that selection for Question #12?
    a. Highest mAs
    b. Highest modulation transfer function
    c. Lowest kVp
    d. Smallest focal-spot size
    e. Smallest pixel size

14. Which of the above contrast-detail curves represents best contrast resolution?
    A
    B
    C
    D
    E

15. Why did you make that selection for Question #14?
    a. Attenuation coefficient (u)
    b. Detective quantum efficiency
    c. Effective dose
    d. Modulation transfer function (MTF)
    e. Proton density, T1, T2

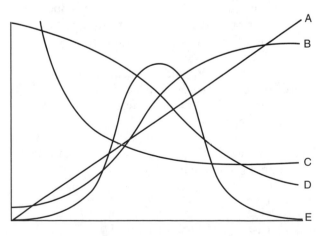

The adoption of digital imaging brings with it a new set of required physics skills. In addition to the physics of ionizing radiation, we must have an understanding of the physics of visible light and how it affects image interpretation.

Photometry is the science of visible light, including its emission, reflection, and measurement. The basic unit of photometry is the lumen, which quantifies the intensity of light from a source. A digital image on a digital display device is called *soft copy*, and a screen-film image on a viewbox is referred to as *hard copy*.

A major advantage of digital imaging is that it allows one to preprocess and postprocess the image, to accentuate image detail. Further, the digital image can be viewed by different people in different locations through the Picture Archiving and Communication System (PACS), which is not available with screen-film imaging.

EXERCISES

1. Photometry is the science of the:
   a. Anatomy of human vision
   b. Measurement of light
   c. Quantity of light
   d. Reflection and refraction of light
   e. Response of the human eye to light

2. The postprocessing manipulation called *image inversion* refers to:
   a. Changing from landscape to portrait format
   b. Exchange of images
   c. Reorienting right and left
   d. Reorienting top and bottom
   e. Turning white-black to black-white

3. Photopic vision is associated with:
   a. Color vision
   b. Cone vision
   c. Dim light
   d. Color vision
   e. Rod vision

4. How does one preprocess a digital image to correct for pixel, row, or column defects?
   a. Dark reference correction
   b. Extrapolation algorithms
   c. Interpolation algorithms
   d. Offset correction
   e. Pixel reregistration

5. Which of the following describes the luminous intensity from a light source such as a light bulb?
   a. Cosine law
   b. Illuminance
   c. Luminance
   d. Luminance intensity
   e. Luminous flux

6. What is the approximate illuminance of an indoor tennis court?
   a. 5 fc
   b. 20 fc
   c. 30 fc
   d. 100 fc
   e. 200 fc

7. The luminance of a digital display device is measured in:
   a. Candela
   b. Candela per meter squared

c. Footcandle

d. Lumen

e. Lux

8. What is the matrix array of a 5 MB digital display device?

a. 500 × 1000 pixels

b. 1000 × 1000 pixels

c. 1200 × 1800 pixels

d. 1500 × 2000 pixels

e. 2000 × 2500 pixels

9. Which of the following is characteristic of a CRT but not of an AMLCD?

a. Active matrix address

b. Flat face

c. Light modulating

d. Square pixel

e. Veiling glare

10. What unit is used to describe illuminance, the intensity of light incident on a surface?

a. Candela

b. Candela per meter squared

c. Footcandle

d. Lumen

e. Lux

11. The luminance of a mammography viewbox must be uniform and at least 3000 nit. What is a nit?

a. Candela per foot squared

b. Candela per meter squared

c. Lumen per foot squared

d. Lumen per meter squared

e. Lumen per steradian

12. With digital radiography, the cosine law applies to:

a. Grayscale imaging

b. Image inversion

c. Inverse square law

d. Off-axis viewing

e. Reduced spatial resolution

13. Compared with photopic vision, scotopic vision:

a. Has better spatial resolution

b. Involves cones

c. Is bright light vision

d. Is more color vision

e. Occurs at shorter wavelengths

14. An active matrix liquid crystal display is better than a cathode ray tube display because:

a. Of its light-emitting property

b. Of its phosphor face

c. It has a curved face

d. It is a light-modulating device

e. It uses a scanning electron beam

15. Liquid crystals are:

a. Linear organic molecules

b. Phosphor grains

c. Photo-detecting devices

d. Thin film transistors

e. Solid grains embedded in glass

16. The aperature ratio refers to the:

a. Ability to control individual pixels

b. Percent of light transmission

c. Size of a pixel

d. Size of the liquid crystals

e. Viewing of an image off-axis

17. Ergonomics is the study of:

a. Hospital information systems

b. Human factors applied to system design

c. Light levels in work areas

d. Light illumination of workstations

e. Picture Archiving and Communications Systems

30-1

AAPM TG-18

Quality control programs supporting screen-film radiography are directed to wet chemistry processing and viewbox illumination, among other activities. Times are changing, and rapidly. Similar quality control activities associated with digital imaging are associated with image receptor response and digital display devices used for image interpretation.

Digital display devices may have a number of deficiencies that can interfere with image interpretation. Several organizations have developed electronic test patterns to assess the image quality of a digital display device.

The American Association of Physicists in Medicine (AAPM) has taken the lead in developing electronic test patterns for quality control procedures for digital display devices. These test patterns are designed to be used regularly to evaluate characteristics of digital monitors such as geometric distortion, reflection, resolution, noise, and other features. Users should now use these test patterns in an ordered program of quality control.

EXERCISES

1. Which of the following organizations never developed electronic test patterns for digital display quality control?
   a. ANSI
   b. AAPM
   c. NEMA
   d. SMPTE
   e. VESA

2. GSDF stands for:
   a. Grand source of detected features
   b. Grayscale display function
   c. Great seal of dynamic function
   d. Gross scale of dynamic factors
   e. Ground source determined factor

3. Luminance response of a digital display device is properly accomplished with a:
   a. Charge-coupled device
   b. Densitometer
   c. Illuminator
   d. Photometer
   e. Sensitometer

4. This is the AAPM TG-18 QC test pattern. What is it used to evaluate?

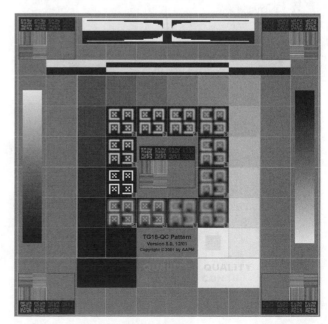

TG18-QC Pattern
Version 8.0, 12/01
Copyright © 2001 by AAPM

a. Artifacts
b. Contrast resolution
c. Geometric distortion
d. Noise
e. Spatial resolution

5. This is the AAPM TG-18 AD test pattern. What is it used to evaluate?

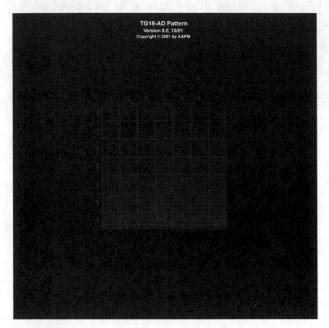

a. Artifacts
b. Contrast resolution
c. Diffuse reflection
d. Geometric distortion
e. Noise

6. This is the AAPM TG-18 CT test pattern that contains 16 shades of gray. What is it used to evaluate?

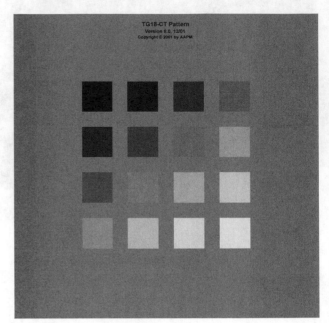

a. Contrast resolution
b. Diffuse reflection
c. Geometric distortion
d. Luminance response
e. Noise

7. This is the AAPM TG-18 LN test pattern that contains three images. What is it used to evaluate?

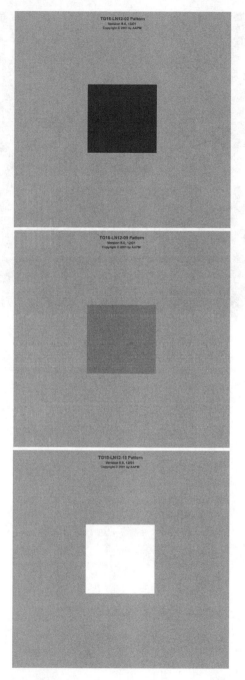

8. This is the AAPM TG-18 UN test pattern that contains three nine-section images. What is it used to evaluate?

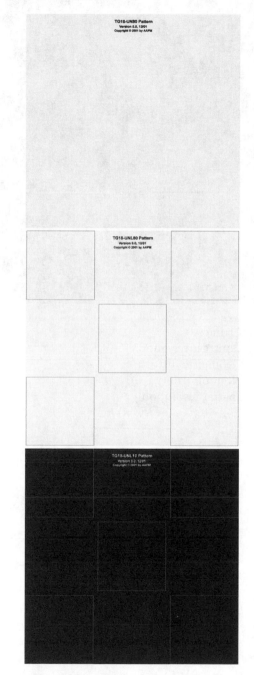

a. Artifacts
b. Contrast resolution
c. Diffuse reflection
d. Luminance
e. Noise

a. Contrast resolution
b. Diffuse reflection
c. Geometric distortion
d. Luminance
e. Nonuniformity

9. This is the AAPM TG-18 CX test pattern. What is it used to evaluate?

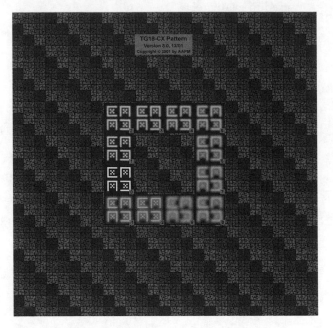

a. Artifacts
b. Contrast resolution
c. Geometric distortion
d. Nonuniformity
e. Spatial resolution

10. This is the AAPM TG-18 PX test pattern with a rather uniform intensity. What is it used to evaluate?

a. Contrast resolution
b. Diffuse reflection
c. Noise
d. Nonuniformity
e. Resolution uniformity

11. This is the AAPM TG-18 AFC test pattern that
    contains low-contrast squares. What is it used
    to evaluate?

TG18-AFC Pattern
Version 8.0, 12/01
Copyright © 2001 by AAPM

a. Artifacts
b. Contrast resolution
c. Luminance
d. Noise
e. Nonuniformity

An artifact is any feature on an image that does not truly represent tissue. Artifacts can interfere with diagnosis and obscure lesions or normal anatomy.

Digital imaging artifacts can be classified into three categories: image receptor artifacts, object artifacts, and processing artifacts. The radiologic technologist must be able to identify the source of an artifact.

Artifacts associated with pixel failure are easily identified but may be difficult to correct. Environmental radiation or previous exposure of computed radiography image receptors can produce ghost images. These are easily corrected. Preprocessing and postprocessing artifacts also are easily corrected, and the correction is automatic.

In general, digital artifacts are easier to correct than screen-film artifacts.

EXERCISES

1. Which of the following is NOT a digital imaging artifact?
   a. Alignment
   b. Collimation
   c. Density difference
   d. Image compression
   e. Partition

2. When does the radiologic technologist have to be concerned with processing artifacts?
   a. When compression is employed
   b. When image histograms are used
   c. When images are printed
   d. When partition is involved
   e. When software is corrupted

3. Ghost images can appear when:
   a. Radiation fatigue is present.
   b. Dust remains on the image receptor.
   c. A CR image receptor has not been erased in 24 hours.
   d. A DR image receptor is not completely read out.
   e. A proper QC program is not instituted.

4. Which of the following should be presented to the radiologist for interpretation?
   a. For-compression image
   b. For-extrapolation image
   c. For-interpolation image
   d. For-presentation image
   e. For-processing image

5. Flatfielding is a preprocessing feature used to apply:
   a. Contrast resolution correction
   b. Geometric distortion correction
   c. Equalize response program
   d. Noise reduction algorithms
   e. Spatial resolution enhancement

6. What level of image compression is considered acceptable?
   a. 3:1
   b. 5:1
   c. 8:1
   d. 10:1
   e. 20:1

7. What does this artifact represent?

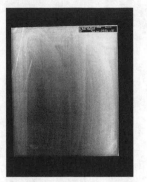

   a. Damaged imaging plate
   b. Debris on imaging plate
   c. Inadequate erasure
   d. Postprocessing artifact
   e. Preprocessing artifact

8. What does this artifact represent?
   a. Inadequate erasure
   b. Inappropriate reconstruction algorithm
   c. Improper alignment
   d. Improper collimation
   e. Improper partition

9. What does this artifact represent?

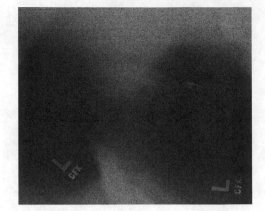

   a. Ghost image
   b. Improper collimation
   c. Improper partition
   d. Inadequate erasure
   e. Preprocessing artifact

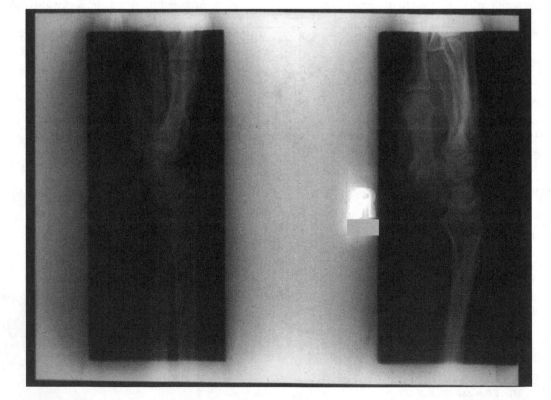

10. What is the cause of this artifact?

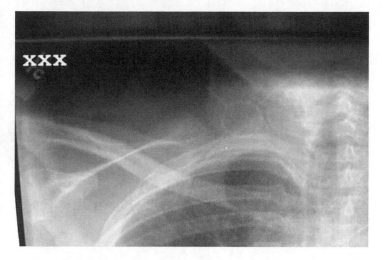

a. Debris on image receptor
b. Ghost image
c. Improper alignment
d. Improper collimation
e. Improper partition

32-1 Human Radiation Response Composition of the Body

An understanding of how radiation affects biologic tissue is essential to the radiologic technologist's task of producing high-quality x-ray images with a minimum of radiation exposure. The composition of the human body has its basis in atoms, and it is at the atomic level that radiation interacts.

The atomic composition of the body determines the character and degree of the radiation interaction, and molecular and tissue composition defines the nature of the radiation response.

The following list summarizes the atomic composition of the body and shows that more than 85% of the body is hydrogen and oxygen.

- 0.1% phosphorus
- 0.1% sulfur
- 0.2% calcium
- 0.8% trace elements
- 2.4% nitrogen
- 10.7% carbon
- 25.7% oxygen
- 60.0% hydrogen

EXERCISES

1. The effects of fetal irradiation include all of the following **except**:
   a. Childhood malignancy
   b. Congenital malformation
   c. Diminished growth and development
   d. Erythema
   e. Neonatal death

2. Which of the following human responses to ionizing radiation would be categorized as a late effect?
   a. Central nervous system syndrome
   b. Gastrointestinal syndrome
   c. Eye damage
   d. Extremity damage
   e. Hematologic depression

3. Anton van Leeuwenhoek:
   a. Accurately described a living cell in 1673 on the basis of microscopic observations
   b. Described atoms as having eyes and hooks
   c. Described the molecular structure of DNA in 1953
   d. First named the cell in 1665
   e. Showed conclusively that all plants and animals contain cells as their basic functional units

4. Schlieiden and Schwann:
   a. Accurately described a living cell in 1673 on the basis of microscopic observations
   b. Described the molecular structure of DNA in 1953
   c. Developed the original periodic table
   d. First named the cell in 1665
   e. Showed conclusively that all plants and animals contain cells as their basic functional units

5. Watson and Crick:
   a. Accurately described a living cell in 1673 on the basis of microscopic observations
   b. Described the molecular structure of DNA in 1953

c. Discovered x-ray crystallography
d. First named the cell in 1665
e. Showed conclusively that all plants and animals contain cells as their basic functional units

6. Approximately what percentage of the body is water?
   a. 20
   b. 35
   c. 50
   d. 65
   e. 80

7. "Crossing over":
   a. Is a process that occurs during meiosis, resulting in changes in genetic constitution and inheritable traits
   b. Is characterized by the disappearance of structural chromosomes into a mass of DNA
   c. Is the final phase of mitosis
   d. Is the period of cell growth between divisions
   e. Is the phase of the cell cycle during which the nucleus swells and the DNA becomes more prominent and begins to take structural form

8. Ribosomes:
   a. Are called the workhorses of the cell
   b. Are helpful in the control of intracellular contaminants
   c. Are sites of protein synthesis that are essential to normal function
   d. Are small, pea-like sacs that are capable of digesting cellular fragments and even the cell itself
   e. Digest macromolecules to produce energy for the cell

9. Lysosomes:
   a. Are called the workhorses of the cell
   b. Are sites of protein synthesis that are essential to normal cellular function
   c. Contain enzymes capable of digesting cell fragments
   d. Deliver energy to target molecules
   e. Digest macromolecules to produce energy for the cell

10. The production of large molecules from small is called:
    a. Anabolism
    b. Catabolism
    c. Hormesis

d. Metabolism
e. Mitosis

11. Which of the following are present in all tissues of the body and are the structural components of cell membranes?
    a. Carbohydrates
    b. Lipids
    c. Nucleic acids
    d. Proteins
    e. Sugar

12. The chief function of carbohydrates in the body is to:
    a. Assist in maintaining body temperature.
    b. Exercise regulatory control over functions such as growth and metabolic rate.
    c. Provide a defense mechanism against infection and disease.
    d. Provide fuel for cell metabolism.
    e. Provide structure and support.

13. During which of the following subphases of meiosis does each chromosome split at the centromere, so that two chromatids are connected by a fiber to the poles of the nucleus?
    a. Anaphase
    b. Metaphase
    c. Prophase
    d. Telophase
    e. None of the above

14. Which of the following is the concept of the relative constancy of the internal environment of the human body?
    a. Homeostasis
    b. Hormesis
    c. Meiosis
    d. Molecular composition
    e. Radiation hormesis

15. RNA:
    a. Contains all the hereditary information that represents a cell
    b. Is a principal component of a hormone
    c. Is located principally in the cytoplasm of the cell
    d. Is located principally in the nucleus of the cell
    e. Serves as the command or control molecule for all functions

32-2

From Molecules to Humans
Human Biology

To understand the effects of radiation on the human body, one must have a basic knowledge of human anatomy and physiology. The body is an extremely organized system, but it is composed mostly of water. Radiation interactions at the atomic level are transferred through the various levels of organization and can result in visible radiation effects.

The single most important molecule in the body is deoxyribonucleic acid (DNA). DNA contains all of the genes and is responsible for controlling the body's growth, development, and function.

It is assumed that the principal type of radiation damage is inflicted on the cell's control center—the DNA—and results in errors in metabolism that can produce a visible radiation effect.

EXERCISES

1. Which of the following is an example of a macromolecule?
   a. A free radical
   b. A lipid
   c. An amino acid
   d. Salt
   e. Water

2. The breaking down of macromolecules into water and carbon dioxide is:
   a. Anabolism
   b. Catabolism
   c. Homeostasis
   d. Hormesis
   e. Metabolism

3. In the human cell:
   a. Both the cytoplasm and the nucleus are surrounded by membranes.
   b. Lysosomes contain nucleic acid.
   c. Macromolecules are digested in the ribosomes.
   d. Macromolecules are synthesized in the mitochondria.
   e. The DNA passes through the endoplasmic reticulum.

4. Which of the following is part of interphase?
   a. DNA synthesis phase
   b. G_0 phase
   c. Prophase
   d. Protein synthesis phase
   e. Telophase

5. The body is organized in such a way that:
   a. Differentiated cells are immature.
   b. Epithelial cells usually are found inside organs.
   c. Mature cells are called stem cells.
   d. Organs combine to form tissues.
   e. Tissues and organs form an organ system.

6. Which of the following molecules is a protein?
   a. A lipid
   b. A nucleic acid
   c. A salt
   d. An amino acid
   e. An enzyme

7. Lipids are:
   a. An energy storehouse
   b. Electrical conductors

   c. Inorganic compounds
   d. Micromolecules
   e. The site of protein synthesis

8. At metaphase, the chromosomes:
   a. Are visible in the microscope
   b. Line up at the poles of the cell
   c. Ooze through the cellular membrane
   d. Remain dominant
   e. Split apart and replicate

9. Lipids store which of the following?
   a. Antibodies
   b. Enzymes
   c. Fat
   d. Salt
   e. Sugar

10. At what phase in mitosis are the chromosomes **most** visible?
   a. Anaphase
   b. Interphase
   c. Metaphase
   d. Prophase
   e. Telophase

11. Messenger RNA (mRNA) moves from:
   a. Cytoplasm to mitochondria
   b. Cytoplasm to nucleus
   c. Nucleus to lysosome
   d. Nucleus to mitochondria
   e. Nucleus to ribosome

12. Which element is **most** abundant in the body?
   a. Calcium
   b. Carbon
   c. Hydrogen
   d. Nitrogen
   e. Oxygen

13. Organic molecules:
   a. Contain calcium
   b. Contain carbon
   c. Contain nitrogen
   d. Include all nucleic acids
   e. Include DNA

14. Which of the following is a principal component of protein?
   a. Amino acid
   b. Enzyme
   c. Lipid
   d. Peptide bond
   e. Sugar

15. Which molecule is **most** abundant in the body?
   a. Carbohydrate
   b. Lipid
   c. Nucleic acid
   d. Protein
   e. Water

16. The general formula ($C_nH_nO_n$) represents which of the following?
   a. Amino acids
   b. Carbohydrates
   c. Genes
   d. Nucleic acids
   e. Proteins

17. Polysaccharides are which of the following?
   a. Carbohydrates
   b. Free radicals
   c. Lipids
   d. Nucleic acids
   e. Proteins

18. Which of the following base pairs is allowed for DNA?
   a. Adenine-cytosine
   b. Adenine-guanine
   c. Cytosine-thymine
   d. Guanine-cytosine
   e. Thymine-guanine

19. The nucleolus in particular contains which of the following?
   a. Amino acids
   b. DNA
   c. Lipids
   d. Proteins
   e. RNA

20. Homeostasis refers to what property of the body?
   a. Atomic composition
   b. Constancy of the internal environment
   c. Molecular composition
   d. Resistance to radiation
   e. Water content

21. Which of the following is the nitrogenous organic base found in RNA but **not** in DNA?
   a. Adenine
   b. Cytosine
   c. Guanine
   d. Thymine
   e. Uracil

22. The nucleic acids of the cell:
    a. Are found only in the nucleus
    b. Are macromolecules
    c. Consist of DNA and RNA
    d. Have a backbone of peptide bonds
    e. Store energy

23. Most radiobiologic research is conducted with animals. Approximately how many human population groups have shown radiation effects?
    a. None
    b. Fewer than 5
    c. 5 to 10
    d. 10 to 20
    e. More than 20

24. Human responses to radiation that do **not** appear for years are called:
    a. Large effects
    b. Late effects
    c. Latent response
    d. Law effects
    e. Linear effects

25. Which of the following tissues is most radiosensitive?
    a. Bone marrow
    b. Brain
    c. Breast
    d. Muscle
    e. Skin

26. Which of the following is the first step in producing a radiation response?
    a. Ionization
    b. Latent effect
    c. Manifestation of a lesion
    d. Molecular alteration
    e. Removal and isolation of a lesion

27. During which of the following subphases of meiosis do the chromosomes appear and line up along the equator of the nucleus?
    a. Anaphase
    b. Metaphase
    c. Prophase
    d. Telophase
    e. None of the above

28. Which of the following make(s) up the bulk of the cell and contain(s) all of the molecular components in great quantity?
    a. Cellular inclusions
    b. Cytoplasm
    c. Endoplasmic reticulum
    d. Membranes
    e. Nucleus

29. Which of the following searches the cytoplasm for the amino acid for which it is coded, attaches to that amino acid, and then carries it to the ribosome?
    a. A codon
    b. DNA
    c. mRNA
    d. The endoplasmic reticulum
    e. tRNA

30. Meiosis:
    a. Is characterized by these four subphases: prophase, metaphase, anaphase, and telophase
    b. Is the process of division and reduction that occurs in genetic cells
    c. Is the process of division that occurs in somatic cells
    d. Results in the formation of two genetically identical daughter cells that look precisely like the parent cell
    e. None of the above

Law of Bergonie and Tribondeau
Physical Factors That Affect Radiosensitivity

 Linear energy transfer (LET) expressed in keV/μm is the rate at which energy is transferred from ionizing radiation to tissue. In general, high LET radiation is more damaging than low-LET radiation.

Different types of ionizing radiation have different LET, and the efficiency for producing a given response is related to LET. Such efficiency is measured by the relative biologic effectiveness (RBE), which is determined experimentally.

$$RBE = \frac{\text{Dose of standard radiation necessary to produce a given effect}}{\text{Dose of test radiation necessary to produce the same effect}}$$

EXERCISES

1. Which of the following is a part of the law of Bergonie and Tribondeau?
   a. A fetus is less radiosensitive than an adult.
   b. Stem cells are radiosensitive.
   c. The more mature a cell is, the more radiosensitive it is.
   d. When metabolism is high, radiosensitivity is low.
   e. When proliferation rate is high, so is radioresistance.

2. The law of Bergonie and Tribondeau states that:
   a. Mature cells are more sensitive than stem cells.
   b. Metabolic activity results in radioprotection.
   c. Radiosensitivity increases with increasing hypoxia.
   d. Radiosensitivity increases with proliferation rate.
   e. The older a cell is, the more radiosensitive it is.

3. The response of tissue to radiation is principally a function of which of the following?
   a. Dose
   b. Fractionation
   c. LET
   d. Oxygen enhancement ratio (OER)
   e. RBE

4. The RBE:
   a. Describes tissue radiosensitivity
   b. Increases as x-ray energy increases
   c. Is a descriptor of the type of radiation
   d. Is equal to 3 keV/μm for alpha particles
   e. Is equal to 3 keV/μm for diagnostic x-rays

5. The law of Bergonie and Tribondeau relates to which of the following?
   a. Radiocurability and tumor size
   b. Radioresistance and cell lethality
   c. Radioresistance and oxygenation
   d. Radiosensitivity and cellular differentiation
   e. Radiosensitivity and oxygenation

6. The RBE:
   a. Has a value of 1 to 100
   b. Is a ratio of effects needed to produce a given dose
   c. Is a ratio of effects produced at a given dose
   d. Is higher for high-LET radiation than for low-LET radiation
   e. Refers to type of effect

7. LET is measured in which of the following?
   a. Gray
   b. keV/rad
   c. keV/μm
   d. rad
   e. rad/μm

8. Which of the following has the highest LET?
   a. Alpha particles
   b. Cobalt-60 gamma rays
   c. Diagnostic x-rays
   d. Neutrons
   e. Protons

9. The maximum value of RBE is approximately:
   a. 0.5
   b. 1
   c. 2
   d. 3
   e. 10

10. Dose fractionation is less effective than a single dose because:
    a. Dose fractionation has a low LET.
    b. Dose fractionation has a low OER.
    c. Fractionated doses are lower.
    d. Recovery occurs between doses.
    e. The RBE is less.

11. The OER:
    a. Has a maximum value of about 10
    b. Is higher for protons than for photons
    c. Is highest for high-LET radiation
    d. Is highest for low-LET radiation
    e. Is independent of LET

12. LET is useful for expressing radiation:
    a. Dose
    b. Production
    c. Quality
    d. Quantity
    e. Response

13. What is related to radiation protection as LET is related to radiobiology?
    a. Dose
    b. Quantity factor
    c. Radiation weighting factor (WR)
    d. Response
    e. Tissue weighting factor (WT)

14. Which of the following has the lowest LET?
    a. Alpha particles
    b. Cobalt-60 gamma rays
    c. Diagnostic x-rays
    d. Fast neutrons
    e. Protons

15. Dose protraction relates principally to which of the following?
    a. Dose
    b. Dose accumulation
    c. Dose integration
    d. Dose rate
    e. Dose response

16. Which of the following is considered a physical dose-modifying factor?
    a. Age
    b. Cell progression
    c. Dose protraction
    d. Oxygen
    e. Recovery

17. Which of the following is considered a biologic dose-modifying factor?
    a. Dose per fraction
    b. Dose protraction
    c. Geometry
    d. LET
    e. The oxygen effect

18. Dose fractionation is less effective than an equal single dose because of which of the following?
    a. Cellular recovery
    b. Oxygenation and proliferation
    c. RBE and LET
    d. Reduced LET
    e. Reduced OER

19. Why do we develop radiation dose-response relationships?
    a. To establish benefit-risk coefficients
    b. To establish estimates of diagnostic accuracy
    c. To predict the harmful effects of radiation after an accident
    d. To predict the therapeutic value of an occupational exposure
    e. To predict the value of a radiologic examination

WORKSHEET 33-2

Biologic Factors That Affect Radiosensitivity
Radiation Dose-Response Relationships

Tissue irradiated in the presence of oxygen (aerobic) responds to radiation more than does tissue irradiated under reduced levels of oxygen or in the absence of oxygen (hypoxic, anoxic, or anaerobic). The magnitude of this ratio in response is called the **oxygen enhancement ratio (OER)**.

$$OER = \frac{\text{Radiation dose necessary to produce an effect under anaerobic conditions}}{\text{Radiation dose necessary to produce same effect under aerobic conditions}}$$

Most radiobiologic research is designed to establish the nature of radiation dose-response relationships. Such relationships generally can be classified as **linear** or **nonlinear** and **threshold** or **nonthreshold**. Knowledge of the precise nature of the radiation dose-response relationship allows one to predict human response after a given dose of radiation.

EXERCISES

1. Radiation-induced damage in tissue:
   a. Is caused by interaction at the tissue level
   b. Is greater in the presence of oxygen
   c. Is greater with protracted delivery
   d. Is irreversible
   e. Results in only latent effects

2. When one considers the biologic modifying factors to radiation response:
   a. Age is a factor.
   b. Nitrogen pressure is a factor.
   c. Pharmaceutical agents are capable only of protection.
   d. Pharmaceutical agents are capable only of sensitization.
   e. Sex is a factor.

3. Why is the linear, nonthreshold dose-response relationship used as a model for radiation protection guides?
   a. Because a linear response is directly proportional to the dose
   b. Because in a nonthreshold dose-response relationship, any dose is expected to produce a response
   c. Because of ALARA
   d. Because such guides are concerned exclusively with the early effects of radiation exposure
   e. Because such guides are concerned exclusively with the late effects of radiation exposure

4. The **least** sensitive time in life to radiation exposure is which of the following?
   a. Adulthood
   b. Childhood
   c. In utero
   d. Old age
   e. There is no least sensitive time.

5. Which of the following effects exhibits a threshold type of radiation dose-response relationship?
   a. Cataracts
   b. Leukemia
   c. Life span shortening
   d. Lung cancer
   e. Thyroid cancer

6. When a radiation dose-response relationship intercepts the response axis at a positive value:
   a. That response is acute.
   b. That response is not related to radiation.
   c. The radiation has a high LET.
   d. The relationship is linear.
   e. The relationship is nonlinear.

7. Which of the following effects follows a nonlinear, threshold type of dose-response relationship?
   a. Breast cancer
   b. Death
   c. Leukemia
   d. Life span shortening
   e. Tissue atrophy

8. Dose limits (DLs) are based on which type of radiation dose-response relationship?
   a. Linear, nonthreshold
   b. Linear, quadratic
   c. Linear, threshold
   d. Nonlinear, nonthreshold
   e. Nonlinear, threshold

9. The late effects of diagnostic x-rays probably follow which type of radiation dose-response relationship?
   a. Linear, nonthreshold
   b. Linear, quadratic
   c. Linear, threshold
   d. Nonlinear, nonthreshold
   e. Nonlinear, threshold

10. A wide error bar on a graphic data point indicates which of the following?
    a. A late effect
    b. Great confidence
    c. High LET
    d. Little confidence
    e. Low LET

11. The LET, OER, and RBE are interrelated. Therefore, which of the following statements is **true**?
    a. Diagnostic x-rays are considered low LET, OER, and RBE.
    b. Diagnostic x-rays have a lower LET than cobalt-60 gamma rays.
    c. Diagnostic x-rays have an LET of 3.0 keV/μm and an OER of 3.
    d. High-LET radiation has low RBE.
    e. High-RBE radiation has high OER.

12. Which of the following factors has no influence on response to radiation exposure?
    a. Age
    b. Dose protraction
    c. Occupation
    d. Oxygen tension
    e. Sex

13. Which of the following have the highest OER?
    a. Alpha particles
    b. Cobalt-60 gamma rays
    c. Diagnostic x-rays
    d. Neutrons
    e. Protons

14. Humans are **most** sensitive to radiation:
    a. At no special time
    b. During childhood
    c. During old age
    d. During preconception
    e. In utero

15. When an irradiated cell dies before the next mitosis, this is called:
    a. Clonal death
    b. Cytogenetic death
    c. Interphase death
    d. Metaphase death
    e. Mitotic death

16. A linear, nonthreshold dose-response relationship:
    a. Describes most early effects
    b. Has a maximum response followed by a minimum response
    c. Is shaped like an "S"
    d. States that there is a range of very low doses that are totally safe
    e. Suggests that even the smallest dose may be risky

17. When a linear, nonthreshold dose-response relationship intersects the response axis at zero dose, this means that:
    a. It is not really linear.
    b. It is really threshold.
    c. Recovery and repair have occurred.
    d. There is a natural incidence of the response.
    e. There is no natural incidence of the response.

18. The genetically significant dose (GSD):
    a. Depends on the average gonadal dose for various procedures
    b. Is more than the annual dose from environmental sources
    c. Is more than the average dose for medical procedures
    d. Is that dose expected to double the natural mutation rate
    e. Is the dose that results in a significant number of mutations in the next generation

Irradiation of Macromolecules
Radiolysis of Water
Direct and Indirect Effects

When irradiated in vitro (outside the body), molecules are relatively resistant to radiation damage. However, when irradiated in vivo (inside the body), even relatively minor molecular damage can produce visible and sometimes significant effects at the whole-body level.

Irradiation of macromolecules can result in main-chain scission, cross-linking, or point lesions. The macromolecule of principal importance in vivo is DNA.

Irradiation of water produces free radicals, hydrogen peroxide (H_2O_2), and the hydroperoxyl radical (HO_2), each of which is considered a harmful molecular byproduct.

If radiation interacts with a macromolecule of importance, the subsequent effect is said to be **direct.** Alternatively, if radiation interacts with water, thereby creating one of the harmful byproducts, which then diffuses through the cell to the macromolecule, the effect is said to be **indirect.**

EXERCISES

1. After a low radiation dose, most cellular radiation damage that results in a late total-body effect occurs because of which of the following?
   a. Cross-linking
   b. In vitro effects
   c. Main-chain scission
   d. Point lesions
   e. Reduced viscosity

2. The biologically reactive molecular byproducts formed during radiolysis of water are thought to be which of the following?
   a. H_2O
   b. H* and OH*

   c. O_2 and H_2
   d. O and H
   e. SH compounds

3. Radiation may interfere with DNA synthesis by:
   a. Causing cells to omit some phases of the cell cycle
   b. The G_1 effect, which is the failure to commence DNA synthesis because of damage that occurs during the G_1 period
   c. The G_2 effect, which is the failure to initiate DNA synthesis because of the blocking of preceding mitosis
   d. The M effect, which is interference with DNA synthesis in progress
   e. The S effect, which is interference with mitosis in progress

4. Which of the following may occur in DNA molecules as a result of irradiation?
   a. Free radical formation
   b. Hydrogen bond breakage
   c. H_2O_2 formation
   d. A double-strand break
   e. Peroxy radical formation

5. When water is irradiated, products of the **initial** interaction are which of the following?
   a. H_2O_2
   b. H_2O and e^-
   c. HOH^+ and e^-
   d. OH* and e^-
   e. OH* and H*

6. Which of the following is an example of anabolism?
   a. Hormesis
   b. Main-chain scission
   c. Protein synthesis
   d. Radiolysis of water
   e. Transfer RNA

7. Radiation-induced changes in DNA that result in genetic damage follow which type of dose-response relationship?
   a. Linear, nonthreshold
   b. Linear, quadratic
   c. Linear, threshold
   d. Nonlinear, nonthreshold
   e. Nonlinear, threshold

8. Which of the following is a free radical?
   a. e^-
   b. H_2O_2
   c. HO_2^*
   d. HOH^+
   e. HOH^-

9. When molecules are irradiated:
   a. Directly, it is with x-rays
   b. In solution in vitro, they are in free radicals
   c. In suspension, they are irradiated in solution
   d. In suspension, they are irradiated in vivo
   e. Inside the cell or body, they are irradiated in vitro

10. Radiation effects at the total-body level occur mainly because of which of the following?
    a. Alterations in viscosity
    b. Direct effect
    c. Increased radiosensitivity
    d. Indirect effect
    e. Irradiation in vitro

Ionization of water yields the following:

$$H_2O \quad\quad Energy \quad\quad H_2O^+ + e^-$$

H_2O^+ is unstable and instantly produces two subunits as follows:

$$H_2O^+ \quad\quad H^+ + OH^*$$
$$(A) \quad\quad\quad (B) \quad (C)$$

and

$$H_2O + e^- \quad H_2O^-$$
$$(D) \quad\quad (E) \quad (F)$$

followed by

$$H_2O^- \quad H^* + OH^-$$
$$(G) \quad\quad (H) \quad\quad (I)$$

Match the ionization products given above (labeled A through I) with the description below:

11. Which of the above is the hydrogen ion?
    a. A
    b. B
    c. C
    d. H
    e. I

12. Which of the above is the hydroxyl free radical?
    a. B
    b. C
    c. G
    d. H
    e. I

13. Which of the above is positively ionized water?
    a. A
    b. B
    c. C
    d. D
    e. F

14. Which of the above is the hydroxyl ion?
    a. B
    b. C
    c. G
    d. H
    e. I

15. Which of the above is the hydrogen free radical?
    a. E
    b. F
    c. G
    d. H
    e. I

Target Theory
Cell Survival Kinetics
Linear Energy Transfer, Relative Biologic Effectiveness, and Oxygen Enhancement Ratio

Radiation effects at the total-body level occur because of radiation damage to cells. Cellular damage, in turn, occurs because of molecular responses to radiation.

It is thought that certain critical molecules constitute sensitive targets within the cell, each of which must be inactivated to produce the ultimate response—cell lethality. This is the **target theory.**

The radiation dose-response relationship for cell lethality is **nonlinear** and **nonthreshold.** Cell survival follows the single-target, single-hit model or the multitarget, single-hit model of radiation-induced lethality. These models are the consequence of target theory and incorporate parameters useful for measuring the efficiency of various conditions of irradiation and the sensitivity of different types of cells.

D_{37} = Radiation dose after which 37% of cells will survive, whereas, conversely, 63% will die

D_O = Mean lethal dose; similar to D_{37} but applicable only to the straight-line portion of the multitarget, single-hit model

n = Extrapolation number

D_Q = Threshold dose or shoulder dose

EXERCISES

1. If undifferentiated cells are irradiated in vivo, such cells are:
   a. Difficult to replace
   b. Easy to replace
   c. Resistant to radiation
   d. Sensitive to radiation
   e. Very abundant

2. Which of the following phases of the cell cycle is considered **most** resistant?
   a. Early S phase
   b. G_1 phase
   c. G_2 phase
   d. Late S phase
   e. M phase

3. When cell-survival curves are used, the measure of cell radiosensitivity is which of the following?
   a. D_O
   b. D_Q
   c. n
   d. O_{37}
   e. RBE

4. When irradiated with high-LET radiation, human cells follow which of the following models?
   a. The linear, quadratic model
   b. The multitarget, multihit model
   c. The multitarget, single-hit model
   d. The single-target, multihit model
   e. The single-target, single-hit model

5. The probability of human cell death can be computed:
   a. If only D_O is known
   b. If only D_Q is known
   c. If only n is known
   d. Using the normal distribution
   e. Using the Poisson distribution

6. If a dose equal to D_{37} were **uniformly** distributed, what percentage of cells would survive?
   a. 0%
   b. 37%
   c. 50%
   d. 63%
   e. 100%

7. Which of the following is the mean lethal dose?
   a. D_O
   b. D_Q
   c. D_{37}
   d. D_n
   e. n

8. The multitarget, single-hit model:
   a. Contains D_O, which is the threshold dose
   b. Contains n, which is the mean lethal dose
   c. Is characterized by D_{37}
   d. Is not a part of target theory
   e. Presumes a threshold

9. The difference in generation time among different types of cells is due mainly to the length of which of the following?
   a. The G_1 phase
   b. The G_2 phase
   c. The G_O phase
   d. The M phase
   e. The S phase

10. Which of the following factors does **not** affect the radiation response of mammalian cells?
    a. Dose rate
    b. LET
    c. Presence of oxygen
    d. Sex of the cell
    e. Stage of the cell in its cycle

11. In cellular radiobiology:
    a. A cell colony is considered to exist after the first cell division.
    b. Cell colonies require two divisions to view.
    c. In vitro studies use cells grown and irradiated in the body.
    d. Only cells irradiated inside the body can be used.
    e. Single cells are allowed to grow into colonies.

12. According to the multitarget model of cell lethality:
    a. Cells have more than one critical target, each of which has to be inactivated for cell death.
    b. Cells have one critical target and several secondary targets.

c. Only cell death can be measured with accuracy.
d. The cell can accumulate radiation dose.
e. The critical target is considered to be the RNA.

13. In the following graph, which shows two cell-survival curves?

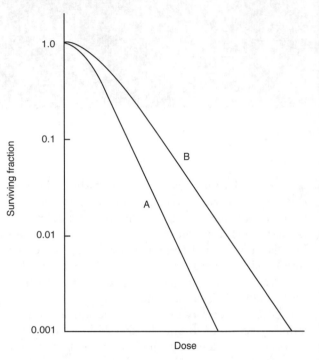

a. Both curves have the same D_{37}.
b. Both curves have the same D_Q.
c. Both curves have the same mean lethal dose.
d. Curve A could represent oxygenated cells if curve B represented anoxic cells.
e. Curve A could represent protracted exposure if curve B represented single exposure.

14. According to target theory:
    a. A hit can occur only by direct effect.
    b. A hit can occur only by indirect effect.
    c. Radiation favors the target molecule.
    d. Radiation interacts randomly.
    e. Radiation interacts uniformly.

15. When irradiated with x-rays, human cells follow which of the following models?
    a. The linear, quadratic model
    b. The multitarget, multihit model
    c. The multitarget, single-hit model
    d. The single-target, multihit model
    e. The single-target, single-hit model

16. To explain radiation effects on living cells, target theory states that:
    a. A target can receive a hit by direct or indirect effect.
    b. Once hit, targets can be replaced.
    c. Only one target exists within the cell.
    d. Only one target must be hit to cause cell death.
    e. There is only one type of target.

17. If a dose equal to D_{37} were randomly distributed, what percentage of cells would die?
    a. 0%
    b. 37%
    c. 50%
    d. 63%
    e. 100%

18. Of the various macromolecules that are sensitive to radiation, the **most** sensitive is/are:
    a. DNA
    b. Free radicals
    c. Proteins
    d. RNA
    e. Water

19. Usually, radiation interacts with DNA:
    a. And causes cell death
    b. And causes irreversible damage
    c. Directly
    d. Indirectly
    e. Slowly

20. Free radical ions are associated with biologic injury induced by which of the following types of radiation?
    a. Diagnostic x-rays
    b. Laser radiation
    c. Microwave radiation
    d. Radiofrequency
    e. Ultrasound

21. A reactive atom or molecule that has an unpaired electron in its outer shell is called a/an:
    a. Bremsstrahlung atom
    b. Free radical
    c. Ion pair
    d. Recoil proton
    e. Transformed molecule

22. The genetic code of DNA:
    a. Consists of codons only at S phase
    b. Consists of sets of five base pairs
    c. Is duplicated during G_2 phase
    d. Is transcribed by mRNA
    e. Is transferred to RNA

23. Which of the following is an effect of radiation on molecular DNA?
    a. Cross-linking
    b. Free radical formation
    c. H_2O_2 formation
    d. Increased viscosity
    e. The induction of radioactivity

35-1

Acute Radiation Lethality Local Tissue Damage

The degree of radiation effect is related to the radiation dose and is predicted by a dose-response relationship. These conclusions are drawn from experimentation with animals and from observations of humans irradiated both accidentally and intentionally.

Effects of radiation exposure at the whole-body level that occur within weeks of exposure are referred to as acute, or early, effects of radiation exposure. These effects include radiation lethality and radiation effects on local tissues. They are generally due to the death of many cells within the tissue.

EXERCISES

1. The $LD_{50/60}$ for humans is closest to which of the following?
   a. 100 rad
   b. 250 rad
   c. 350 rad
   d. 450 rad
   e. 600 rad

2. A whole-body dose equivalent of 3000 rem (30 Sv) would probably cause death in 4 to 10 days by which of the following mechanisms?
   a. Central nervous system death
   b. Gastrointestinal death
   c. Hemopoietic death
   d. Latent effects
   e. Prodromal syndrome

3. With regard to the radiation exposure of mammalian gonads:
   a. A linear, nonthreshold dose-response relationship prevails for sterility.
   b. Effects are apparently independent of LET.
   c. Germ cell depression has been measured at as low as 10 rad.
   d. Sterility is induced at doses as low as 100 rad.
   e. The spermatocyte represents the most sensitive stage in the male.

4. The minimum testicular dose for transient infertility is approximately:
   a. 5 rad
   b. 10 rad
   c. 50 rad
   d. 200 rad
   e. 500 rad

5. The $LD_{50/30}$ refers to a:
   a. Lethal dose delivered within 30 to 50 days
   b. Lethal dose of total-body radiation for 30% of the people so exposed in 50 days
   c. Lethal dose of total-body radiation for 30% to 50% of the people so exposed
   d. Lethal dose of total-body radiation for 50% of the people so exposed in 30 days
   e. Lovely dance for half the people younger than 30 years

6. Which of the following is considered an early response to radiation exposure?
   a. Cataracts
   b. Cytogenetic damage
   c. Genetic damage
   d. Leukemia
   e. Shortened life span

7. The $LD_{50/60}$ represents the dose:
   a. Equivalent to 37% cell survival (D37)
   b. Required to kill 50% of the cells in 60 days
   c. Required to kill 60% of the cells in 50 days
   d. Resulting in 60% human death within 2 months
   e. That will kill half the people in 60 days

8. Human radiation lethality follows which dose-response relationship?
   a. Linear, quadratic
   b. Linear, nonthreshold
   c. Linear, threshold
   d. Nonlinear, nonthreshold
   e. Nonlinear, threshold

9. Which dose range, applied to both ovaries, is needed to induce permanent sterility?
   a. 10 to 100 rad
   b. 100 to 200 rad
   c. 300 to 800 rad
   d. 900 to 1200 rad
   e. 1200 rad

10. Which syndrome has a mean survival time that is independent of dose?
    a. Central nervous system
    b. Gastrointestinal
    c. Hematologic
    d. Latent
    e. Prodromal

11. The dose of x-rays necessary to produce erythema in half of those exposed is approximately:
    a. 50 rad
    b. 100 rad
    c. 300 rad
    d. 500 rad
    e. 1000 rad

12. The acute radiation syndrome consists of all of the following **except**:
    a. Central nervous syndrome
    b. Gastrointestinal syndrome
    c. Hematologic syndrome
    d. Latent injury syndrome
    e. Latent period

13. Which of the following is **not** an early response to radiation exposure?
    a. Breast cancer
    b. Chromosome aberrations
    c. Epilation
    d. Intestinal distress that occurs 1 week after exposure
    e. Skin erythema that occurs 2 weeks after exposure

14. Which of the following is a delayed local tissue effect?
    a. Cataracts
    b. Epilation
    c. Moist desquamation
    d. Skin erythema
    e. Transient sterility

15. Three days after a dose of 1000 rad (10 Gy_t) is received, physiologic alterations in the small intestine include all of the following **except**:
    a. Crypt cell death
    b. Diarrhea
    c. Epilation
    d. Leakage of proteins from the intestinal lumen
    e. Loss of electrolytes and water

16. The acute radiation syndrome:
    a. Begins at a threshold dose of 50 rad
    b. By gastrointestinal death indicates a mean survival time of about 4 to 10 days
    c. Can occur after high doses administered over a short time or over several months
    d. Includes the gastrointestinal syndrome, which occurs after doses of approximately 5000 to 10,000 rad
    e. Includes the most sensitive of the syndromes— the gastrointestinal syndrome

17. The mean survival time for mammals after a single whole-body dose of radiation is:
    a. Dependent on dose (~200 to 1000 rad)
    b. Dependent on repair mechanisms
    c. Independent of dose
    d. Independent of the type of death
    e. The same for all species

18. Death caused by a single dose of total-body irradiation primarily involves damage to which of the following?
    a. Bone marrow
    b. Endocrine system
    c. Respiratory system
    d. Skeletal system
    e. Skin

19. The mean survival time after a lethal radiation dose is constant:
    a. Between 200 and 1000 rad
    b. For gastrointestinal death
    c. For hematologic death
    d. With increasing dose >5000 rad
    e. With increasing dose >10,000 rad

All of the acute radiation effects observed at the whole-body level have been studied thoroughly in experimental animals. Most have been observed in human populations, including atomic bomb survivors, radiation accident victims, and patients with radiation-induced cancer.

Blood is a body tissue that has received considerable attention as a biologic in vivo radiation dosimeter. Because blood is radiosensitive and is easy to sample, it often is used to predict the likely outcome of an unknown radiation exposure.

Cell counts and cytogenetic analysis of lymphocytes are conducted on all radiation accident victims to determine the aggressiveness of supportive therapy and to help guide treatment.

EXERCISES

1. Which of the following cell types is mostly severely depressed by radiation?
   a. Erythrocytes
   b. Granulocytes
   c. Lymphocytes
   d. Megakaryocytes
   e. Neurons

2. The normal human karyotype consists of:
   a. 23 chromosomes
   b. 23 chromosome pairs
   c. 42 autosomes
   d. 46 autosomes
   e. Two sex chromosome pairs

3. Of the following chromosome aberrations, which requires a karyotype for analysis?
   a. Chromatid deletion
   b. Dicentric chromosome
   c. Isochromatid fragments
   d. Reciprocal translocation
   e. Ring chromosome

4. Which of the following blood observations is **most** appropriate during monitoring for radiation response?
   a. Erythrocyte count
   b. Granulocyte count
   c. Hematocrit
   d. Lymphocyte count
   e. Thrombocyte count

5. A whole-body radiation dose of 25 rad (0.25 Gy_t) is **most** likely to produce which of the following?
   a. Cytogenetic damage
   b. Depletion of oogonia
   c. Epilation
   d. Erythrocyte depression
   e. Skin erythema

6. Which of the following is **not** a mature blood cell?
   a. Cystocyte
   b. Erythrocyte
   c. Granulocyte
   d. Lymphocyte
   e. Thrombocyte

7. Radiation effects on the hematologic system:
   a. Are first observed as a lymphocyte depression
   b. Are measurable at whole-body doses as low as 5 rad
   c. Are permanent
   d. Cannot result in a late response
   e. Suggest that radiation workers should undergo routine blood analysis

8. Which of the following blood observations is **most** appropriate for routine monitoring of radiation workers?
   a. Erythrocyte count
   b. Lymphocyte count
   c. Shilling differential
   d. Thrombocyte count
   e. None of the above

9. Which of the following chromosome aberrations obeys a linear, nonthreshold dose-response relationship?
   a. Chromatid break
   b. Dicentric
   c. Reciprocal translocation
   d. Ring chromosome
   e. Tricentric

10. Which cells are involved in the human immune response?
    a. Erythrocytes
    b. Granulocytes
    c. Lymphocytes
    d. Spermatocytes
    e. Thrombocytes

11. Which cells are **most** sensitive to radiation exposure?
    a. Cystocytes
    b. Erythrocytes
    c. Granulocytes
    d. Lymphocytes
    e. Thrombocytes

12. What phase of the cell cycle has the **most** variable length?
    a. G_0
    b. G_1
    c. G_2
    d. M
    e. S

13. Which of the following is the precursor to a thrombocyte?
    a. Cystocyte
    b. Lymphocyte
    c. Megakaryoblast
    d. Myeloblast
    e. Reticulocyte

14. Which two cell lines are the **most** radiosensitive?
    a. Granulocytes, lymphocytes
    b. Granulocytes, oogonia
    c. Granulocytes, spermatogonia
    d. Spermatogonia, lymphocytes
    e. Spermatogonia, oogonia

15. Which of the following human cells are **most** often used for cytogenetic analysis?
    a. Lymphocytes
    b. Oogonia
    c. Skin cells
    d. Spermatogonia
    e. Thrombocytes

16. How long after radiation exposure do chromosome aberrations first appear in peripheral blood cells?
    a. Hours
    b. Months
    c. Years
    d. Decades
    e. Never

17. The principal response of the blood to radiation exposure is:
    a. A decrease in cell number
    b. Stimulation of cell proliferation
    c. Cellular transformation
    d. Fragmentation of chromosomes
    e. Rearrangement of chromosomes

18. After radiation exposure, the first blood cells to respond are the:
    a. Cystocytes
    b. Erythrocytes
    c. Granulocytes
    d. Lymphocytes
    e. Thrombocytes

19. A chromosomal karyotype is:
    a. A description of the radiation response
    b. A point mutation
    c. An analysis of chromosome fragments
    d. An orderly map of chromosomes
    e. Unrestrained growth of chromosomes

20. In a mutation, the following cells can be passed on for a lifetime:
    a. Leydig cell
    b. Sertoli cell
    c. Spermatocyte
    d. Spermatid
    e. Spermatogonia

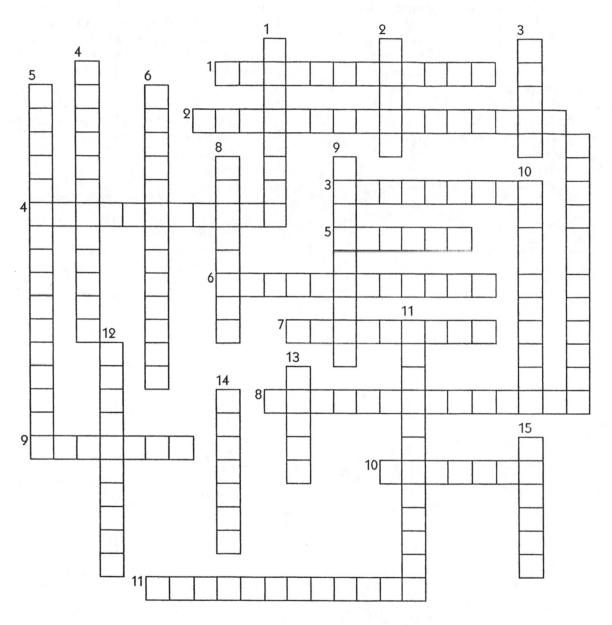

ACROSS

1. Platelets involved in blood clotting
2. Syndrome produced by radiation doses of approximately 1000 to 5000 rad
3. Syndrome of acute clinical symptoms that occur within hours of exposure and continue for up to a day or two
4. Reduction in the number of immune response cells
5. Intermediate layer of connective tissue in the skin
6. Red blood cells that are the transportation agents for oxygen
7. Loss of hair
8. Rapid rise in scavenger cells
9. Effect of cell death, resulting in reduction in size of tissue or organ
10. Stem cells of the ovaries
11. Scavenger cells used to fight bacteria

DOWN

1. Sunburn-like reddening of the skin
2. Syndrome represented by the sequence of events after high-level radiation exposure that leads to death within days or weeks
3. Stem cells in the lowest layer of the skin that mature as they slowly migrate to the surface of the epidermis
4. Ulceration and denudation of the skin
5. Rapid decrease, then slower decrease, in scavenger cells
6. Development of germ cells by both ovaries and testes that occurs at varying rates and times
8. _____ illness refers to the acute radiation lethality stage, including hematologic, gastrointestinal, and neuromuscular symptoms.
9. Outer layer of the skin
10. White cells
11. Platelets
12. Reduction in white cells of the peripheral blood
13. Soft x-rays once used to treat skin diseases such as ringworm
14. Ovarian stem cells encapsulated by primordial follicles during late fetal life
15. Period during which a subject exposed to radiation is free of visible effects

Delayed or late responses to radiation exposure include genetic effects and those somatic effects that require months or even years to develop. Radiobiologists rely heavily on data extrapolated from observations of humans who have suffered high radiation doses or on large-scale epidemiologic studies.

These late effects generally follow low doses of radiation. Precise dose-response relationships are seldom possible to determine; therefore, radiation scientists resort to various estimates of risk.

Principal late effects of concern are the induction of malignant disease and genetic effects. Each of these is presumed to follow a linear, nonthreshold dose-response relationship. Late local tissue effects are for the most part threshold in nature.

EXERCISES

1. Which of the following is an example of a linear, nonthreshold, dose-response relationship?
   a. Cataracts
   b. CNS syndrome
   c. Epilation
   d. Lethality
   e. Leukemia

2. Which of the following statements about radiation-induced cataracts after a CT examination of the head is **most** appropriate?
   a. Cataracts are possible because there is no threshold.
   b. Lens shields should be used.
   c. The dose is certainly below the threshold for such an effect.

d. The dose is probably in the neighborhood of the threshold for such an effect.
   e. The probability of cataracts is high.

3. The best estimate for radiation-induced life span shortening is:
   a. 10 hours/rad
   b. 10 days/rad
   c. 24 hours/rad
   d. 24 days/rad
   e. 1 month/rad

4. Diagnostic x-rays have been shown to produce which of the following?
   a. Cataracts
   b. Chromosome aberrations
   c. Leukemia
   d. Organ atrophy
   e. Shortening of life

5. Supporting evidence for radiation carcinogenesis comes from:
   a. British radiologists
   b. Fluoroscopic monitoring of patients with tuberculosis
   c. ^{131}I therapy for hyperthyroidism
   d. Pelvimetry
   e. People living in areas with high background radiation (e.g., Denver)

6. If the incidence of cancer is 1:5000, what is the relative risk if an irradiated population shows an incidence of 4:10,000?
   a. 2:1
   b. 4:1

c. 10:1
d. 1000:1
e. 4000:1

7. Which of the following groups has suffered a harmful radiation effect?
   a. Patients receiving diagnostic x-rays
   b. Nuclear power plant workers
   c. Radiologic technologists
   d. Radium watch-dial painters
   e. The last generation of radiologists

8. Radiation-induced cataracts:
   a. Appear on the posterior pole of the lens
   b. Exhibit a threshold to x-rays of approximately 10 rad
   c. Follow a linear, nonthreshold type of dose-response relationship
   d. Follow a nonlinear, threshold type of dose-response relationship
   e. Have a latent period of approximately 1 year

9. Approximately how many Americans will die of malignant disease from natural causes?
   a. 5%
   b. 10%
   c. 20%
   d. 40%
   e. 50%

10. Significant gonadal radiation exposure occurs:
    a. In whole-body MRI
    b. Only when no collimator is used
    c. When radiation is scattered from other parts of the body
    d. When radiation is scattered internally
    e. When the gonads are in the primary beam

11. Epidemiology is the study of which of the following?
    a. Early radiation effects
    b. Late radiation effects
    c. Populations
    d. Radiation
    e. Statistics

12. Radiation-induced chromosome aberrations are which of the following?
    a. Early or late effects
    b. Observable following 1 rad
    c. Only early effects
    d. Only late effects
    e. Present only after whole-body irradiation

13. The average latent period for radiation-induced cataracts is:
    a. 5 years
    b. 15 years
    c. 30 years
    d. 50 years
    e. Life

14. The approximate acute x-ray dose required to produce a 100% incidence of cataracts is:
    a. 1 Gy_t
    b. 10 Gy_t
    c. 100 Gy_t
    d. 1000 Gy_t
    e. 10,000 Gy_t

15. When engaged in a busy fluoroscopy schedule, who should wear protective lens shields?
    a. Both radiologists and technologists
    b. Neither radiologists nor technologists
    c. Not enough information
    d. Only radiologists
    e. Only technologists

16. Which of the following has the greatest loss-of-life expectancy?
    a. Accidents
    b. Being male
    c. Cancer
    d. Occupation
    e. Radiation

17. Protective lens shields for patients should be used:
    a. Always
    b. Never
    c. When the lens is in the primary beam and such use does not interfere with the examination
    d. Whenever the lens is in the primary beam
    e. Not enough information is given.

18. Breast cancer is observed in 30 of 450 patients. If the normal incidence is 2:1000, what is the approximate relative risk in these patients?
    a. 10:1
    b. 30:1
    c. 50:1
    d. 100:1
    e. 300:1

Radiation-Induced Malignancy
Total Risk of Malignancy
Radiation and Pregnancy

It is undeniable that humans are most sensitive to the harmful effects of radiation while in utero. Furthermore, the fetus is most radiation-sensitive early in pregnancy. Radiation effects include prenatal and postnatal mortality, congenital abnormalities, and latent malignant disease.

Low-dose irradiation (e.g., 10 rad [0.1 Gy_t]) has never caused such effects in humans. Only epidemiologic studies such as the Oxford survey have suggested an increased risk of latent malignant disease after low-dose in utero irradiation.

No direct evidence of radiation-induced genetic effects has been found in humans.

Observations of flies and mice, however, have shown the following:

1. Radiation-induced genetic mutations follow a linear, nonthreshold dose-response relationship.
2. The passage of time leads to some recovery from the genetic effects of radiation.
3. Radiation does not induce specific genetic mutations but rather increases the incidence of already existing mutations.
4. Radiation-induced genetic mutations are usually recessive.
5. For humans, the doubling dose is approximately 50 rad (0.5 Gy_t).

EXERCISES

1. The relative risk of leukemia after low-dose radiation in utero is approximately:
   a. 0.5
   b. 1.5
   c. 3.5
   d. 5.0
   e. 10

2. The generally accepted absolute risk factor for radiation-induced breast cancer is:
   a. 0.06 cases/10^6/rad/yr
   b. 0.6 cases/10^6/rad/yr
   c. 6 cases/10^6/rad/yr
   d. 60 cases/10^6/rad/yr
   e. 600 cases/10^6/rad/yr

3. Radiation-induced leukemia:
   a. Can be reversed
   b. Does not occur after long-term, low-level radiation exposure
   c. Follows a linear, threshold dose-response relationship
   d. Has been demonstrated in both animals and humans
   e. Probably does not occur at doses of less than approximately 25 rad

4. Which of the following dose-response relationships best describes radiation-induced lung cancer?
   a. Linear, nonthreshold
   b. Linear, quadratic
   c. Linear, threshold
   d. Nonlinear, nonthreshold
   e. Nonlinear, threshold

5. Which of the following numbers approximates the total cases of leukemia observed in the 100,000 atomic bomb survivors?
   a. 50
   b. 150
   c. 500
   d. 1500
   e. 5000

6. Which of the following statements about the development of radiation-induced liver cancer in Thorotrast-injected patients is **true?**
   a. The findings are negative.
   b. The findings are positive and statistically significant.
   c. The findings are positive but not statistically significant.
   d. The radiation source was iodine.
   e. The suspected principal radiation dose comes from beta emission.

7. After a dose of 10 rad at 6 weeks of gestation, the increase in congenital abnormalities is approximately:
   a. 0.1%
   b. 1%
   c. 10%
   d. 25%
   e. 50%

8. The latent period of radiation-induced leukemia is considered to be:
   a. 1 year
   b. 1 to 3 years
   c. 4 to 7 years
   d. 8 to 12 years
   e. >12 years

9. Analysis of the survivors of the atomic bomb shows that the induction of leukemia:
   a. Does not exist
   b. Peaked 10 years after the bomb
   c. Principally implicates chronic lymphocytic leukemia

d. Suggests a threshold of 300 rad
   e. Supports a linear, nonthreshold dose-response relationship

10. Which of the following populations has shown an increased incidence of leukemia after radiation exposure?
    a. American radiologic technologists
    b. Atomic bomb survivors
    c. Chernobyl survivors
    d. Diagnostic imaging patients
    e. Radium watch-dial painters

11. Which of the following types of cancer has **not** been demonstrated in humans after irradiation?
    a. Breast
    b. Colon
    c. Liver
    d. Lung
    e. Skin

12. Which type of radiation-induced cancer exhibits a threshold dose-response relationship?
    a. Bone
    b. Breast
    c. Liver
    d. Lung
    e. Skin

13. The radiation dose-response relationship for genetic mutations is:
    a. Exponential
    b. Independent of dose
    c. Linear
    d. Nonlinear
    e. Threshold

14. The relative risk of leukemia after irradiation in utero:
    a. Is approximately 50
    b. Is approximately 100
    c. Is less than 1.0 at zero dose
    d. Would equal 1.0 if there were no risk
    e. Would equal 100 if there were no risk

15. Which of the following radiation responses in utero is **most** likely when exposure occurs during organogenesis?
    a. Childhood cancer
    b. Congenital abnormalities
    c. Leukemia
    d. Neonatal death
    e. Prenatal death

16. With regard to radiation-induced genetic mutations:
    a. The dose-response relationship is nonlinear.
    b. The dose-response relationship is threshold.
    c. The doubling dose is approximately 50 to 250 rad.
    d. The male is more sensitive than the female.
    e. The most frequent types are dominant.

17. The data and conclusions of the Oxford survey:
    a. Are based on exposure of mice
    b. Show a 100% incidence of effects after an exposure of 200 rad
    c. Suggest a relative risk of approximately 8:1 during the first trimester of pregnancy
    d. Suggest a threshold for cataracts of approximately 200 rad
    e. Suggest a shortening of the life span by 10 days/rad

Cardinal Principles of Radiation Protection Dose Limits

Time and experience have led to a body of rules, regulations, and recommendations known as the principles of radiation protection. Exposure levels considered to be safe have been established, and these have been supplemented by the concept of **ALARA** (*as low as reasonably achievable*). Procedures and techniques have been developed to maintain occupational exposure below recommended limits and to ensure that all exposures are ALARA.

The cumulative **dose limit (DL)** is the dose that, if received each year during a 40-year occupational span, would result in an acceptable risk of injury.

Three principles of radiation control are known as the cardinal principles:

1. Keep the time of radiation exposure as short as possible.
2. Increase the distance from the source.
3. Place shielding between the source and the person who is being shielded.

These cardinal principles of radiation protection must be applied. Nearly all of the protective procedures and devices that are used in diagnostic radiology incorporate some aspect of these principles.

EXERCISES

1. Half-value layer (HVL) is related to which of the following principles of radiation protection?
   a. Distance
   b. Exposure
   c. Monitoring
   d. Shielding
   e. Time

2. If all other factors remain constant, radiation dose is related to x-ray beam-on time:
   a. By the inverse square
   b. Directly
   c. Exponentially
   d. Geometrically
   e. Inversely

3. If all other factors remain constant, radiation dose is related to source-to-object distance (SOD):
   a. By the inverse square
   b. Directly
   c. Exponentially
   d. Inversely
   e. Proportionately

4. If all other factors remain constant, radiation dose is related to shielding:
   a. By the inverse square
   b. Directly
   c. Exponentially
   d. Inversely
   e. Proportionately

5. One tenth-value layer (TVL) is defined as:
   a. $\frac{1}{10}$ the initial dose
   b. $\frac{1}{10}$ the initial shielding
   c. 10 times the HVL
   d. The shielding necessary to reduce exposure to $\frac{1}{10}$
   e. The shielding that will produce 10 times the dose

6. One TVL is equal to approximately how many HVLs?
   a. 2.0
   b. 2.2
   c. 3.3
   d. 5.0
   e. 10.0

7. During radiography, the best position for the radiologic technologist is:
   a. Behind the operating console barrier
   b. Down the hall
   c. Holding the patient
   d. In the examination room and as far from the patient as practical
   e. In the examination room and next to the patient

8. The HVL for 70 kVp is greater:
   a. For long exposure time than for short exposure time
   b. Than that for 90 kVp
   c. Than the TVL for 70 kVp
   d. With high filtration than with low filtration
   e. With single-phase power than with three-phase power

9. The exposure rate from a point source is 100 mR/hr at 120 cm. If a radiologic technologist moves to within 30 cm of the source of radiation, how many HVLs would be needed to reduce the exposure rate to 100 mR/hr?
   a. 1
   b. 2
   c. 4
   d. 6
   e. 8

10. If a survey meter reads 25 mR/hr, how long can a person stay at that location before receiving an exposure of 100 mR?
    a. 1 hour
    b. 2 hours
    c. 4 hours
    d. 6 hours
    e. 8 hours

11. If the exposure rate 1 m from a source is 9000 mR/hr, what is the exposure rate at 3 m from the source?
    a. 100 mR/hr
    b. 900 mR/hr
    c. 1000 mR/hr
    d. 3000 mR/hr
    e. 9000 mR/hr

12. The exposure rate alongside a fluoroscopic table (distance = 60 cm from the source) is 400 mR/hr. Therefore, if the radiologic technologist:
    a. Completed a 3-minute barium enema, the exposure would be 20 mR
    b. Completed a procedure at a distance of 120 cm, the total exposure would be 40 mR
    c. Completed a procedure that required 10 minutes, the exposure would be 40 mR
    d. Moved 60 cm farther from the table, the exposure rate would be 200 mR/hr
    e. Moved 60 cm farther from the table, the exposure rate would be increased

13. The DL for a radiologic technologist is:
    a. 100 mrem per year
    b. 500 mrem per 9 months
    c. 500 mrem per year
    d. 5000 mrem per 9 months
    e. 5000 mrem per year

14. You are a 17-year-old radiologic technologist student. How much occupational exposure are you allowed?
    a. 100 mrem per 9 months
    b. 100 mrem per year
    c. 500 mrem per 9 months
    d. 500 mrem per year
    e. 5000 mrem per year

15. During fluoroscopy, the exposure rate at the technologist's position is 350 mR/hr. How much x-ray beam-on time is allowed before the technologist reaches a weekly DL?
    a. 8 minutes
    b. 17 minutes
    c. 35 minutes
    d. 1 hour
    e. 2 hours

16. The cumulative DL is computed as follows:
    a. 5 to 18N
    b. 5(N − 18)
    c. 5N − 18
    d. 10 mSv × N
    e. 50 mSv × N

17. A protective apron is equivalent to 2 HVLs. How much more time does such an apron allow the radiologic technologist to remain during fluoroscopy than without the apron?
    a. Half as much time
    b. Twice as much time
    c. Four times as much
    d. Eight times as much
    e. Not enough information

38-1 Design of X-Ray Apparatus
Design of Protective Barriers

Designers of x-ray facilities and equipment exercise considerable care and attention. Much of this attention results from the need for radiation protection.

X-ray imaging systems have filters, collimators, and shields to reduce radiation exposure to patients and personnel. Attention is given to proper design and calibration of kVp, mA, and exposure timers so that radiographic techniques can be accurately and consistently used. This accuracy reduces the number of reexaminations, which in turn reduces human exposure. This is why periodic radiation control surveys and performance evaluation of x-ray apparatus are recommended.

Nearly all diagnostic x-ray rooms have lead in the walls. Sometimes, floor and ceiling barriers also require lead shielding.

EXERCISES

1. Every diagnostic x-ray tube housing must be sufficiently shielded to limit the level of exposure 1 m from the housing to:
   a. 10 mR/hr
   b. 100 mR/hr
   c. 1000 mR/hr
   d. A factor that varies according to kVp
   e. A factor that varies according to use

2. During mammography, at tube potentials less than 30 kVp, the minimum acceptable total equivalent filtration is:
   a. 0.05 mm Al
   b. 0.1 mm Al
   c. 0.25 mm Al
   d. 0.5 mm Al
   e. 2.5 mm Al

3. The minimum permissible filtration for general purpose radiographic or fluoroscopic tubes is:
   a. 0.05 mm Al
   b. 0.1 mm Al
   c. 0.25 mm Al
   d. 0.5 mm Al
   e. 2.5 mm Al

4. The fluoroscopic tube should **not** be positioned closer than 38 cm to the tabletop because the:
   a. Bucky slot would interfere
   b. Geometric unsharpness would increase
   c. Heat load on the tube would increase
   d. Patient radiation dose would be excessive
   e. Resultant magnification would be objectionable

5. Which of the following is regulated in a controlled area?
   a. Patient flow
   b. Public access
   c. Radiation exposure
   d. Type of procedure
   e. X-ray operation

6. Radiographic work load (W) has units of:
   a. mAmin/wk
   b. mR/mAmin
   c. mR/mAs
   d. R/mAmin/wk
   e. R/wk

7. The radiographic workload in a busy R&F room is approximately:
   a. 10 mAmin/wk
   b. 50 mAmin/wk
   c. 100 mAmin/wk
   d. 500 mAmin/wk
   e. 5000 mAmin/wk

8. Which of the following locations in a hospital should have the highest occupancy factor (T)?
   a. Laboratory
   b. Elevator
   c. Corridor
   d. Restroom
   e. Waiting room

9. Which of the following usually is considered to be a secondary protective barrier?
   a. All walls
   b. Chest wall
   c. Control booth barrier
   d. Floor
   e. Lateral wall

10. Fluoroscopic x-ray units must:
    a. Be image-intensified
    b. Have at least 2.5 mm Al equivalent filtration
    c. Have spot-film capability
    d. Limit leakage radiation to 1000 mR/hr at 1 m from the tube
    e. Never exceed 10 R/min at the tabletop

11. Which of the following contributes to the exposure of radiologic personnel?
    a. Off-focus radiation
    b. Primary radiation
    c. Remnant x-rays
    d. Scatter radiation
    e. Useful beam

12. The design limit for exposure of occupants in controlled areas is:
    a. 1 mrem/wk
    b. 10 mrem/wk
    c. 100 mrem/wk
    d. 500 mrem/wk
    e. 1000 mrem/wk

13. The use factor (U):
    a. Applies only to radiography, not fluoroscopy
    b. Describes the use of the room
    c. Describes the use of the x-ray tube
    d. Is always 1 for secondary barriers
    e. Takes on values from 0 to 10

14. All fluoroscopes have a 5-minute reset timer:
    a. Because no patient shall ever receive more than 5 minutes of x-ray beam-on time
    b. To allow image receptor change
    c. To permit a tube cool-down period
    d. To protect the patient
    e. To protect the x-ray tube

15. A test to ensure that radiation intensity is doubled when radiographic mA is doubled is called a test of:
    a. Alignment
    b. Coincidence
    c. Linearity
    d. Reproducibility
    e. Uniformity

16. When the fluoroscopic x-ray tube is mounted farther under the table, what is reduced?
    a. Beam alignment
    b. Filtration
    c. Image receptor speed
    d. Patient dose
    e. Scatter radiation

17. Which of the following would definitely be a secondary barrier?
    a. All walls of a dedicated chest room
    b. Any wall in a CT room
    c. The chest wall in an R&F room
    d. The door
    e. The floor

18. What is the weekly workload if 20 patients are examined each day at an average of 78 kVp/60 mAs per view and 3.4 views per patient?
    a. 68 mAmin/wk
    b. 340 mAmin/wk
    c. 442 mAmin/wk
    d. 500 mAmin/wk
    e. >700 mAmin/wk

19. A dedicated chest examination room is used to image 40 patients per day, two views per patient, and the PA technique is 110 kVp/1.5 mAs; the LAT technique is 120 kVp/3 mAs. What is the workload?
    a. 5 mAmin/wk
    b. 15 mAmin/wk
    c. 30 mAmin/wk
    d. 65 mAmin/wk
    e. 100 mAmin/wk

Radiation Detection and Measurement

For many years, film was the only type of detector available to indicate the presence of x-radiation. As a radiation detector, photographic emulsion has many advantages, but it also has many disadvantages. Its advantages continue to qualify it for personnel radiation monitoring—the film badge.

Other methods of radiation detection and measurement are now available, and some of them are more sensitive, more accurate, and more applicable for certain situations.

Gas-filled detectors are used for x-ray output calibration and radiation monitoring of areas for exposure levels. Thermoluminescent dosimetry (TLD) and optically stimulated luminescence (OSL) are used for personnel monitoring and patient dose estimation. Scintillation detectors are used principally in nuclear medicine imaging apparatus such as the gamma camera.

Instruments that incorporate nearly all of these methods can be designed for many different uses. To apply the best possible instrumentation to a given situation, one must understand the basic operating principles of each method and the associated characteristics of sensitivity, accuracy, range, and type of radiation detected.

EXERCISES

1. Which of the following is a characteristic of the ionization chamber survey meter?
   a. Geiger-Mueller counter
   b. Detection of individual ionizations
   c. Highly sensitive, 0.01 mR/hr
   d. Narrow range, 0 to 50 mR/hr
   e. Wide range, 0 to 1000 mR/hr

2. Gas-filled radiation detectors are used:
   a. As a proportional counter to measure the output of an x-ray machine
   b. As an integration type of ionization chamber
   c. Because they are more sensitive than scintillation detectors
   d. For occupational radiation monitoring
   e. In the Geiger region to map the radiation exposure levels in fluoroscopy

3. If each stage of a photomultiplier tube has a gain of approximately 4, a 10-stage photomultiplier tube will have a gain of approximately:
   a. 10^4
   b. 4^9
   c. 4^{10}
   d. 40
   e. 400

4. Which of the following is used in thermoluminescent dosimetry?
   a. Barium fluorochloride
   b. Cadmium tungstate
   c. Calcium tungstate
   d. Lithium fluoride
   e. Polyester

5. Which of the following detectors can be used to identify an unknown gamma emitter?
   a. Geiger-Mueller counter
   b. Ionization chamber
   c. Lithium fluoride
   d. Multichannel crystal spectrometer
   e. Photographic emulsion

6. Which of the following normally operates in the rate mode?
   a. A proportional counter
   b. A thermoluminescence dosimeter
   c. An ion chamber
   d. Photographic emulsion
   e. Photoluminescence dosimeter

7. Operation in which region of a gas-filled chamber results in the lowest output:
   a. Continuous discharge
   b. Geiger-Mueller region
   c. Ionization chamber
   d. Proportional
   e. Recombination

8. The resolving time of a radiation detector is the time required:
   a. For the meter to respond
   b. To detect sequential ionizations
   c. To identify different types of radiation
   d. To read the meter
   e. To reset the meter

9. The amount of light emitted by a scintillation phosphor is proportional to what feature of photon energy?
   a. Absorbed
   b. Attenuated
   c. Incident
   d. Scattered
   e. Transmitted

10. In thermoluminescence dosimetry, a plot of output intensity versus temperature is called a:
    a. Glow curve
    b. Glow worm
    c. Pulse height
    d. Pulse height analysis
    e. Pulse height spectrum

11. Which of the following statements correctly applies to the voltage response plot of the ideal gas-filled detector?
    a. Instrument sensitivity is highest in the Geiger-Mueller region.
    b. The ionization region is most sensitive.
    c. The lowest voltage of operation corresponds to the Geiger-Mueller region.
    d. Voltage is higher in the proportional region than in the Geiger-Mueller region.
    e. The curve has three distinct regions.

12. Which of the following is a gas-filled detector?
    a. Film badge
    b. Geiger-Mueller counter

c. Recombination chamber
d. Scintillation counter
e. Thermoluminescent dosimeter

13. When an accurate measurement of radiation exposure is made in the air, which should be used?
    a. Film badge
    b. Geiger-Mueller counter
    c. Ionization chamber
    d. Scintillation detector
    e. TLD

14. Which of the following is characteristic of a Geiger-Mueller counter?
    a. For laboratory use only
    b. Measures counts per minute
    c. Measures integrated radioactivity
    d. Useful personal monitor
    e. Wide range (1 to 10^4 mR/hr)

15. Which of the following is characteristic of scintillation detectors that are used as survey instruments?
    a. Can detect individual photons
    b. Are independent of energy
    c. Need extremely high voltage
    d. Suffer from saturation effects
    e. Have very low detection efficiency

16. Sodium iodide is a good gamma ray detector because:
    a. It has a high Z.
    b. It has excellent energy resolution.
    c. It is gas-filled.
    d. Photoelectrons are easily collected.
    e. The resultant charge is stored.

17. Compared with Geiger-Mueller counters, scintillation counters:
    a. Are more sensitive to gamma rays
    b. Are sensitive to beta particles
    c. Have a lower background counting rate
    d. Make better occupational radiation monitors
    e. Will count longer

18. The signal detector of a gas-filled radiation detector is the:
    a. Central electrode
    b. Chamber case
    c. Ionization region
    d. Planchet
    e. Scintillation crystal

WORKSHEET 39-1 — Patient Radiation Dose Reduction of Unnecessary Patient Dose

In diagnostic radiology, radiation control procedures are designed to maintain patient radiation dose ALARA while producing quality images. This requires measurement and estimation of patient dose.

Patient dose is expressed in three ways. The first, entrance skin exposure (ESE), can be measured easily. One can directly measure the output intensity of an x-ray unit at the source-to-skin distance (SSD), or one can position dosimeters such as those used in thermoluminescence dosimetry (TLD) on the skin of the patient for direct measurement during examination.

The second method of expressing patient dose is to state the radiation dose to the bone marrow. This dose, of course, cannot be measured directly; it must be computed from phantom exposures and skin measurements. The marrow dose is used to estimate the population **mean marrow dose,** which is considered to be an indication of the leukemogenic radiation hazard.

A third method of expressing patient dose relates to organ dose and usually to gonad dose. Gonad dose can be directly measured in males, but it can only be estimated in females. This is an important patient dose quantity because from it is estimated the **genetically significant dose (GSD).** The GSD is the dose of radiation that, if received by the entire population, would result in the same dose to the gene pool that is actually received by those irradiated.

EXERCISES

1. To protect a patient from soft radiation, one should use which of the following?
   a. Cone
   b. High-speed screen
   c. Small focal spot
   d. Increased filtration
   e. Tighter collimation

2. The GSD from medical radiation exposure depends on all of the following **except** the:
   a. Average gonad dose per examination
   b. Future childbearing expectancy of the population during any given year
   c. Number of people examined during any given year
   d. Occupational exposure
   e. Total population

3. Which of the following units is **most** appropriate when patient dose is expressed?
   a. Coulombs/kilogram
   b. Gray
   c. Rem
   d. Roentgen
   e. Sievert

4. Which of the following procedures helps to reduce patient dose during radiographic examination?
   a. Cones
   b. Digital detectors
   c. Filtration
   d. Grids
   e. Single-emulsion film

5. In the production of an acceptable radiograph, patient dose increases as _____ increases.
   a. Added filtration
   b. The grid ratio
   c. Image receptor speed

d. kVp
e. The SID

6. Which of the following is **most** important in determining patient dose during radiography?
   a. Grid ratio
   b. SID
   c. Single-phase or three-phase power
   d. Size of the field exposed
   e. Size of the focal spot

7. Which of the following procedures might result in an ESE that exceeds 100 mGy$_a$?
   a. 5 minutes of fluoroscopy
   b. A 10-minute sonogram
   c. A mammogram
   d. An intravenous pyelogram
   e. Spiral CT

8. The GSD is:
   a. A radiation dose that will produce chromosome aberrations
   b. An index of radiation received by the gene pool
   c. Determined from A-bomb survivor data
   d. The radiation dose considered to be the threshold for genetic mutations
   e. Used to predict the level of genetic damage

9. The mean marrow dose is:
   a. Approximately 200 mrad/yr
   b. Considered an important indicator of somatic radiation hazard
   c. Greater than the gonad dose for examinations of the abdomen and pelvis
   d. An index of radiation response
   e. That which results in leukemia

10. In the United States, the GSD from medical radiation exposure is approximately:
    a. 5 mrad/yr
    b. 20 mrad/yr
    c. 50 mrad/yr
    d. 200 mrad/yr
    e. 500 mrad/yr

11. If a 26-year-old female undergoes KUB (radiography of the *k*idneys, *u*reters, and *b*ladder) examination, which will be highest?
    a. Bone marrow dose
    b. Gonad dose
    c. Kidney dose
    d. Mean marrow dose
    e. Skin dose

12. Which of the following examinations results in the highest ESE?
    a. Abdomen
    b. Cervical spine
    c. Lateral chest
    d. Lateral skull
    e. Lumbar spine

13. If the skin dose from a single CT image is compared with that from multiple images:
    a. The dose will be the same for both.
    b. The multiple-image dose will be proportionally higher in relation to the number of images.
    c. The multiple-image dose will be slightly higher.
    d. The multiple-image dose will be twice as high.
    e. The single-image dose will be slightly higher.

14. Which of the following devices is designed specifically for patient protection purposes?
    a. Dental pointer cone with an integral diaphragm
    b. Fixed diaphragm
    c. Positive beam-limiting (PBL) system
    d. Fluoroscopic shutters
    e. 2.5 mm Al added filtration

15. At 70 kVp, 10 mAs, the patient dose is 50 mrad. What is it at 86 kVp, 5 mAs?
    a. 25 mrad
    b. 31 mrad
    c. 38 mrad
    d. 151 mrad
    e. 172 mrad

16. In radiography of the lumbar spine, which of the following techniques would provide the **least** patient ESE?
    a. 84 kVp, 100 mAs
    b. 90 kVp, 100 mAs
    c. 95 kVp, 50 mAs

WORKSHEET

39-2

X-Rays and Pregnancy

Exposure to radiation during diagnostic radiology, whether as a patient or as a technologist, is extremely low. Nevertheless, because of the increased sensitivity of the fetus to radiation, the portion of a radiation safety program that deals with x-rays and pregnancy requires some extra effort.

Pregnant patients should be alerted by information posted in the waiting area. Pregnant technologists should be assigned a second personnel radiation monitor with instructions that it be worn under the protective apron at waist level.

If, after a radiologic examination, a patient is found to be pregnant, the extent of the examination should be reviewed, the fetal dose should be estimated, and the time of gestation at which the dose was delivered should be determined. **Termination of pregnancy is rarely indicated.** However, should the fetal dose exceed 25 rad, such termination should be seriously considered.

The pregnant technologist should inform her supervisor as soon as she knows of her condition so that a second monitor can be provided. The dose limit to the fetus is 50 mrem/mo (0.5 mSv/mo).

EXERCISES

1. If an AP examination of the pelvis results in an ESE of 300 mR, the approximate fetal dose will be:
   a. 5 mrad
   b. 50 mrad
   c. 100 mrad
   d. 200 mrad
   e. 300 mrad

2. When a second radiation monitor is provided to a pregnant radiologic technologist:
   a. It should be worn at collar position.
   b. It should be worn outside the apron at waist level.
   c. It should be worn under the apron at waist level.
   d. She should alternate wearing the two.
   e. She should wear both under the apron at waist level.

3. What could a radiologic technologist do to reduce the radiation dose to the fetus of a pregnant patient?
   a. Decrease kVp and increase mAs.
   b. Increase OID.
   c. Increase SID and mAs.
   d. Reduce exposure time.
   e. Use specific area shields if appropriate.

4. A patient is to undergo radiographic examination because of low back pain. As she is being positioned, she asks whether this will affect her current pregnancy. What should the radiologic technologist do?
   a. Ignore the patient.
   b. Reassure her and proceed with the examination.
   c. Refuse to do the examination.
   d. Seek advice from the radiologist before proceeding.
   e. Use a high-kVp technique and a gonad shield.

5. Which of the following techniques results in the lowest exposure to the fetus?
   a. 60 kVp, 80 ms, 100 mA
   b. 85 kVp, 200 ms, 300 mA
   c. 90 kVp, 200 ms, 100 mA
   d. 100 kVp, 200 ms, 100 mA
   e. 120 kVp, 100 ms, 100 mA

6. After a skull series, a brain scan, a barium enema, and an intravenous pyelogram, it is discovered that the patient is pregnant. What is the **correct** course of action?
   a. Estimate the fetal dose.
   b. Do nothing.
   c. Perform a hysterosalpingogram.
   d. Reassure the patient and send her home.
   e. Terminate the pregnancy.

7. Radiation dose to the fetus from radiographic procedures is usually:
   a. <1 rad
   b. 2 to 4 rad
   c. 5 to 10 rad
   d. 10 to 20 rad
   e. >20 rad

8. What effects of diagnostic radiation exposure are possible in a newborn?
   a. Chromosome aberrations
   b. Extrauterine growth retardation
   c. IUGR
   d. Microcephaly
   e. Neonatal death

9. A patient who is 2 months pregnant is to undergo intravenous pyelography. Which of the following is **correct**?
   a. No more than two radiographs should be made.
   b. Normal precautions are adequate because fetal damage is least likely during this period of gestation.
   c. Order a pregnancy test first.
   d. The examination should be delayed if possible.
   e. The possibility of spontaneous abortion is high.

10. The greatest nonlethal radiation hazard to an embryo or fetus occurs:
    a. During the first 2 weeks of gestation
    b. At 2 to 8 weeks of gestation
    c. At 8 to 15 weeks of gestation
    d. During the second trimester
    e. During the third trimester

11. The National Council on Radiation Protection and Measurements (NCRPM) recommends a therapeutic abortion if the fetal dose exceeds:
    a. 1 rad
    b. 5 rad
    c. 10 rad
    d. 25 rad
    e. No recommendation is made.

12. In pelvic radiography, a dose to the shielded female gonads is primarily due to the:
    a. Characteristic x-rays released by high-atomic-number atoms in the pelvis
    b. Internally scattered x-rays
    c. Leakage radiation and air scatter
    d. Secondary electrons scattered out of the x-ray field
    e. X-rays scattered from nearby objects

13. When a radiologic technologist becomes pregnant, she should be:
    a. Counseled on proper radiation safety
    b. Fired
    c. Given a temporary leave of absence
    d. Given an additional lead apron
    e. Reassigned to nonfluoroscopy work

14. For a pregnant radiologic technologist, required radiation protection practice includes which of the following?
    a. Assignment to a low-exposure job
    b. No fluoroscopy
    c. Providing an additional apron
    d. Providing two radiation monitors
    e. Use of a gonad shield

15. Which of the following is needed to calculate the dose received by a fetus after a radiographic procedure?
    a. Fetal sex
    b. Gestation period
    c. Grid ratio
    d. Image receptor speed
    e. X-ray output

16. The fetal dose below which termination of pregnancy need **not** be considered is approximately:
    a. 2 rad
    b. 5 rad
    c. 10 rad
    d. 20 rad
    e. 50 rad

Occupational Exposure Reduction in Occupational Exposure

The dose limit (DL) applies only to occupationally exposed persons—not to patients. The DL is the dose of radiation below which the probability of harmful somatic or genetic effects is negligibly small, even when the DL is received each year of a working career.

Personnel monitoring is a program designed to measure the occupational exposure of workers. The quantity measured is the dose equivalent (DE), and the unit of DE is the rem (sievert).

Fluoroscopy is responsible for nearly all occupational radiation exposure among radiology personnel. Consequently, fluoroscopy requires maximum care with attention to good radiation safety practices. When a protective apron is worn, the monitor should be positioned above the apron in the collar region.

EXERCISES

1. What is the approximate annual occupational exposure received by a radiologic technologist?
   a. 50 mrem
   b. 100 mrem
   c. 300 mrem
   d. 1000 mrem
   e. 3000 mrem

2. Which of the following should **not** be part of a personnel radiation monitoring program?
   a. Film badges
   b. Optically stimulated luminescence (OSL)
   c. Photoluminescence dosimetry (PLD)
   d. Routine blood examination
   e. Thermoluminescence dosimeter (TLD)

3. To reduce occupational exposure during mobile x-ray examination:
   a. The patient should be given a film badge.
   b. The patient should be given a protective apron.
   c. The radiographic tube head should have a photoluminescence dosimeter.
   d. The radiologic technologist should wear a personnel monitor.
   e. The radiologic technologist should wear a protective apron.

4. In evaluation of a personnel monitoring report:
   a. Beta radiation is considered to contribute to the whole-body dose.
   b. Extremity dose is most limiting.
   c. Lens dose is most limiting.
   d. The skin dose is considered the sum of the whole-body dose and the extremity dose.
   e. Whole-body dose is usually highest.

5. Which of the following is required on the personnel monitoring report?
   a. Activity in millicuries
   b. Birthdate
   c. Cumulative annual skin exposure
   d. Occupational position
   e. Position of monitor

6. Recommendations proposed for mobile x-ray imaging systems state that the exposure cord length should be at least:
   a. 1 m
   b. 1.5 m
   c. 1.8 m
   d. 3 m
   e. 5 m

7. Personnel monitoring is required:
   a. For all radiology employees
   b. Only for radiologic technologists and radiologists
   c. When a pregnant patient is deliberately examined
   d. When it is likely that one will receive $\frac{1}{10}$ the DL
   e. When it is likely that one will receive the DL

8. A nurse is 3 feet to the patient's side during a portable chest x-ray exposure. What is likely to be her exposure?
   a. <1 mR
   b. 1 to 5 mR
   c. 5 to 10 mR
   d. 10 to 25 mR
   e. >25 mR

9. Which of the following personnel monitors can be worn the longest?
   a. Film badge
   b. Geiger-Mueller tube
   c. Pocket ionization chamber
   d. Scintillation monitor
   e. TLD device

10. During fluoroscopy, the personnel radiation monitor should be worn:
    a. Anywhere; it really does not matter
    b. At waist level, outside the apron
    c. At waist level, under the apron
    d. On the chest
    e. On the collar, outside the apron

11. Personnel monitoring must be conducted at least:
    a. Every 2 weeks
    b. Monthly
    c. Every 2 months
    d. Quarterly
    e. Annually

12. A 0.5 mm Pb equivalent apron attenuates a 75 kVp x-ray beam by approximately:
    a. 10%
    b. 30%
    c. 70%
    d. 90%
    e. 99%

13. Which of the following people is the **most** appropriate choice to hold a patient during a radiologic examination?
    a. Nurse
    b. Orderly
    c. Radiologic technologist
    d. Radiology secretary
    e. Relative

14. Which of the following statements about the use of protective apparel is **true**?
    a. Aprons are required even when a technologist is behind a protective barrier.
    b. During pregnancy, two aprons should be worn.
    c. Gloves should be worn by all who hold patients during the x-ray examination.
    d. It is unnecessary during mobile radiography.
    e. It is unnecessary while in the room during CT.

15. Which of the following personnel radiation monitors is **most** sensitive?
    a. Film badge
    b. Geiger-Mueller tube
    c. Pocket ionization chamber
    d. Scintillation detector
    e. TLD device

16. Which of the following is an advantage of film over TLD for personnel monitoring?
    a. Can be reused
    b. Can be used for longer periods
    c. Is cheaper
    d. Is less energy-dependent in the diagnostic range
    e. Is less sensitive to heat and humidity

17. Personnel monitoring of the extremities is necessary:
    a. During angiointerventional procedures
    b. During contrast injections
    c. During mobile radiography
    d. When the dose to the hands may exceed $\frac{1}{10}$ the DL
    e. When the dose to the hands may exceed 5000 mrem/yr

18. Filters are used in film badges to:
    a. Correct for film fog.
    b. Correct for length of wear.
    c. Estimate radiation energy.
    d. Identify the wearer.
    e. Increase the sensitivity.

19. For radiologists, protective eyewear:
    a. Is unnecessary
    b. Must be used for C-arm fluoroscopy
    c. Must be used with fluoroscopy with no protective curtain
    d. Must have 0.5 mm Pb equivalent shielding
    e. Must have side shields for scatter

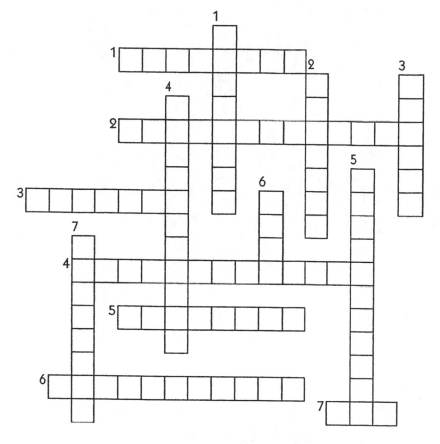

ACROSS

1. Proper unit for measuring occupational exposure
2. Proper unit for measuring radiation exposure
3. Monitoring periods and associated exposure records must not exceed a calendar _____.
4. Biologic effectiveness of radiation energy absorbed (2 words)
5. Term that refers to radiation intensity in air
6. The population gonad dose of importance is the _____ significant dose.
7. The unit of effective dose used for radiation protection purposes; usually applied to occupationally exposed persons

DOWN

1. Proper unit for measuring radiation dose
2. The _____ monitor is used to measure background exposure during transportation, handling, and storage.
3. One of the factors considered when GSD is computed
4. Diagnostic x-ray procedure that leads to one of the highest occupational exposures
5. Exposure to the skin (ESE) (2 words)
6. Measures radiation energy absorbed as a result of radiation exposure during patient examinations
7. The GSD is a _____-average gonad dose.

MATH TUTOR

Contributed by Quinn B. Carroll, MEd, RT

Working With Decimal Timers

Name _____

Date _____

EXERCISE 1:
CALCULATING TOTAL mAs VALUES

One of the first things you will learn in any radiographic imaging course is the relationship between milliamperage (mA) and exposure time (s) in producing a total mAs. The total mAs value is very important because it directly relates to how dark the radiograph will be. Exposure time cannot be considered alone, nor can mA, when it comes to controlling the *total* density of the resultant image.

A key point to remember is that mA is a *rate*. It tells us how many x-rays are emitted from the x-ray tube per second or, to phrase it another way, how "fast" they are coming out.

The speedometer in your car measures a rate as well. It does not tell you what the end result of your trip will be. For example, to determine when you will arrive in Dallas, you must also know how long you will be driving at that rate. You must multiply the miles per hour (the rate) by the number of hours (the time) to find the total miles you will travel. It makes no difference whether you go 50 mph for 2 hours or 25 mph for 4 hours—the end result will be the same distance covered.

Likewise, whether the x-ray tube emits 1 million x-rays per second for 1 second or 0.5 million x-rays per second for 2 seconds, the resultant total exposure to the film will be the same. As a radiologic technologist, your first concern is to produce adequate density on the film for a visible image. This depends on how "fast" the x-rays are being emitted *and* how long the tube is left on. It depends on the mA multiplied by the time—the total mAs.

Because many combinations of mA and time can be used to achieve the same total mAs, radiologic technologists must become skilled at computing these numbers so they can adapt to different equipment and different situations. Some would argue that mAs conversion charts are often available on the wall in the control booth and that all you have to do is look this information up. However, such charts are almost never found on mobile (portable) machines or in surgery, and often they do not match the equipment in the department.

Suppose you normally use 400 mA and $\frac{1}{80}$ second for an ankle radiograph in the department and you are called to do a portable ankle radiograph using a mobile unit with a maximum of 300 mA available. It is a time-saving and repeat-avoiding skill to be able to quickly and mentally determine the total mAs value to be 5 mAs and by doing so to realize that for this value to be obtained at 300 mA, a time of $\frac{1}{60}$ second is needed.

Such mental math should be second nature to every radiologic technologist. It is not as hard as you might think; it just requires practice. The drills that follow are designed to provide the practice needed to develop that skill.

This section first focuses on total mAs conversions using decimals (because most modern equipment uses decimal timers); then several drills on conversions using fractional times are provided. After that, conversion of fractions to decimals—and vice versa—is reviewed. This is helpful because radiologic technologists often must adjust from equipment that uses decimal timers to equipment that uses fractional timers and then back again.

On x-ray machines, the most used mA stations are provided in multiples of 100. On the exposure timers, the most used decimal times consist of two digits after the decimal, that is, they are "hundredths" (e.g., 0.25, 0.05). This provides an easy starting point for practicing decimal conversions: All you must do to figure the total mAs is to get into the habit of moving the decimal point on the exposure time two places to the right in your mind's eye; then ignore the two zeros on the mA station while multiplying. You are simply cancelling the hundreds with hundredths.

For example, find the total mAs for the following:

200 mA at 0.05 s

Moving the time decimal two places to the right, you have 5. Ignoring the two zeros on the mA, you have 2. This is simply 2 × 5, or 10 mAs.

Think of 300 mA at 0.080 second (ignore the last zero) as simply 3 × 8, which is 24 mAs; 100 mA at 0.025 second is 1 × 2.5, or 2.5 mAs. Examine these three examples carefully before going on.

If three digits follow the decimal, as in 0.008 second, you will use the same method, but you will still be dealing with a decimal when multiplying. For example, 200 mA at 0.008 second should be thought of as 2 × 0.8, which gives a total of 1.6 mAs. However, relatively few time settings on x-ray machines are given in the thousandths like this.

If there is only one digit behind the decimal point, such as 0.4 second, again move the decimal two places over. This time it will add a zero to your time number, so you will consider 0.4 as 40. Hence, 200 mA at 0.4 second will be thought of as 2 × 40, for a total of 80 mAs. Think of 100 mA at 0.2 second as 1 × 20, or 20 mAs; 500 at 0.8 is 5 × 80, or 400 mAs.

If two nonzero numbers are present after the decimal, you will simply ignore the decimal. That is, 0.16 will be thought of as 16. Three positive numbers after the decimal keep the decimal in the problem: 300 mA at 0.125 is thought of as 3 × 12.5. Multiply 3 × 12 first for 36, and then add 3 halves for a total of 37.5 mAs.

On most x-ray machines, a repeating pattern is available in the time settings. Note for example the following times from one common brand of equipment, in order: .002 s, .003, .004, .005, .007, .01, .015, .02, .025, .03, .035, .05, .07, .1, .15, .2, .25, .3, .35, .5, .7, 1, 2, and 4. One pattern you will see is that between a 5 and a 1, there is always a 7. Table MT-1 simply reorganizes these numbers so you can see the repetition.

Consider the recurring sevens on this machine: .007, .07, and .7. Once you become familiar with mAs values at, for example, the .07 time, you can easily do figuring with the other two "seven" times by simply moving the decimal point in your answer.

TABLE MT-1 Decimal exposure times available on a typical x-ray machine			
	.01	.1	1
.015	.15		
.002	.02	.2	2
	.025	.25	
.003	.03	.3	
	.035	.35	
.004			4
.005	.05	.5	
.007	.07	.7	

As was previously discussed, you should be thinking of 200 mA at 0.07 second as 2 × 7, for 14 mAs total.

Think of 200 mA at 0.007 also as 2 × 7, only with a decimal added in the answer: 1.4 mAs.

Think of 200 mA at 0.7 second as 2 × 7 with a zero added, or 2 × 70, for 140 mAs.

The act of writing down something helps you to remember it, even if you never again refer to your note. An excellent exercise for memorizing mAs values on a particular machine is to jot down the available times in just the format shown in Table MT-1. Write at the top the mA station you use most often, perhaps 200 or 300 mA, and then write to the side of each time setting the total mAs produced at that mA station. When you are through, look at the pattern of mAs values. Note the repeating patterns.

Do the following part of this exercise on your own, calculating total mAs values mentally. If you get stuck on one, review the instructions above for help. Do not check your answers after each question; do the whole exercise first, figuring the problems in your head and then writing the answer down. When you have completed the exercise, check your answers and correct the ones you missed.

To benefit from this drill, *do not figure your calculations on paper—do them mentally,* and then write down your answer. Do not look at the answers after trying each question; try the entire exercise, write your answers down, and then check all your answers with the Math Tutor Answer Key.

Name _____

Date _____

Working With Decimal Timers

EXERCISE 1:
CALCULATING TOTAL mAs VALUES

mA	×	Time(s)	=	mAs
1. 100	@	0.05	=	_____
2. 100	@	0.064	=	_____
3. 100	@	0.019	=	_____
4. 100	@	0.125	=	_____
5. 100	@	0.8	=	_____
6. 200	@	0.02	=	_____
7. 200	@	0.05	=	_____
8. 200	@	0.064	=	_____
9. 200	@	0.15	=	_____
10. 200	@	0.015	=	_____
11. 200	@	0.125	=	_____
12. 200	@	0.3	=	_____
13. 200	@	0.4	=	_____
14. 200	@	0.008	=	_____
15. 200	@	0.003	=	_____
16. 200	@	0.035	=	_____
17. 300	@	0.03	=	_____
18. 300	@	0.07	=	_____
19. 300	@	0.7	=	_____
20. 600	@	0.05	=	_____
21. 600	@	0.25	=	_____
22. 600	@	0.8	=	_____
23. 600	@	0.006	=	_____
24. 600	@	0.008	=	_____
25. 300	@	0.1	=	_____

mA	×	Time(s)	=	mAs
26. 300	@	0.3	=	_____
27. 300	@	0.04	=	_____
28. 300	@	0.015	=	_____
29. 300	@	0.25	=	_____
30. 300	@	0.025	=	_____
31. 300	@	0.15	=	_____
32. 300	@	0.006	=	_____
33. 300	@	0.004	=	_____
34. 400	@	0.01	=	_____
35. 400	@	0.04	−	_____
36. 400	@	0.07	=	_____
37. 400	@	0.16	=	_____
38. 400	@	0.016	−	_____
39. 400	@	0.33	=	_____
40. 400	@	0.8	=	_____
41. 400	@	0.7	−	_____
42. 400	@	0.007	=	_____
43. 500	@	0.08	=	_____
44. 500	@	0.03	=	_____
45. 500	@	0.2	=	_____
46. 500	@	0.7	=	_____
47. 500	@	0.007	=	_____
48. 500	@	0.125	=	_____

Be sure to review those problems you answered incorrectly and to go back to the instructions just given, if necessary.

Name _____

Date _____

Working With Fractional Timers

EXERCISE 2:
THE 100 mA STATION

Exposure timers that read in fractions are becoming rare. They are somewhat more difficult to convert mentally than those that read in decimals, but they also tend to follow patterned sequences. If you memorize just a few pairs of numbers, you can do most of them.

For this unit, we will do practice drills for each mA station separately. At each mA station, certain pairs of numbers always go together. For example, at the 100 mA station, fives and twos always go together:

100 mA at ½ s 50 mAs
100 mA at ⅕ s 20 mAs
100 mA at 1/50 s 2 mAs
100 mA at 1/20 s 5 mAs

Note that these numbers are rounded up or down to make it easier to memorize them. For example, 100 mA at ⅙ second is actually 16.67 mAs and would normally round up to 17. However, it is easier to remember 16 because the mind associates the sixes in ⅙ with those in 16. The results are close enough for any radiographic technique. Likewise, ⅛ of 100 is actually 12.5, and 1/12 of 100 is actually 8.33. In these units on fractions, all answers will be rounded out. The goal is for you to *mentally* derive a good estimated technique, not an exact answer.

Memorizing the pairs of numbers will not tell you where to put any decimal points—you will have to learn that by practice.

It is important to solve these problems mentally, not on paper. After you have completed this entire exercise, check your answers and review the questions you missed.

Zero may be added or a decimal point moved, but a time fraction that uses a 5 will always result in a total mAs involving a 2, and vice versa.

At the 100 mA station, the following pairs of numbers always go together; commit them to memory before you go on. The best way to memorize them is to get a study partner to drill you as if it were an oral test: 3 and 33 × 4 and 25 × 5 and 2 × 6 and 16 × 7 and 15 × 8 and 12.

mA	×	Time(s)	=	mAs
1. 100	@	½	=	_____
2. 100	@	1/20	=	_____
3. 100	@	1/50	=	_____
4. 100	@	⅕	=	_____
5. 100	@	⅛	=	_____
6. 100	@	1/80	=	_____
7. 100	@	1/12	=	_____
8. 100	@	1/120	–	_____
9. 100	@	⅐	=	_____
10. 100	@	1/15	=	_____
11. 100	@	1/40	=	_____
12. 100	@	⅓	=	_____
13. 100	@	1/30	=	_____
14. 100	@	⅙	=	_____
15. 100	@	1/60	=	_____
16. 100	@	⅔	=	_____

Name _____

Date _____

Working With Fractional Timers

EXERCISE 3:
THE 200 mA AND 50 mA STATIONS

Having memorized the number pairs for the 100 mA station, you can figure the total mAs for most time settings at the 200 mA station simply by doubling the answer you would get at 100 mA. For example, once it becomes second nature to you that 100 mA at $\frac{1}{60}$ second is 1.7 mAs, whenever you see 200 mA at $\frac{1}{60}$ second, you can simply double 1.7 in your mind for a total of 3.4 mAs.

You can cope with the 50 mA station in a similar fashion: Simply cut in half the answer you would get at the 100 mA station. If 100 mA at $\frac{1}{30}$ second is 3.3 mAs, 50 mA at $\frac{1}{30}$ second will be approximately 1.6 or 1.7 mAs.

Practice these conversions for typical fractions in this exercise. Carefully correct and review your answers with the Math Tutor Answer Key after you have completed the entire exercise.

	mA	$\times$	TIME(S)	=	mAs
1.	200	@	$\frac{1}{8}$	=	_____
2.	50	@	$\frac{1}{20}$	=	_____
3.	200	@	$\frac{1}{5}$	=	_____
4.	200	@	$\frac{1}{50}$	=	_____
5.	50	@	$\frac{1}{8}$	=	_____
6.	200	@	$\frac{1}{80}$	=	_____
7.	200	@	$\frac{1}{12}$	=	_____
8.	200	@	$\frac{1}{120}$	=	_____
9.	50	@	$\frac{1}{12}$	=	_____
10.	50	@	$\frac{1}{120}$	=	_____

	mA	$\times$	TIME(S)	=	mAs
11.	50	@	$\frac{1}{7}$	=	_____
12.	200	@	$\frac{1}{15}$	=	_____
13.	200	@	$\frac{1}{40}$	=	_____
14.	50	@	$\frac{1}{3}$	=	_____
15.	50	@	$\frac{1}{30}$	=	_____
16.	200	@	$\frac{1}{3}$	=	_____
17.	200	@	$\frac{1}{30}$	=	_____
18.	200	@	$\frac{1}{6}$	=	_____
19.	200	@	$\frac{1}{60}$	=	_____
20.	200	@	$\frac{2}{3}$	=	_____
21.	50	@	$\frac{1}{6}$	=	_____
22.	50	@	$\frac{1}{60}$	=	_____
23.	50	@	$\frac{1}{80}$	=	_____
24.	200	@	$\frac{1}{7}$	=	_____

Name _____

Date _____

Working With Fractional Timers

EXERCISE 4:
THE 300 mA STATION

The 300 mA station is a different number and produces its own unique number pairs when a fractional timer is used. For example, at the 300 mA station, fives and sixes always go together: $\frac{1}{5}$ second yields 60 mAs total, whereas $\frac{1}{6}$ second produces 50 mAs. The following pairs of numbers always go together when 300 mA is used. Commit these to memory, and drill with a study partner if you can:

5 and 6
15 and 20
12 and 25

Remember that at the 100 mA station, sevens always pair with fifteens. One seventh of 100 is about 15. So think of this as the following:

3 sets of 15
= Approximately 45 mAs
= 300 mA at $\frac{1}{8}$ s

Remember that at the 100 mA station, eights always pair with twelves. So think of this as the following:

= 3 sets of 12
= Approximately 36 mAs

Other combinations can be made, but these three pairs are very common. For other times, such as $\frac{1}{8}$ second or $\frac{1}{7}$ second, it is easier to simply use the paired number you memorized for the 100 mA station and then triple that number. Here are some examples:

300 mA at $\frac{1}{7}$ s

With these tips and with the previous exercises completed, you should be able to figure most mAs values for the 300 mA station in your head.

Proceed to solve the following problems mentally and write only your answer down. Check and review your answers using the Math Tutor Answer Key.

	mA	×	TIME(S)	=	mAs
1.	300	@	$\frac{1}{5}$	=	_____
2.	300	@	$\frac{1}{6}$	=	_____
3.	300	@	$\frac{1}{50}$	=	_____
4.	300	@	$\frac{1}{60}$	=	_____
5.	300	@	$\frac{1}{20}$	=	_____
6.	300	@	$\frac{1}{2}$	=	_____
7.	300	@	$\frac{1}{15}$	=	_____
8.	300	@	$\frac{1}{12}$	=	_____
9.	300	@	$\frac{1}{120}$	=	_____
10.	300	@	$\frac{1}{25}$	=	_____
11.	300	@	$\frac{1}{4}$	=	_____
12.	300	@	$\frac{1}{40}$	=	_____
13.	300	@	$\frac{1}{8}$	=	_____
14.	300	@	$\frac{1}{80}$	=	_____
15.	300	@	$\frac{1}{7}$	=	_____
16.	300	@	$\frac{2}{30}$	=	_____

Name _____

Date _____

Working With Fractional Timers

EXERCISE 5:
THE 400, 500, AND 600 mA STATIONS

Number pairs also can be made for these higher (400, 500, and 600) mA stations, but once you become comfortable with fractions at those stations up to 300 mA, this would be unnecessary. For the 600 mA station, the total mAs values learned at the 300 mA station can simply be doubled. The same thing can be done with the 400 mA station by doubling the results from the 200 mA station.

Any of these can be solved by going back to the number pairs you memorized for the 100 mA station. Whenever you get stuck, use the approach of solving for the 100 mA station and then multiplying the result by the first digit of the mA. Take the following example:

500 mA at $\frac{1}{20}$ s

You may recognize right away that the answer is 25 mAs. Or, you may mentally remove a zero from both the mA and the time, yielding the following:

= 50 at $\frac{1}{2}$ s
= 25 mAs

But *if you are not comfortable* with these other approaches, *go back to the 100 mA number pairs* you memorized. Remembering that 2 and 5 always go together and that $\frac{1}{20}$ of 100 is 5, think of this problem as follows:

500 mA at $\frac{1}{20}$ s
= 5 *sets of* 5
= 25 mAs

Proceed to the following questions, and then check and review your answers using the Math Tutor Answer Key.

	mA	×	Time(s)	=	mAs
1.	400	@	$\frac{1}{20}$	=	_____
2.	500	@	$\frac{1}{20}$	=	_____
3.	600	@	$\frac{1}{20}$	=	_____
4.	400	@	$\frac{1}{5}$	=	_____
5.	600	@	$\frac{1}{5}$	=	_____
6.	100	@	$\frac{1}{50}$	=	_____
7.	600	@	$\frac{1}{50}$	=	_____
8.	500	@	$\frac{1}{4}$	=	_____
9.	600	@	$\frac{1}{4}$	=	_____
10.	500	@	$\frac{1}{40}$	=	_____
11.	600	@	$\frac{1}{40}$	=	_____
12.	600	@	$\frac{1}{30}$	=	_____
13.	400	@	$\frac{1}{30}$	=	_____
14.	400	@	$\frac{1}{60}$	=	_____
15.	400	@	$\frac{1}{7}$	=	_____
16.	400	@	$\frac{2}{8}$	=	_____
17.	400	@	$\frac{1}{80}$	=	_____
18.	500	@	$\frac{1}{8}$	=	_____
19.	600	@	$\frac{1}{12}$	=	_____
20.	600	@	$\frac{1}{120}$	=	_____
21.	500	@	$\frac{1}{12}$	=	_____
22.	400	@	$\frac{1}{120}$	=	_____
23.	400	@	$\frac{1}{15}$	=	_____
24.	500	@	$\frac{1}{15}$	=	_____
25.	400	@	$\frac{1}{25}$	=	_____
26.	500	@	$\frac{1}{25}$	=	_____
27.	600	@	$\frac{1}{25}$	=	_____
28.	400	@	$\frac{1}{3}$	=	_____

Name _____

Date _____

Working With Fractional Timers

EXERCISE 6:
COMPLEX FRACTIONS

If you have completed all of the previous sections, you are ready to move on to fractional times that involve numerators other than "1" on the top, such as $2/5$ or $7/20$. These are not as hard as they might seem at a glance. You must do them in two steps: First, divide the bottom (denominator) into the mA station, and then think of the top number as the number of "sets."

To solve the following example:

200 mA at $2/5$ s

First, consider the top (numerator) of the fraction as a "1," in other words, find $1/5$ of 200. When you have this number, multiply it by the top of the fraction, thinking in "sets," as follows:

$1/5$ of 200 = 40
2 sets of 40 = 80 mAs

Think of 200 mA at $7/20$ second as 7 sets of 10, and think of 300 mA at $3/15$ second as 3 sets of 20. Using this approach, solve all of the following problems mentally, and then check and review your answers.

mA	×	Time(s)	=	mAs
1. 100	@	$2/5$	=	_____
2. 100	@	$2/15$	=	_____
3. 100	@	$3/15$	=	_____
4. 100	@	$3/20$	=	_____
5. 100	@	$7/20$	=	_____
6. 200	@	$3/4$	=	_____
7. 200	@	$2/5$	=	_____
8. 200	@	$3/5$	=	_____

mA	×	Time(s)	=	mAs
9. 200	@	$4/5$	=	_____
10. 200	@	$3/10$	=	_____
11. 200	@	$7/10$	=	_____
12. 200	@	$2/15$	=	_____
13. 200	@	$3/15$	=	_____
14. 200	@	$3/20$	=	_____
15. 200	@	$7/20$	=	_____
16. 400	@	$2/5$	=	_____
17. 400	@	$3/5$	=	_____
18. 400	@	$4/5$	=	_____
19. 400	@	$3/10$	=	_____
20. 400	@	$7/10$	=	_____
21. 300	@	$2/3$	=	_____
22. 300	@	$2/5$	=	_____
23. 300	@	$3/5$	=	_____
24. 300	@	$4/5$	=	_____
25. 300	@	$3/10$	=	_____
26. 300	@	$7/10$	=	_____
27. 300	@	$2/15$	=	_____
28. 300	@	$3/15$	=	_____
29. 300	@	$3/20$	=	_____
30. 400	@	$3/20$	=	_____
31. 400	@	$7/20$	=	_____
32. 500	@	$2/5$	=	_____
33. 500	@	$3/10$	=	_____
34. 500	@	$7/10$	=	_____
35. 500	@	$3/20$	=	_____
36. 600	@	$2/5$	=	_____
37. 600	@	$3/5$	=	_____
38. 600	@	$3/10$	=	_____
39. 600	@	$3/20$	=	_____
40. 600	@	$3/15$	=	_____

Name _____

Date _____

Timers: Converting Fractions Into Decimals and Vice Versa

EXERCISE 7: CONVERTING FRACTIONS INTO DECIMALS

A radiologic technologist who is used to working with decimal timers should be able to quickly adapt to an x-ray machine that employs a fractional timer. The reverse is also true, and both types of machines are commonly found. It turns out that the mathematics used for doing this is very similar to the mathematics used for mAs conversions.

For example, in converting the fraction ⅙ into a decimal number, 6 is simply divided into 1.00 for an answer of 0.16. Note how similar this operation is to taking ⅙ second at 100 mA to obtain 16 mAs. The only difference is the placement of the decimal point.

You should recall from "Working With Fractional Timers" that certain number pairs always go together; one of these pairs was 6 and 16. When fractions are converted to decimals and back, these number pairs always apply: ⅙ = 0.16, 1/16 = 0.6. (Although the sixteens are actually 16.6666, we are rounding down rather than up because this results in an easy memory device: associating the sixes.) Once again, the list of number pairs that always go together is as follows:

> 3 and 33
> 4 and 25
> 5 and 2
> 6 and 16
> 7 and 15
> 8 and 12

Committing these number pairs to memory will be of great help in solving technique problems in your head.

To change a fraction into a decimal, simply divide the numerator (top) by the denominator (bottom).

However, you first need to place a decimal point to the right of the numerator and then add as many zeros as needed to complete the division. For example, to find the decimal equivalent for ³⁄₂₀, you need to complete the following steps.

Temporarily remove the decimal, and remove the extra zeros:

> = 1.5

Now, "replacing" the decimal moves it one place to the left in the answer:

> = 0.15

If you are comfortable with the mA station exercises in "Working With Decimal Timers" and "Working With Fractional Timers," you will find it even easier to pretend that the numerator is an mA station, in multiples of 100. The following example illustrates.

Think of the numerator (3.0) as the 300 mA station (recall from "Working With Fractional Timers" that at 300 mA, 15 and 20 always go together):

> = 15

Now, since you added two zeros to the numerator above, you must move the decimal two places to the left in your answer:

> = 0.15

In this exercise, convert each fraction listed into its decimal equivalent. Rely as much as you can on the skills developed in "Working With Decimal Timers" and "Working With Fractional Timers." For unusual fractions or where these skills do not apply, simply divide the numerator by the denominator. Do the entire exercise, and then review your answers using the Math Tutor Answer Key.

	FRACTION		DECIMAL		FRACTION		DECIMAL
1.	$\frac{3}{4}$	=	_____	16.	$\frac{1}{80}$	=	_____
2.	$\frac{2}{3}$	=	_____	17.	$\frac{1}{100}$	=	_____
3.	$\frac{1}{4}$	=	_____	18.	$\frac{1}{200}$	=	_____
4.	$\frac{1}{5}$	=	_____	19.	$\frac{7}{10}$	=	_____
5.	$\frac{1}{6}$	=	_____	20.	$\frac{2}{15}$	=	_____
6.	$\frac{1}{7}$	=	_____	21.	$\frac{3}{20}$	=	_____
7.	$\frac{1}{8}$	=	_____	22.	$\frac{2}{5}$	=	_____
8.	$\frac{1}{12}$	=	_____	23.	$\frac{3}{5}$	=	_____
9.	$\frac{1}{15}$	=	_____	24.	$\frac{4}{5}$	=	_____
10.	$\frac{1}{20}$	=	_____	25.	$\frac{1}{3}$	=	_____
11.	$\frac{1}{25}$	=	_____	26.	$\frac{3}{15}$	=	_____
12.	$\frac{1}{30}$	=	_____	27.	$\frac{7}{20}$	=	_____
13.	$\frac{1}{40}$	=	_____	28.	$\frac{1}{150}$	=	_____
14.	$\frac{1}{50}$	=	_____	29.	$\frac{3}{8}$	=	_____
15.	$\frac{1}{60}$	=	_____	30.	$\frac{5}{16}$	=	_____

Name _____

Date _____

Timers: Converting Fractions Into Decimals and Vice Versa

EXERCISE 8: CONVERTING DECIMALS INTO FRACTIONS

Converting a decimal number into a fraction requires three steps. First, find the numerator (top of the fraction) by simply writing out all of the nonzero figures to the right of the decimal point. Then, to find the denominator (bottom of the fraction), write 1 for the decimal point and a zero for each decimal place after it. For example, to find the fractional equivalent for 0.0125, the following steps are needed:

For the numerator, write out nonzero figures to the right of the decimal point: 125 is the numerator.

For the denominator, write a 1 in place of the decimal point. There are four figures or decimal places to the right of the decimal point (0.0125), so you will write four zeros after the 1: 10,000 is the denominator. The fraction is as follows:

$$\frac{125}{10,000}$$

Finally, reduce the fraction (if possible) to its lowest common denominator. In the preceding example, 125 and 10,000 do not have a lower common denominator, and the fraction cannot be reduced. Following is an example of a decimal number that can be reduced after it is converted into a fraction:

0.6

For the numerator, write the nonzero figures to the right of the decimal point: 6 is the numerator. For the denominator, write a 1 for the decimal point and a zero for each place after it: 10 is the denominator. The fraction is as follows:

$\frac{6}{10}$

Six and ten share a common denominator: They are both divisible by 2. Reduce the fraction by dividing both numbers by 2:

$\frac{3}{5}$

This fraction cannot be further reduced, and it is the final answer.

In this exercise, convert the decimal numbers listed into equivalent fractions. Some of these problems are easily solved by computing them, whereas *others are better solved by simply recognizing the number pairs listed in Exercise 2.* Do the entire exercise, and then check and review your answers using the Math Tutor Answer Key.

	DECIMAL		FRACTION
1.	0.05	=	_____
2.	0.0333	=	_____
3.	0.2	=	_____
4.	0.75	=	_____
5.	0.025	=	_____
6.	0.6667	=	_____
7.	0.143	=	_____
8.	0.002	=	_____
9.	0.08	=	_____
10.	0.167	=	_____
11.	0.125	=	_____
12.	0.6	=	_____
13.	0.0625	=	_____
14.	0.00833	=	_____

Finding mA and Time Combinations for Desired mAs

Name _____

Date _____

EXERCISE 9:
WARM-UP CALCULATIONS

Common mathematics problems that a radiologic technologist faces in daily practice include the following:

1. Having a desired total mAs in mind and trying to mentally determine an mA-time combination that will yield that total
2. Mentally applying the 15% rule for kVp to adjust techniques
3. Mentally applying the inverse square law for distance changes

The following exercises will help you to develop the ability to do all three of these types of problems in your head. If you have trouble following the instructions on any of these, you may wish to review "Part One: Basic mAs and Time Conversions."

Probably the most common mathematics problem a radiologic technologist faces every day is that of having a desired total mAs in mind and trying to mentally determine an mA-time combination that will yield that total.

This is exactly the reverse of the exercises in Part One, and if you have completed the previous exercises, you will see how they help you in this one. The same number pairs are used. The only difference is that now you must decide whatever mA station your desired total mAs will divide into easily. With a little practice, the correct time fraction will then come to mind.

One unique thing about fractions (and something that you will not find when working with decimals) is that some of the answers can be found only in "complex fractions" as we have defined them. To solve these, you must again learn to think in "sets," such as using two sets of 20 mAs to obtain 40 mAs.

For example, how would you obtain 80 mAs using the 200 mA station? Because 80 does not divide *evenly* into 200, no usable fraction with a "1" on top as the numerator can be found. If you simply divide it out, you will get 2.5 as the denominator, resulting in a fraction of $\frac{1}{2.5}$; this is a complex fraction that will not be found on the timer knob. However, if you learn to recognize that 80 is 2 sets of 40, you can find a usable time.

First, divide 40 mAs into 200 mA. This will equal 5, and 5 is the denominator of your fraction.

In other words, the fraction used to obtain 40 mAs is $\frac{1}{5}$.

Now, simply go back and take *2 sets* of $\frac{1}{5}$ by changing the numerator to 2.

> The answer is $\frac{2}{5}$ second.
> 80 mAs = 200 mA at $\frac{2}{5}$ second
> (80 mAs = 2 sets of 40 mAs)

This exercise will "warm you up" for finding these sets of numbers. For each total mAs listed, express it as so many sets of a smaller number that will easily divide into one of the typical mA stations. There are *one* or *two* answers to each problem but no more because for that smaller number, you must choose a number that does not require further reduction. For example:

> 120 mAs can be expressed as _____ sets of _____.

If you use 6 sets of 20, this ratio can then be reduced to 3 sets (of 40), so 6 sets of 20 is not a good answer. One good answer is *3 sets of 40*, because this number of sets cannot be further reduced. Another good answer is *2 sets of 60*, because again, this number of sets cannot be further reduced. (One set of 120 is absurd, because there is no 120 mA station available.)

Note that sets of 40 will be evenly divisible into the 200 mA station, whereas sets of 60 will be divisible into the 300 mA station.

It sounds complicated at first, but try the following part of this exercise and you will find it is not as hard as you might have expected.

1. 80 mAs can be expressed as _____ sets of ____.
2. 45 mAs can be expressed as _____ sets of ____.
3. 66 mAs can be expressed as _____ sets of ____.
4. 75 mAs can be expressed as ____ sets of _____.
5. 180 mAs can be expressed as ____ sets of ____.
6. 120 mAs can be expressed as ____ sets of ____
   or as _____ sets of _____.
7. 160 mAs can be expressed as ____ sets of _____
   or as _____ sets of ____.
8. 240 mAs can be expressed as ____ sets of _____
   or as _____ sets of ____.
9. 90 mAs can be expressed as ____ sets of _____.
10. 320 mAs can be expressed as ____ sets of ____.

Check your answers in the Math Tutor Answer Key.

In Exercises 10 and 11, the total mAs desired is given, along with the mA station to be used. You must mentally decide which time to use. Use only those times that are available on most x-ray machines. In Exercise 10, your times must be expressed as fractions. In Exercise 11, use decimals. Do the exercises mentally, and then check your answers.

Name _____

Date _____

Finding mA and Time Combinations for Desired mAs

EXERCISE 10:
CALCULATIONS USING FRACTIONS

TOTAL mA	=	mA	×	SECONDS
1. 4 mAs	=	100 mA	×	_____
2. 2.5 mAs	=	100 mA	×	_____
3. 66 mAs	=	100 mA	×	_____
4. 7 mAs	=	100 mA	×	_____
5. 17 mAs	=	100 mA	×	_____
6. 8 mAs	=	100 mA	×	_____
7. 3.3 mAs	=	100 mA	×	_____
8. 1.7 mAs	=	100 mA	×	_____
9. 1.25 mAs	=	100 mA	×	_____
10. 0.8 mAs	=	100 mA	×	_____
11. 40 mAs	=	100 mA	×	_____
12. 5 mAs	=	150 mA	×	_____
13. 2.5 mAs	=	50 mA	×	_____
14. 25 mAs	=	50 mA	×	_____
15. 25 mAs	=	200 mA	×	_____
16. 40 mAs	=	200 mA	×	_____
17. 120 mAs	=	200 mA	×	_____
18. 5 mAs	=	200 mA	×	_____
19. 2.5 mAs	=	200 mA	×	_____
20. 14 mAs	=	200 mA	×	_____
21. 50 mAs	=	300 mA	×	_____
22. 6 mAs	=	300 mA	×	_____
23. 20 mAs	=	300 mA	×	_____
24. 2.5 mAs	=	300 mA	×	_____
25. 45 mAs	=	300 mA	×	_____
26. 180 mAs	=	300 mA	×	_____
27. 240 mAs	=	300 mA	×	_____
28. 75 mAs	=	300 mA	×	_____
29. 80 mAs	=	400 mA	×	_____
30. 240 mAs	=	400 mA	×	_____

Name _____

Date _____

Finding mA and Time Combinations for Desired mAs

EXERCISE 11:
CALCULATIONS USING DECIMALS

Total mA	=	mA	×	Seconds
1. 4 mAs	=	100 mA	×	_____
2. 2.5 mAs	=	100 mA	×	_____
3. 66 mAs	=	100 mA	×	_____
4. 7 mAs	=	100 mA	×	_____
5. 16 mAs	=	100 mA	×	_____
6. 8 mAs	=	100 mA	×	_____
7. 3.3 mAs	=	100 mA	×	_____
8. 1.7 mAs	=	100 mA	×	_____
9. 40 mAs	=	100 mA	×	_____
10. 2.5 mAs	=	50 mA	×	_____
11. 1.25 mAs	=	50 mA	×	_____
12. 25 mAs	=	200 mA	×	_____
13. 40 mAs	=	200 mA	×	_____
14. 120 mAs	=	200 mA	×	_____
15. 5 mAs	=	200 mA	×	_____
16. 2.5 mAs	=	200 mA	×	_____
17. 14 mAs	=	200 mA	×	_____
18. 50 mAs	=	300 mA	×	_____
19. 6 mAs	=	300 mA	×	_____
20. 21 mAs	=	300 mA	×	_____
21. 180 mAs	=	300 mA	×	_____
22. 75 mAs	=	300 mA	×	_____
23. 80 mAs	=	400 mA	×	_____
24. 240 mAs	=	400 mA	×	_____

Name _____

Date _____

Technique Adjustments

EXERCISE 12:
APPLYING THE 15% RULE FOR KVP, APPLYING THE RULE IN STEPS, APPLYING THE RULE IN PORTIONS

Radiologic technologists often must adjust techniques using the 15% rule for kVp to increase penetration or change the contrast on the radiograph while maintaining overall density. The ability to make these adjustments mentally should be second nature to the radiologic technologist. It is not very difficult to develop this ability, but it does require practice and repetition. The following drills will help you develop this ability.

The rule states that a 15% adjustment in kVp will change the resultant image density by a *factor of 2*. A 15% increase will double the film density, and a 15% reduction will cut the image density to one-half the original. This is an approximation, but it works very well and is the only practical rule of thumb for predicting the effects of kVp on the ultimate darkness of the radiograph.

To find 15% of the original kVp mentally, think of the operation as taking 10% first and then adding half as much again. For example, to find 15% of 80 kVp:

$80 \times 10\% = 8$	Take 10% of the kVp.
$8/2 = 4$	Figure one half of 8.
$8 + 4 = 12$	Add these two numbers.
$80 \times 15\% = 12$	

Fifteen percent of 60 kVp would be $6 + 3 = 9$. Fifteen percent of 120 would be $12 + 6 = 18$. This number is added to the original kVp to double film density, and it is subtracted to obtain one half of the original density.

In the above example that uses 80 kVp, what new total kVp would compensate for cutting the mAs to one half? The answer is 92 kVp ($80 + 12$). What would the new kVp be if, because of overpenetration, a radiograph turned out twice to be too dark and you wished to cut the density in half? The answer is 68 kVp.

You should also become comfortable with applying the 15% rule in steps and in portions.

A common misconception is that an adjustment of 10 kVp changes density by a factor of 2. This stems from the fact that 15% of 70 is 10.5, and 70 may be considered an "average" kVp for radiographic procedures. However, a 10 kVp change in the range of 40 kVp will almost double the density twice, whereas a 10 kVp change in the range of 100 kVp is only two thirds of the change needed to double or halve the density. For accuracy, it is important to use the 15% rule as prescribed rather than the "10 kVp rule."

Sometimes the desired adjustment in image density is much greater than a doubling or halving. Suppose you need to repeat an extremely light radiograph caused by underpenetration and the density has to be increased fourfold. Always translate the desired changes into terms of doubling (factors of two), and you can apply the rule.

To produce a radiograph that is four times darker, think of this change as two doublings. To obtain two doublings, you will need to increase 15% kVp *in two steps*. (It is not as accurate to simply make a 30% change, and the greater the change, the less accurate this approach is.) For example, if the original radiograph was exposed using 80 kVp:

$80 \times 15\% = 12$
Step 1: Increase by 15% of the original kVp.
$80 + 12 = 92$
This increase achieves the first doubling.
$92 \times 15\% = 14$
Step 2: Increase by 15% of the *adjusted kVp, not the original kVp.*
$92 + 14 = 106$
This increase achieves the second doubling.

A fourfold increase in image density will result from 106 kVp. This would also compensate for a reduction of mAs to one fourth of the original.

Only rarely is kVp adjusted by more than 1 set of 15%, especially for reductions that might result in an underpenetrated radiograph, regardless of increases in mAs. It is to be emphasized that mAs, not kVp, is the primary density control for radiographs, and that kVp is changed only to adjust for penetration, scatter radiation levels, image contrast, or grayscale. Nonetheless, when such adjustments are made, the mAs often must be compensated to maintain density, and the 15% rule comes into play.

One practical example of a kVp adjustment made using two steps of 15% is found in deriving a barium technique (upper gastrointestinal [GI] or solid column barium enema) from a routine abdomen technique. If the technique for an anteroposterior (AP) projection of the abdomen were 30 mAs and 80 kVp, the following calculations would allow adequate penetration of the same abdomen when the gastrointestinal tract is filled with barium:

30 mAs @ 80 kVp
Routine AP abdomen.
15 mAs @ 92 kVp
First step: Increase of 15% (12 kVp), accompanied by one-half the mAs to maintain a density of 15 mAs @ 92 kVp
Second step: Increase (14 kVp) is 15% of 92, with another halving of the mAs to 7.5 mAs.

For a solid column barium procedure (not air contrast), approximately 7 mAs at about 110 kVp would provide good penetration through the barium while keeping overall image density at an optimum level. (For an air contrast technique, simply reduce by 10 to 15 kVp, with the mAs still at about 7.)

The image density on a radiograph must be changed by at least one third (about 30%) for the human eye to detect any difference. In practice, efforts to increase overall radiographic technique by less than 50% or to decrease it by less than 30% are wasted. Changes such as these can be made with the use of the 15% rule in portions.

Suppose you wish to reduce the density but decide that cutting it in half would be too much. You must reduce overall technique by at least one third to make any visible difference. Taking one third of 15%, we can derive a kVp change of about 5%. The kVp must be reduced by a minimum of 5% to lighten up the image. To find 5% of the original kVp, think of it as one half of 10%. For this problem, if the original kVp was 120 kVp, the solution would be as follows:

120 × 10% = 12
Figure 10% of the kVp.
12 × ½ = 6
Take one half of that amount.
120 − 6 = 114

Subtract this number from the original kVp.

The kVp must be reduced at least to 114 for the density to be visibly lightened up in this case.

Although a 2 kVp adjustment may visibly change image density in the 40 kVp range, the same adjustment will not make a visible difference in higher ranges. The change must be at least 5%.

Consider an increase in density of 50% (1.5 times denser than the original). You will recall the recommendation to think of technique changes in terms of doublings or halvings. In this context, such a 50% increase should be thought of as *halfway to doubling*. (Similarly, a 25% reduction in overall technique would be thought of as *halfway to cutting it in half*.) Because a 15% increase in kVp will double the density, one half of 15% should bring the density halfway to a doubling. In other words, to increase the density by 50%, increase the kVp by one half of 15%.

For example, suppose a radiograph taken at 80 kVp comes out a bit light. Doubling the density would be too much. You decide to increase the density by about one half (50%):

80 × 15% = 12
Find 15% of the kVp.
12 × ½ = 6
Find one half of that amount.
80 + 6 = 86
Add this number to the original kVp.
For a radiograph that is 50% darker, increase kVp to 86.

Complete the following exercise using the 15% rule. Some problems will require you to apply the rule in sequential steps, and in some, the rule will have to be applied in portions of one third or one half of 15%. Finish the entire exercise, and then check and review your answers using the Math Tutor Answer Key.

1. What is 5% of 120?
2. What is 5% of 90?
3. What is 5% of 80?
4. What is 5% of 50?
5. What is 5% of 60?
6. What is 15% of 70?
7. What is 15% of 40?
8. What is 15% of 60?
9. What is 15% of 110?
10. What is one half of 15% of 40?
11. What is one half of 15% of 70?
12. What is one half of 15% of 80?
13. What is one half of 15% of 50?
14. What is one half of 15% of 90?
15. What is one half of 15% of 120?

16. Starting at 120 kVp, what new kVp would result in a density that is one-half as dark as the original?

17. Starting at 40 kVp, what new kVp would result in a density that is twice as dark as the original?

18. Starting at 60 kVp, what new kVp would result in a density that is 50% darker than the original (halfway to double the original)?

19. Starting at 80 kVp, what new kVp would result in a density that is about 75% (halfway to one half) of the original?

Name _____

Date _____

Technique Adjustments

EXERCISE 13:
ADJUSTING FOR DISTANCE CHANGES, THE INVERSE SQUARE LAW, THE SQUARE LAW: RULES OF THUMB FOR DISTANCE CHANGES

As described in the textbook, radiologic technologists should be completely familiar with the inverse square law. It describes the relationship between radiation quantity or intensity in the x-ray beam and distance from the x-ray tube. Because the x-ray beam "fans out" over larger areas with increasing distance, the concentration of x-rays decreases at a rate inversely proportional to the square of the distance. The formula is as follows:

$$I_2 = I_1 \left(\frac{D_1}{D_2} \right)^2$$

where I_1 is the original quantity or concentration of x-rays, I_2 is the new radiation quantity after the distance change, and $D1$ and $D2$ are the old and new distances (source-to-image receptor distances [SIDs]), respectively.

The inverse square law can be used to predict radiation exposure to the patient, operator, or film. Because the density produced on the film is generally directly proportional (or "reciprocal") to the exposure, the inverse square law can be used to predict image density changes when distance is altered. Some of the questions in the following exercise apply this formula.

However, this section also focuses on two derivations from the inverse square law that are extremely helpful in daily practice: the "square law" and rules of thumb for distance changes.

Whereas the inverse square law is used to predict image density, the square law is used to compensate technique so that density is maintained when distance changes. The formula for the square law is as follows:

$$mAs = mAs_1 \left(\frac{D_2}{D_1} \right)^2$$

where *mAs1* is the original mAs used at D1 (the original SID), and *mAs2* is the new mAs needed to maintain equal density if the SID is changed to D2.

When the original mAs is not given or known, place a 1 in the formula for "mAs1" and solve for mAs2. The resulting number will be the *factor* by which mAs should be changed. A result of 2.0 would indicate that the original mAs, whatever it was, should be doubled. A result of 0.5 would indicate that it should be cut in half, and so forth.

As an example, suppose the distance (SID) is increased from the usual 40 inches to 60 inches. The technique chart is written for 40 inches. What change would have to be made in the overall technique taken from the chart to maintain adequate image density at 60 inches?

Because the actual mAs is not given, use a 1 for "mAs1." D1 is 40 inches, and D2 is 60 inches.

> First, square the distances.
> 1600(mAs2) = 3600 (mAs₁)
> Then cross-multiply.
> Isolate mAs2 by dividing both sides of the equation by 1600.
> mAs2 = 2.25 (mAs₁)

This makes 2.25 the *factor* by which mAs should be changed.

The 40-inch technique should be increased 2.25 times to maintain density at 60 inches SID.

The solutions to square law problems are always the inverse of those for solving inverse square law problems. For example, if a distance change would result in twice as dark a film by the inverse square law, then the technique that would be required to maintain the original density at the new distance would be one-half the mAs. If the density change can be predicted, simply invert this change to find the technique adjustment.

Although the inverse square law is important to understand, in practice, radiologic technologists rarely use a calculator or a pencil to apply it accurately. Rather, when doing a mobile procedure at

60 inches SID, for example, they will likely make a mental estimate of the increase in technique required as compared with the usual 40-inch SID. This section provides some simple rules of thumb that, if committed to memory, will greatly improve your accuracy in making this kind of technique adjustment.

A handful of distances (30, 40, 60, 72, and 96 inches) can be applied to more than 95% of radiographic procedures. By taking the most commonly used 40 inches as a standard and comparing the others with it, rules of thumb are easily derived and learned.

It helps to think of distance changes in factors of two, that is, doublings and halvings. For example, the square law formula shows that if SID is increased from 40 inches to 80 inches (a doubling), the technique must be increased by four times to maintain density. However, by thinking of this quadrupling of the technique as two doublings, rules of thumb can be formulated for other distance changes.

For example, think of increasing the SID from 40 inches to 60 inches as going halfway to doubling the SID, that is, 60 inches is halfway from 40 to 80. Because 80 inches would require two doublings of technique, 60 inches will require one half of that increase, or one doubling. For a 60-inch projection, double the mAs used at 40 inches.

In a similar manner, 30 inches can be considered as halfway to cutting 40 inches in half. A 20-inch distance would require one fourth of the overall technique, or two halvings. Thus, 30 inches requires only one halving of the 40-inch technique.

Table MT-2 summarizes these rules of thumb for the most often used distances. A column listing the actual solution based on the square law formula is provided as well, so you can see how close these rules of thumb are for accuracy. If you keep in mind that density must be changed by at least 30% for a visible difference to be seen, the rules of thumb are clearly accurate enough for practical use.

By far the most useful of these rules of thumb will be those for 60 inches and 72 inches because these distances are frequently used in mobile procedures and in the radiology department. For mobile procedures, the rules of thumb can be taken one step further to derive a technique for 50 inches SID.

If you consider 50 as halfway to 60, the technique would be increased halfway to a doubling, or increased by 50%. By the square law formula, the needed increase is 1.57 times the original. The rule of thumb rounds it to 1.5 times. *Radiologic technologists assigned to mobile units should remember that, compared with the usual 40-inch technique, a 50-inch SID requires a 50% increase in overall technique (preferably using mAs), a 60-inch distance requires a doubling, and a 72-inch distance requires a tripling.*

Because chest radiography is commonly performed with the 72-inch SID, it is important to emphasize that the 72-inch distance requires three times the 40-inch technique, and that a 40-inch distance requires one third of the 72-inch technique. This relationship is frequently encountered when upright or decubitus abdomen radiographs are taken along with chest radiographs. *Remember that the relationship between a 40-inch SID and a 72-inch SID is a factor of 3.*

These rules of thumb also can be used to solve for density problems if you remember to invert them (make fractions out of them). For example, if the distance is increased from 40 inches to 72 inches and the technique is not compensated for this change, how dark will the radiograph be? Simply invert the factor for 72 inches that is found in Table MT-2. The answer is that the new radiograph will have one-third the density of the original. A radiograph taken at 60 inches without compensating technique would be one-half as dense, and so forth.

Complete the following exercise as directed. The first 13 questions should be done mentally, using rules of thumb. Note that those starting at 60 inches or 30 inches also can be solved in your head if you analyze the distance changes as doubling, halving, halfway to doubling, or halfway to halving. Questions 14 to 25 employ the square law to find a new mAs that will compensate for the change in distance.

After completing the entire exercise, carefully check and review your answers using the Math Tutor Answer Key.

TABLE MT-2 Rules of thumb for distance changes starting at 40 inches		
New distance (in)	Technique change computed by square law	Rule of thumb technique change
30	0.56	1/2
40	1.0 (standard)	1
60	2.25	2×
72	3.24	3×
80	4.0	4×
96	5.76	6×

Name _____

Date _____

Technique Adjustments

EXERCISE 13:
ADJUSTING FOR DISTANCE CHANGES, THE INVERSE SQUARE LAW, THE SQUARE LAW: RULES OF THUMB FOR DISTANCE CHANGES

Use the technique rules of thumb to solve these problems:

	FROM:	TO MAINTAIN DENSITY:
1.	25 mAs	_____ mAs
	40-in SID	72-in SID
2.	15 mAs	_____ mAs
	40-in SID	60-in SID
3.	7.5 mAs	_____ mAs
	40-in SID	80-in SID
4.	6 mAs	_____ mAs
	40-in SID	96-in SID
5.	60 mAs	_____ mAs
	40-in TFD	20-in TFD
6.	2.5 mAs	_____ mAs
	30-in TFD	60-in TFD
7.	30 mAs	_____ mAs
	40-in TFD	30-in TFD
8.	12.5 mAs	_____ mAs
	30-in TFD	45-in TFD
9.	30 mAs	120 mAs
	80 kVp	_____ mAs
	40-in TFD	60-in TFD

Use the density rules of thumb to solve these problems:

	FROM:	TO:
10.	40-in TFD	20-in TFD
	Density=1	Density=_____
11.	60-in TFD	45-in TFD
	Density=1	Density=_____
12.	40-in TFD	80-in TFD
	Density=1	Density=_____
13.	30-in TFD	45-in TFD
	Density=1	Density=_____

Use the square law to solve these problems:

	FROM:	TO MAINTAIN DENSITY:
14.	10 mAs	_____ mAs
	40-in TFD	100-in TFD
15.	5 mAs	_____ mAs
	60-in TFD	50-in TFD
16.	2.5 mAs	_____ mAs
	72-in TFD	40-in TFD
17.	2.5 mAs	_____ mAs
	60-in TFD	20-in TFD
18.	2.5 mAs	2.5 mAs
	80 kVp	_____ kVp
	60-in TFD	42.5-in TFD
19.	180 mAs	20 mAs
	36-in TFD	_____ TFD
20.	45 mAs	5 mAs
	90 in TFD	_____ TFD
21.	30 mAs	120 mAs
	20-in TFD	_____ TFD
22.	5 mAs	45 mAs
	20-in TFD	_____ TFD
23.	12 mAs	_____ mAs
	96-in TFD	30-in TFD
24.	25 mAs	_____ mAs
	96-in TFD	40-in TFD
25.	40 mAs	_____ mAs
	80-in TFD	36-in TFD

Use the inverse square law to solve these problems:

	FROM:	TO:
26.	40-in TFD	72-in TFD
	Density=1	Density=_____
27.	60-in TFD	72-in TFD
	Density=1	Density=_____
28.	50-in TFD	36-in TFD
	Density=1	Density=_____
29.	72-in TFD	96-in TFD
	Density=1	Density=_____

LABORATORY
EXPERIMENTS

Inverse Square Law

Name _____

Date _____

OBJECT

To demonstrate the effect that distance from the x-ray source has on x-ray intensity.

DISCUSSION

X-rays are emitted isotropically (i.e., with equal intensity in all directions) from the target of the x-ray tube. The anode and diagnostic housing prevent x-rays from exiting in any direction other than through the window of the tube and the port of the housing. The collimator or other beam-restricting devices further define the useful x-ray beam.

The intensity of the x-ray beam decreases as the square of the distance from the source increases. If the distance from the source is doubled, the intensity will be reduced to one-fourth its former value. This relationship, known as the inverse square law, is based solely on geometry. It has nothing to do with x-ray absorption. The x-ray intensity (I_1) passing through a unit area at some distance (d_1) from the target will be

$$I_1 = \frac{I_0}{4\pi d_1^2}$$

where I_0 is the total number of x-rays emitted from the target. The intensity (I_2) at any other distance (d_2) from the target will similarly be expressed as follows:

$$I_2 = \frac{I_0}{4\pi d_2^2}$$

Combining these equations:

$$I_0 = \frac{I_0}{4\pi d_1^2} - I_2 = \frac{I}{4\pi d_2^2} \text{ and } I_1 = \frac{I_0}{d_1^2}$$

$$\frac{I_0}{4\pi d_2^2} \quad I_2 \quad \frac{I_0}{d_2^2}$$

results in

$$\frac{I_1}{I_2} = \frac{d_2^2}{d_1^2}$$

MATERIALS REQUIRED

- Radiographic imaging system
- Ionization chamber
- Tape measure
- Linear graph paper
- Semilog graph paper

PROCEDURE

1. The x-ray imager may be used as it is normally filtered. Record the total filtration present if known.
2. Set the tube potential to 70 kVp. This will remain constant throughout the experiment.
3. Locate the position of the source (the target) of x-rays. Many tube housings are marked at the position of the target; if not, assume that the target position is at the middle of the tube housing.
4. Position the ionization chamber on the central ray of the useful beam and as close to the source as possible.

5. Record this distance on the data sheet provided, and take three readings of intensity. If possible, the mA and the exposure time should remain constant throughout this experiment. However, if the response range of the ionization chamber will not accommodate such measurements, either or both may require adjustment.

6. Repeat these measurements at approximately 25 cm intervals to a distance of 200 cm from the source.

7. Express the radiation intensity as exposure rate (mR/mAs) at each distance with use of the following expression:

$$\text{Exposure rate (mR/mAs)} = \frac{\text{Exposure (mR)}}{\text{Tube current (mA) exposure time(s)}}$$

RESULTS

Plot exposure rate (mR/mAs) as a function of distance from the source (cm) on the semilog graph paper provided.

EXERCISES

1. What was the shape of the curve obtained? Why?

2. Calculate the quantity 1 mR/mAs, and plot this as a function of distance from the target on the linear graph paper provided. What is the appearance of this curve and why? Where does the curve intersect the x-axis (distance axis), and where should it have intersected?

3. If the output intensity of an x-ray tube is 2.5 mR/mAs at 100 cm source-to-image receptor distance (SID), what would the intensity be at 150 cm SID?

4. The output intensity is shown to be 150 mR/mAs at 100 SID. At what SID will the intensity be 100 mR/mAs?

DATA SHEET FOR EXPERIMENT 1: INVERSE SQUARE LAW

CONSTANT FACTORS
- 70 kVp
- Filtration: _____ mm Al

Source to ionization chamber distance	Exposure measurement, mR				Tube current, mA	Exposure time, s	mAs	mR/mAs	1 mR/mAs
	First	Second	Third	Average					
25 cm									
50 cm									
75 cm									
100 cm									
125 cm									
150 cm									
175 cm									
200 cm									

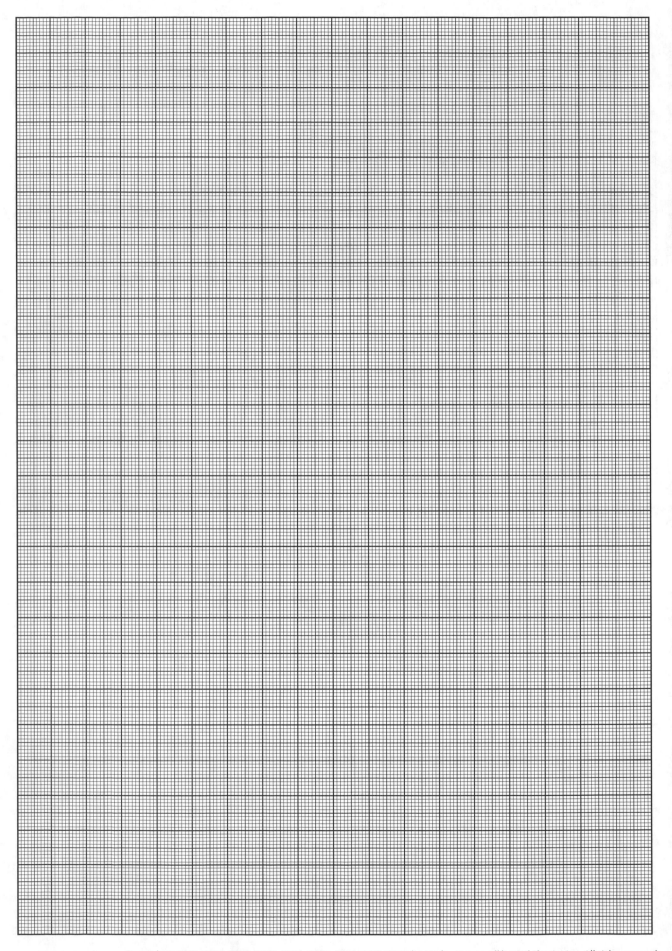

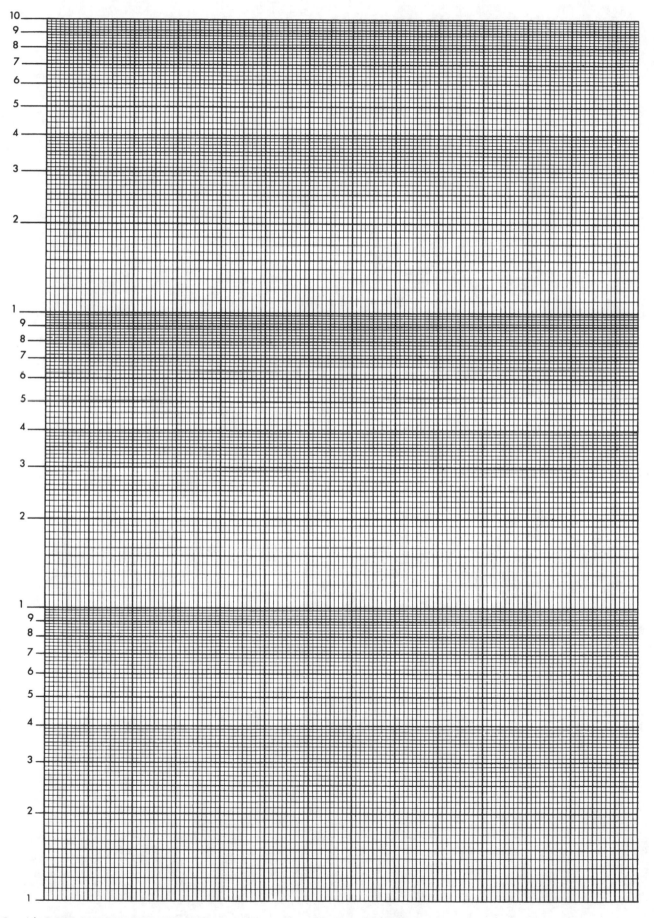

Effect of Source-to-Image Receptor Distance on Optical Density

Name _____

Date _____

OBJECT

To demonstrate the effect of changing the source-to-image receptor distance (SID) on the optical density (OD) of the image.

DISCUSSION

As was demonstrated in Experiment 1, radiation intensity changes inversely with the square of the SID. The intensity of the x-ray beam directly controls the OD of the film; consequently, film responds to the inverse square law.

To maintain a given OD when SID is changed, the technique must be compensated according to the square law. For example, if the SID were reduced to one half, the mAs should be cut to one quarter (one half squared). If this adjustment were not made to compensate for the change in distance, the resultant radiograph would be darker because of higher OD.

MATERIALS REQUIRED

- Radiographic imaging system
- Step-wedge penetrometer
- X-ray film processor
- 400-speed 14 in × 17 in (35 cm × 42 cm) screen-film cassette
- Lead or vinyl lead sheets
- Rectangular sponge approximately 4 inches thick
- Tape measure
- Lead numbers
- Viewbox
- Densitometer

PROCEDURE

1. Warm up the processor if needed, and run a couple of "scrap" films through it to stabilize temperature and circulation.

2. Load and place the cassette on the tabletop. Three exposures will be taken on one film. Collimate the light field to a 3 in × 10 in area crosswise at one end of the film. Use the leaded sheets to mask the adjacent film area.

3. Place the thick, flat sponge over the light field area. This creates a large object-to-image receptor distance (OID), which must be kept constant on all exposures.

4. Place the step-wedge penetrometer crosswise on the sponge, centered to the light field.

5. Number each exposure with a lead marker on the cassette. Take three exposures using the following techniques, or alternate techniques to accommodate your equipment.

   Exposure 1 Carefully set the SID at 100 cm to the tabletop.
   Technique: 100 mA, 100 ms, 50 kVp

   Exposure 2 Carefully set the SID at 50 cm to the tabletop. Be sure to collimate the light field, opening it up to include the entire step wedge if possible.
   Technique: 100 mA, 25 ms, 50 kVp

   Exposure 3 Place the cassette on the floor with the sponge and step wedge over the last third of the film. Carefully measure and set the SID to 180 cm from the cassette. Collimate the light field.
   Technique: 100 mA, 350 ms, 50 kVp

6. Process the film.

7. On resultant images, select a step on the step wedge from which to take OD measurements. On Exposure 1, the selected step should have a medium OD, for example, between 0.2 and 1.0. Using the densitometer, determine the OD at this step for each exposure.

RESULTS

In Table E2-1, record for each exposure the total mAs used at each SID and the measured OD.

TABLE E2-1			
	Total mAs	SID	OD
Exposure 1			
Exposure 2			
Exposure 3			

EXERCISES

1. Compare the relative changes in OD for Exposures 2 and 3 by dividing the OD for Exposure 1 into that for Exposure 2 and by dividing the OD for Exposure 1 into that for Exposure 3. Record here:

   2/1: _____ 3/1: _____

2. Compute the average OD change by summing these two ratios and then dividing by two.

   Average density change ratio: _____

3. Optical density ratio of 1.0 would indicate that the ODs produced by the different techniques are exactly the same. Is your computed average change within 15% of the original?

4. Visually compare Exposure 2 with Exposure 1. In 2, the SID was reduced to one half of the original and, with the square law, the mAs was reduced to one fourth. Did this technique change reasonably maintain image OD?

5. On Exposure 2, if the mAs had not been adjusted, what OD would you predict?

6. If the SID were doubled, what change in mAs would be required to maintain OD?

7. Restate your answer to Exercise 5 in terms of sets of doubling mAs. For example, would you double the original mAs once, twice, three times, or four times to compensate?

8. Now consider a change in SID from 100 cm to 150 cm. This can be thought of as going halfway to doubling the distance. In light of your answer to Exercise 6, how many doublings of mAs would be required at 150 cm to maintain a constant OD?

9. Visually compare Exposure 3 with Exposure 1. The SID for Exposure 3 was 180 cm, roughly halfway between 150 cm and 200 cm. Was OD reasonably maintained? By what ratio was the mAs increased for Exposure 3?

10. As a rule of thumb, by what factor must mAs be changed to compensate for adjustment of the SID from 100 cm to 180 cm?

Effect of Source-to-Image Receptor Distance on Image Blur

Name _____

Date _____

OBJECT

To demonstrate the effect of changing the source-to-image receptor distance (SID) on the degree of blurring of an image.

DISCUSSION

In addition to optical density (OD), distance affects two geometric properties of an image. The amount of focal-spot blur is inversely proportional to the SID. Long SIDs result in less focal-spot blur and increased sharpness. The magnification of the image is reduced with a long SID. Usually, focal-spot blur and magnification are undesirable; therefore, as a rule, the longest practical SID should be used.

MATERIALS REQUIRED

- Radiographic imaging system
- Small dry bone such as a phalanx (or other small object)
- Resolution test pattern (lp/mm)
- X-ray film processor
- 400-speed 14 in × 17 in (35 cm × 43 cm) screen-film cassette
- Lead or vinyl lead sheets
- Rectangular sponge approximately 4 inches thick
- Tape measure
- Lead numbers
- Viewbox

PROCEDURE

1. Warm up processor if needed and run a couple of "scrap" films through it to stabilize temperature and circulation.
2. Load and place the cassette on the tabletop. Two exposures will be taken on one film. Collimate the light field to a 5 in × 10 in area crosswise at one end of the film. Use the leaded sheets to mask the adjacent film area.
3. Place the thick, flat sponge over the light field area to create a large object-to-image receptor distance (OID), which must be kept constant on all exposures.
4. Place the resolution test pattern crosswise on the sponge with the small bone alongside. Pay close attention to the position in which the bone is laid, because you must lay it precisely the same way on subsequent exposures.
5. Number each exposure with a lead marker on the cassette. Take two exposures using the following techniques, or alternate techniques to accommodate available equipment.

   Exposure 1 Carefully set the SID to 50 cm. Open the light field to include the resolution and the bone.
   Technique: 50 mA, 8 ms, 60 kVp
   Exposure 2 Place the cassette on the floor with the sponge, resolution test pattern, and bone over the other half of the image receptor. Carefully measure and set the SID at 180 cm.
   Technique: 50 mA, 100 ms, 60 kVp

6. Process the film.

RESULTS

On the images of the resolution test pattern, scan across the black and white line pairs from thickest to thinnest and determine the first position where they are so blurred that you cannot distinguish separate lines from one another. Note this value of lp/mm. Refer to the test pattern itself or to the table provided by your instructor.

The unit "line pair per millimeter" (lp/mm) is a direct measure of spatial resolution or image blur. The larger the number of lp/mm seen, the better the resolution of the system, and the less blur will be noted in the image. In the table that follows, record each SID and the lp/mm resolved.

When you have completed this, obtain a millimeter rule and measure the length of the bone images on both exposures. Then, taking care to hold the bone as it was placed on the cassette and lining the ruler up precisely to the same points as you did on the radiographs, measure.

TABLE E3-1			
	Total mAs SID	Resolution, lp/mm	Bone image length
Exposure 1			
Exposure 2			

EXERCISES

1. Visually examine the marrow portion of the bone images for fine trabecular details. At which SID is more detail resolved? At which SID does the image appear to have sharper edges, less blur, and better spatial resolution?
2. Refer to Table E3-1. Which SID resolved the greater number of line pairs per millimeter? Is this consistent with your visual observations in Exercise 1?

3. What general rule of thumb can you make for SID to consistently produce radiographs with minimum image blur (best resolution)?
4. From Table E3-1, compute the magnification factor (MF) for the two exposures, using the formula below:

$$MR = \frac{\text{Imaged bone length}}{\text{Actual bone length}}$$

Exposure 1 magnification: _____
Exposure 2 magnification: _____

5. Convert the above magnification factors to percentages by subtracting 1.0 from the ratio and then multiplying the result by 100. (For example, a ratio of 1.33 would be solved as $1.33 - 1.0 = 0.33 \times 100 = 33$. This would be 33% magnification.) Record your answers below:

Exposure 1 percent magnification: _____
Exposure 2 percent magnification: _____

6. Which SID caused the greater percent magnification?
7. What general rule of thumb can you make for SID to consistently produce radiographs with minimum magnification?

Effect of mAs on X-ray Quantity

Name _____

Date _____

OBJECT

To measure the effect of mAs on radiation intensity.

DISCUSSION

The product of x-ray tube current (mA) and exposure times (s) directly controls the radiation intensity (mR) emitted by the x-ray tube. That is, as the mAs is increased, the radiation intensity increases proportionally.

Selection of a certain mA station (e.g., 50, 100, 200 mA) causes a precise current to flow through the filament of the x-ray tube. This change in filament current alters the heating of the filament and changes the tube current accordingly.

The x-ray tube current is the number of electrons accelerated across the tube from cathode to anode per second. When multiplied by exposure time (s), the product (mAs) represents the total number of electrons used for that exposure. As these electrons strike the target of the anode, x-rays are produced. The number of x-rays produced is the x-ray intensity or x-ray quantity.

By following this logic further, one can see that if the number of electrons is increased, the quantity of x-rays is increased proportionally. Tube current is controlled by selecting an appropriate mA station. When energized for a certain exposure time, the total mAs obtained determines the x-ray quantity (mR).

MATERIALS REQUIRED

- Radiographic imaging system
- Ionization chamber
- Tape measure
- Linear graph paper

PROCEDURE

1. Position the ionization chamber 100 cm from the x-ray source.
2. The x-ray imaging system may be used as it is normally filtered. Record the amount of total filtration present, if possible.
3. Adjust the tube potential to 70 kVp. If, as you change mA stations, the kVp drifts, readjust it to 70 kVp so that it will remain constant throughout the experiment.
4. Select the lowest mA station and, using the data sheet provided, record the results of three exposures.
5. The exposure time selected should be held constant throughout these measurements in case of a timer error. However, the response range of the ionization chamber may require that exposure time be reduced as mA is increased. If this occurs, note it on the data sheet.
6. Repeat these measurements for at least four additional mA stations, including the small and the large focal spots. The highest possible mA should be one of these five.
7. Determine the average intensity (mR) at each mAs.
8. Express the x-ray intensity as exposure rate in mR/mAs. The following relationship may be used:

$$\text{Exposure rate (mR/mAs)} = \frac{\text{Exposure (mR)}}{\text{mAs}}$$

RESULTS

Plot exposure rate (mR/mAs) versus mAs on the linear graph paper provided.

EXERCISES

1. What was the shape of the curve obtained? Why?
2. What effect was observed when focal spot size was changed? In a properly designed x-ray imaging system, what should you expect?
3. Calculate the quantity mR/s at each mA station. If these data were graphed, what would be the shape of the curve?
4. If 200 mA, 0.5 s results in an exposure of 50 mR, what exposure would 100 mA, 1 s produce?
5. An x-ray imaging system produces radiation intensity of 4.5 mR/mAs. What radiation exposure would result from the following techniques?
   a. 50 mA, 200 ms
   b. 300 mA, 1.5 s
   c. 800 mA, 16 ms

DATA SHEET FOR EXPERIMENT 4: EFFECT OF mAs ON X-RAY QUANTITY

CONSTANT FACTORS

- 70 kVp
- Filtration: _____ mm Al
- 100 cm source-to-detector distance

Tube current, mA	Exposure time, ms	Exposure, mR			Average exposure, mR	Exposure rate	
		First	Second	Third		mR/mAs	mR/s
Small focal spot							
Large focal spot							

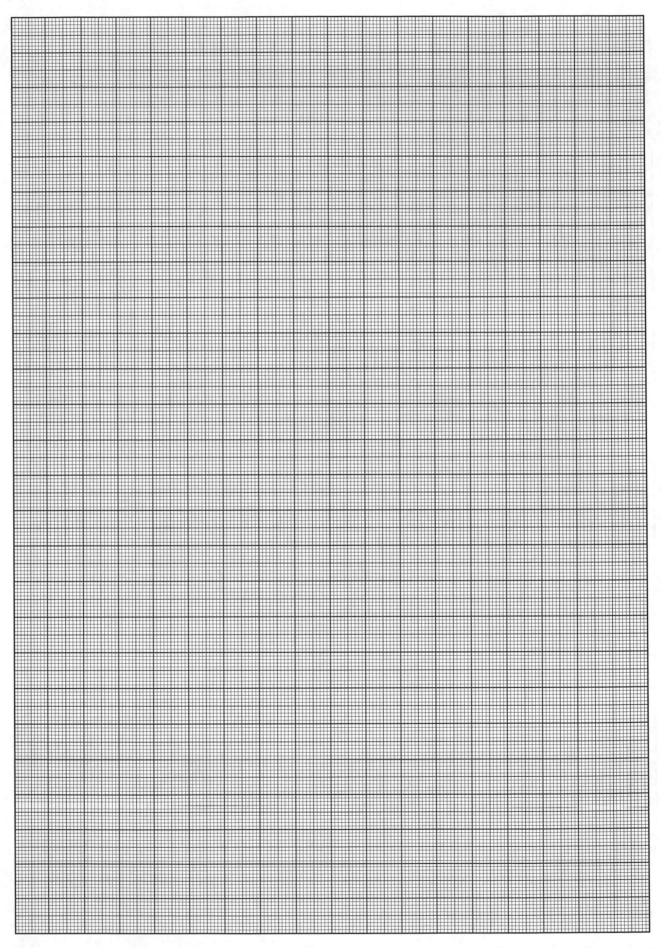

Effect of mAs on Optical Density

Name _____

Date _____

OBJECT

To determine the relationship among mA, exposure time, and total mAs and their combined effect on optical density (OD).

DISCUSSION

When the radiographic imaging system is properly calibrated, the radiation intensity will be directly proportional to the mA and to the exposure time selected. For example, a doubling of mA or exposure time will result in twice as much radiation intensity. Radiographic film responds in a complicated way to radiation exposure. Optical density increases as radiation intensity increases.

The total mAs is the product of the selected mA station and the exposure time. Optical density is related to mAs. To maintain constant OD when the mA is doubled, the exposure time should be cut to one half. Conversely, if the mA is cut to one third its original value, the exposure time should be tripled to maintain constant OD. In other words, mA and exposure time are inversely related to each other when constant mAs and, therefore, constant OD are maintained.

MATERIALS REQUIRED

- Radiographic imaging system
- Step-wedge penetrometer
- X-ray film processor
- 400-speed 14 in × 17 in (35 cm × 43 cm) screen-film cassette
- Lead or vinyl lead sheets
- Lead numbers
- Viewbox
- Densitometer

PROCEDURE

1. Set 50 kVp. This will remain constant throughout the experiment. If the kVp drifts when mA stations are changed, adjust it to remain constant at 50 kVp.
2. Warm up the processor if needed and run a couple of "scrap" films through it to stabilize temperature and circulation.
3. Position the x-ray tube 100 cm from the tabletop.

PART I

1. Load and place the cassette face up on the tabletop. Place the step-wedge penetrometer crosswise at one end of the cassette. Four exposures will be taken on one film. It is important to use one film so that processing conditions will be constant.
2. Collimate the light field to a 4 in × 14 in area, and center over the step wedge. Use the lead sheets to mask the adjacent film area to prevent image fog that may result from scattered radiation.
3. Number each exposure with a lead marker on the cassette. Take four exposures using the techniques listed below, or record any alternate techniques you use. Begin with a very low mA and an exposure time of 50 ms or less that can be exactly doubled at least twice. After the first exposure, move the step wedge to the next quarter of the film, double the time as shown in the technique for Exposure 2 below, and so forth. For the fourth exposure, double the mA station instead of the time. Always use lead sheets to mask the cassette adjacent to either side of the exposure area.

Exposure 1: 50 mA, 50 ms
Exposure 2: 50 mA, 100 ms

Exposure 3: 50 mA, 200 ms
Exposure 4: 100 mA, 200 ms

4. Process the film.
5. On the resultant images, select a step on which to make OD measurements. The step selected must have a measured OD of less than 0.3 on Exposure 1; however, it should be visibly darker on Exposure 2. This will be an extremely light OD on Exposure 1. Using the densitometer, determine the OD for each exposure, taking care to measure the same step each time.

RESULTS

In Table E5-1, record for each exposure the mA and exposure time used, the total resultant mAs, and the measured OD.

TABLE E5-1

	mA	Time	Total mAs	OD
Exposure 1				
Exposure 2				
Exposure 3				
Exposure 4				

EXERCISES

1. Compute the relative OD change for each increase in technique by dividing the OD for Exposure 2 by that for 1, the OD for Exposure 3 by that for 2, and the OD for Exposure 4 by that for 3, and record the results below. You will note that these relative changes vary somewhat because x-ray imaging systems are not perfectly calibrated.

   2/1: _____
   3/2: _____
   4/3: _____

2. Compute an average OD change by summing these three numbers and then dividing by 3:

   Average OD change: _____

   Does this change fall within 15% of a doubling? That is, does it fall between 1.7 and 2.3?

3. If the relationship between total mAs and OD were plotted on linear paper, what would be the appearance of the graph?
4. What term best describes this relationship?
5. In terms of the resultant OD, is there any difference between doubling the mA and doubling the exposure time?

PART II

1. Load and place the cassette face up on the tabletop. Place the step-wedge penetrometer crosswise at one end of the cassette. Three exposures will be taken on one film. It is important to use one film so that processing conditions will be constant.
2. Collimate the light field to a 4 in × 10 in area, and center over the step wedge. Use the lead sheets to mask the adjacent film area to prevent scatter fogging.
3. Number each exposure with a lead marker on the cassette. Take three exposures using the techniques listed below, or record any alternate techniques you use. After the first exposure, move the step wedge to the next third of the film. Double the mA station, but cut the exposure time to exactly one half of the original so that the same total mAs results. For Exposure 3, double the mA and halve the exposure time again. Always use lead sheets to mask the cassette adjacent to either side of the exposure area.

   Exposure 1: 50 mA, 50 ms
   Exposure 2: 50 mA, 100 ms
   Exposure 3: 50 mA, 200 ms
   Exposure 4: 100 mA, 200 ms

4. Process the film.
5. On the resultant images, select a step on which to make OD measurements; the step selected must have a medium gray OD between 0.5 and 1.5 as measured on the densitometer. Determine the OD for each exposure, taking care to measure the same step each time.

RESULTS

In Table E5-2, record for each exposure the mA and exposure time used, the total resultant mAs, and the measured OD.

TABLE E5-2				
	mA	Time	Total mAs	OD
Exposure 1				
Exposure 2				
Exposure 3				

EXERCISES

1. Compute the relative OD changes between these techniques by dividing the OD for Exposure 2 by that for 1, the OD for Exposure 3 by that for 2, and the OD for Exposure 3 by that for 1, and record here:

   2/1: _____
   3/2: _____
   3/1: _____

2. Compute the average OD change by summing these three numbers and then dividing by 3:

   Average OD change: _____

   An OD change ratio of 1.0 would indicate that the ODs produced by the different techniques are exactly the same. Is your computed average change close to 1.0?

3. Visually examine the three images. Is there a substantial difference in OD among them?

4. As long as the total mAs is the same, does the particular mA station or exposure time make any difference in terms of overall OD?

5. In maintaining a given OD, what term would describe the relationship between milliamperage and exposure time?

6. Why should you generally choose short exposure times with high mA stations?

7. When would you choose a very long exposure time with a low mA station?

X-Ray Beam Penetration

Name _____

Date _____

OBJECT

To demonstrate the relationship among kVp, x-ray beam penetration, and the resultant grayscale of the radiographic image.

DISCUSSION

To produce useful optical densities (ODs) on the radiograph, x-rays first must penetrate through each tissue of interest and interact with the image receptor. If the x-ray beam is not sufficiently energetic to penetrate the body part, an inadequate image will result, regardless of the x-ray beam intensity. Therefore, no amount of mAs (which controls only x-ray quantity) will ever compensate for insufficient kVp.

As kVp is increased, more different types of tissue are penetrated and recorded on the image receptor. The image has a longer grayscale because the range of OD is greater.

Tissues that are not penetrated result in white areas on the radiograph. In such areas, no information is recorded; therefore, they are diagnostically useless.

Adequate penetration is essential to the production of a useful radiograph. Penetration is also directly related to the number of different gray shades produced on the image. The penetrating ability of the x-ray beam, often termed *radiation quality*, is controlled primarily by kVp.

MATERIALS REQUIRED

- Radiographic imaging system
- Pelvis phantom or other large phantom
- X-ray film processor
- 400-speed 10 in × 12 in (24 cm × 30 cm) screen-film cassette
- Lead numbers
- Viewbox
- Densitometer

PROCEDURE

1. Warm up the processor if needed, and run a couple of "scrap" films through it to stabilize temperature and circulation.
2. Position the x-ray tube 100 cm from the tabletop.
3. Load and place a cassette lengthwise in the Bucky tray. Place the pelvis phantom on the table in supine position.
4. Collimate the light field to the film size, and center.
5. Number each exposure with a lead marker on the cassette. Take four exposures on separate films using the techniques listed here or alternate techniques to accommodate your equipment.

   Exposure 1: 200 mA, 100 ms, 84 kVp
   Exposure 2: 200 mA, 200 ms, 50 kVp
   Exposure 3: 200 mA, 500 ms, 50kVp
   Exposure 4: 200 mA, 1000 ms, 50 kVp

6. Process the films.

RESULTS

For comparison purposes, Exposure 1 must be of good average OD. If it is not, change the mA station used, but keep the mA constant throughout the experiment.

Visually examine each radiograph and compare it with Exposure 1 to determine the amount of diagnostic information present and the number of different shades of gray produced.

EXERCISES

1. For each succeeding exposure (Exposures 2, 3, and 4), the total mAs was approximately doubled each time, but a very low kVp was used. Note that for Exposure 4, the total mAs is 10 times the mAs used for Exposure 1. Has a satisfactory OD been achieved on Exposure 2, 3, or 4?

2. Would a satisfactory OD be achieved at 40 kVp if the total mAs was increased to 1000 mAs?

3. Explain why this is so in terms of x-ray intensity and beam penetration.

4. Restate your answer from Exercise 3 in terms of mAs and kVp.

5. Count the number of different ODs or shades of gray on Exposures 1 and 2, and record them here:

   Exposure 1: _____
   Exposure 2: _____

6. Which of these two radiographs displays the longest grayscale? Explain why this is so.

Effect of kVp on X-Ray Quantity

Name _____

Date _____

OBJECT

To measure the effect of varying x-ray tube potential (kVp) on radiation intensity.

DISCUSSION

Experiment 4 demonstrated that x-ray quantity is directly related to mAs. X-ray quantity varies more rapidly with changes in kVp. The radiation intensity of an x-ray imaging system increases approximately as the square of the increase in kVp, according to the following relationship:

$$\frac{I_1}{I_2} = \frac{kVp_1{}^2}{kVp_2}$$

where I_1 and I_2 are the x-ray intensities at kVp_1 and kVp_2, respectively, and the exponent 2 is a reasonable approximation.

The number of electrons accelerated from cathode to anode is measured by the mAs. The number of accelerated electrons does not change with increasing tube potential (kVp). However, as kVp is increased, each electron possesses increased kinetic energy, which is transformed into more heat and more x-rays. As kVp is increased, each electron has a higher probability of multiple interactions with target atoms, thereby producing more x-rays. Further, each x-ray so produced will average a higher energy and, therefore, will be more penetrating.

Changing kVp changes x-ray quantity and quality; changing mAs affects only x-ray quantity.

MATERIALS REQUIRED

- Radiographic imaging system
- Tape measure
- Ionization chamber
- Linear graph paper

PROCEDURE

1. Position the ionization chamber 100 cm from the x-ray tube target.
2. The x-ray imaging system may be used as it is normally filtered. Record the amount of total filtration present, if known.
3. Select a low mA station (i.e., less than 100 mA) so that a number of repeat exposures will be possible at all kVp settings without overheating the tube.
4. Beginning at 40 kVp and increasing in 20 kVp increments, record the measured radiation intensity on the data sheet provided. Three measurements should be recorded at each kVp, and the average value should then be calculated. In addition to constant mA, the exposure time should remain fixed if the response range of the ionization chamber will allow; otherwise, the exposure time will have to be reduced with increasing kVp.
5. Determine the average exposure (mR) at each kVp setting.
6. Express the x-ray output intensity as exposure rate in mR/s. The following relationship may be used:

$$\text{Exposure rate (mR/s)} = \frac{\text{Exposure (mR)}}{\text{Exposure time(s)}}$$

RESULTS

Plot exposure rate (mR/s) versus tube potential (kVp) on the linear graph paper provided.

EXERCISES

1. What was the shape of the curve obtained? Why?
2. Calculate the quantity mR/mAs at each kVp selected. If these data were graphed, what would be the shape of the curve?

3. From the data recorded, estimate the actual value of n x-ray imaging system in the following expression:

$$\frac{I_1}{I_2} = \left(\frac{kVp_1}{kVp_2} \right)^n$$

4. From the data obtained, estimate the x-ray quantity that would result from the following factors:
   a. 55 kVp, 100 mA, 50 ms
   b. 73 kVp, 200 mA, 250 ms

c. 96 kVp, 50 mA, 750 ms
d. 124 kVp, 300 mA, 16 ms
e. 114 kVp, 300 mA, 16 ms

5. A useful rule of thumb states that a 15% increase in kVp accompanied by a 50% reduction of mA will result in the same OD and reduced patient exposure. Can this be confirmed by your data? Begin with 70 kVp/50 mAs.

DATA SHEET FOR EXPERIMENT 7: EFFECT OF KVP ON X-RAY QUANTITY

CONSTANT FACTORS
- 100 cm SID
- mA _____
- Filtration: _____ mm Al

kVp	Exposure time, ms	Exposure, mR			Average exposure, mR	Exposure, mR	
		First	Second	Third		mR/mAs	mR/s

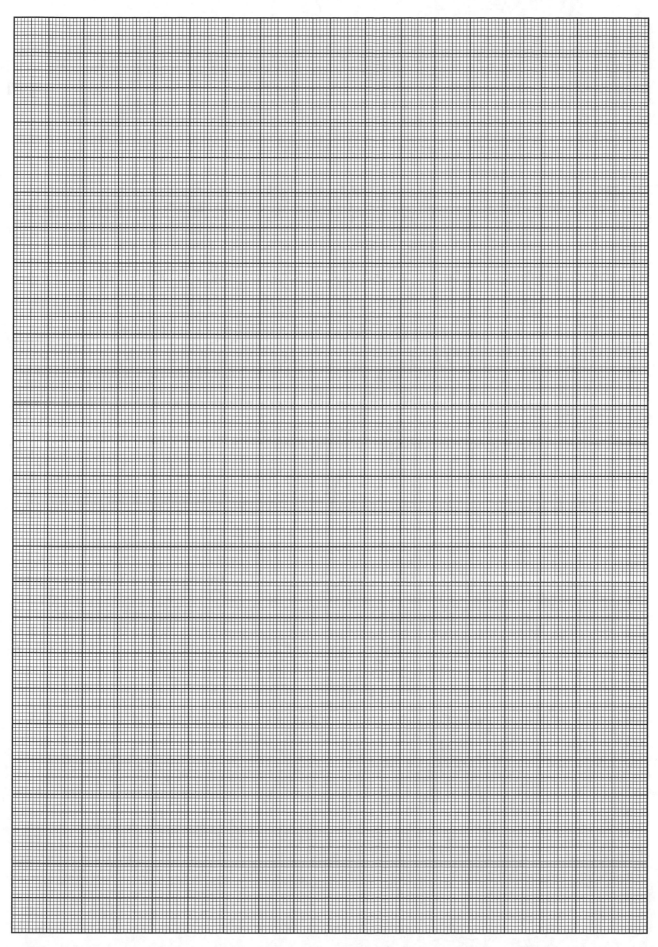

Effect of kVp on Optical Density

Name _____

Date _____

OBJECT

To demonstrate how kVp influences optical density (OD) and the basis for the 15% rule.

DISCUSSION

Peak kilovoltage controls the energy level of the x-ray beam. This property of the x-ray beam is also called **penetrability** or x-ray beam quality. At higher energy, a greater percentage of x-rays penetrate through the anatomy and reach the image receptor, thus contributing to OD. Also, at higher kVp, the x-ray tube emits more x-rays. When this higher radiation intensity is added to the increased penetration, the resultant image becomes much darker, that is, a small change in kVp causes a big change in OD.

When kVp is changed, it is not easy to predict exactly how much OD will change because this depends on two different processes: changing beam intensity and changing beam penetration. However, a rule of thumb traditionally used by radiologic technologists has proved very useful. The **15% rule** states that if the kVp is changed by 15%, the mAs must be changed by a factor of 2 if the same OD is to be maintained. Therefore, a 15% increase in kVp should be accompanied by a 50% reduction in mAs to maintain constant OD.

MATERIALS REQUIRED

- Radiographic imaging system
- Skull phantom, other large phantom, or large step wedge
- X-ray film processor
- 400-speed 10 in × 12 in (24 cm × 30 cm) screen-film cassette
- Lead numbers
- Positioning sponges
- Viewbox
- Densitometer

PROCEDURE

1. Warm up the processor if needed, and run a couple of "scrap" films through it to stabilize temperature and circulation.
2. Position the x-ray tube 100 cm from the tabletop.
3. Load and place a cassette crosswise on the tabletop. Place the anatomic phantom on the cassette in lateral position, using sponges as needed to balance it.
4. Collimate the light field to the film size, and center to the anatomic phantom.
5. Number each exposure with a lead marker on the cassette. Take four exposures on separate films using the techniques listed here, or alternate techniques to accommodate your equipment. If possible, use the same mA station for all exposures. Kilovoltage increases are made in 15% increments. Beginning with Exposure 3, these changes are compensated by cutting the exposure time in half each time.

   Exposure 1: 50 mA, 100 ms, 70 kVp
   Exposure 2: 50 mA, 100 ms, 80 kVp
   Exposure 3: 50 mA, 50 ms, 80 kVp
   Exposure 4: 50 mA, 25 ms, 92 kVp

6. Process the films.
7. On the resultant images, select an area within the bony anatomy that shows a smooth medium-gray OD on Exposure 1. Circle this area and, using the densitometer, determine the OD in this area for each exposure.

RESULTS

In Table E8-1, record for each exposure the total mAs and kVp used and the measured OD.

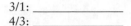

TABLE E8-1

	mA	Time	Total mAs	OD
Exposure 1				
Exposure 2				
Exposure 3				
Exposure 4				

EXERCISES

1. Compute the relative OD change for Exposure 2 by dividing the OD for Exposure 1 into that for 2, and record here:

   2/1: _____

2. Visually compare Exposure 2 with Exposure 1. When kVp is increased without adjustment of any other factors, what happens to overall OD?

3. According to your preceding calculation, how much darker is Exposure 2 as compared with Exposure 1?

4. Compute the relative OD changes for the adjustments in technique made in the subsequent exposures by dividing the OD for Exposure 3 by that for 1 and the OD for Exposure 4 by that for 3, and record here:

   3/1: _____
   4/3: _____

5. Compute an average OD change by summing these two numbers and then dividing by 2.

   Average OD change: _____

6. An OD change ratio of 1.0 would indicate that the ODs produced by the different techniques are exactly the same. Is your computed average change within 15% of the original? That is, does it fall between 0.85 and 1.15?

7. In Exposures 3 and 4, a 15% increase in kVp was accompanied by halving the mAs. Does the 15% rule of thumb work in approximately maintaining overall OD when kVp is changed?

Effect of kVp on Image Contrast

Name _____

Date _____

OBJECT

To demonstrate how image contrast changes when kVp is changed.

DISCUSSION

Kilovoltage affects image contrast for two important reasons. First, at higher energies, the x rays penetrate more tissues and thus lengthen the grayscale recorded. Secondly, at higher x-ray beam energy, fewer photoelectric interactions occur. The fogging of the image from Compton interactions then becomes more apparent. By combining the effects of a longer grayscale with more visible fog, contrast is reduced. Conversely, use of a low kVp will result in higher image contrast.

MATERIALS REQUIRED

- Radiographic imaging system
- Skull phantom, other large phantom, or large step wedge
- X-ray film processor
- 400-speed 10 in × 12 in (24 cm × 30 cm) screen-film cassette
- Lead numbers
- Positioning sponges
- Viewbox
- Densitometer

PROCEDURE

1. Warm up the processor if needed, and run a couple of "scrap" films through it to stabilize temperature and circulation.
2. Position the x-ray tube 100 cm from the tabletop.
3. Load and place a cassette crosswise on the tabletop. Place the anatomic phantom on the cassette in lateral position, using sponges as needed to balance it.
4. Collimate the light field to the film size, and center the anatomic phantom.
5. Number each exposure with a lead marker on the cassette. Take two exposures on separate films using the techniques listed below, or alternate techniques to accommodate your imaging system. If possible, use the same mA station for both exposures.

   Exposure 1: 50 mA, 100 ms, 70 kVp
   Exposure 2: 50 mA, 25 ms, 92 kVp

6. Process the films.
7. On each resultant image, select an area, Area A, within the bony anatomy that shows a uniform light gray optical density (OD) and another area, Area B, that shows a uniform medium gray OD. Circle these areas and, using the densities, determine the OD in each area for each exposure.

RESULTS

In Table E9-1, record for each exposure the kVp used and the measured OD in Area A and Area B.

TABLE E9-1			
	kVp	OD of area A	OD of area B
Exposure 1			
Exposure 2			

EXERCISES

1. Compute the contrast for each exposure by subtracting the optical density (OD) of Area B from the OD of Area A, and record here:

   Exposure 1 contrast (A − B): _____
   Exposure 2 contrast (A − B): _____

2. Compare the computed contrast levels. Even though mAs was compensated for kVp to maintain OD, what happened to the measured contrast for Exposure 2 when a much higher kVp was used?

3. Visually compare Exposure 2 with Exposure 1. When a much higher kVp is used, is the change in contrast visible?

4. The difference between Exposure 1 and Exposure 2 is 22 kVp. Would a difference in contrast be visible for a much smaller change, such as an increase of 4 kVp?

5. Explain why this contrast change occurs at high kVp levels.

Half-Value Layer

Name _____

Date _____

OBJECT

To determine the half-value layer (HVL) of an x-ray beam and observe how it changes with kVp.

DISCUSSION

Half-value layer is defined as that thickness of an absorbing material required to reduce the intensity of the x-ray beam to one half of its original value. Half-value layer is the single most appropriate unit of measure for beam quality. Total filtration, effective energy, and kVp are also useful for describing beam quality. The absorbing material most often used to determine the HVL of diagnostic x-ray imaging systems is aluminum.

MATERIALS REQUIRED

- Radiographic imaging system
- Ionization chamber
- Aluminum absorbers
- Ring stand and clamps
- Linear graph paper

PROCEDURE

1. Position the ionization chamber 100 cm from the x-ray tube target. Place aluminum absorbers approximately midway between the ionization chamber and the x-ray tube target.
2. The x-ray imaging system may be used as it is normally filtered. Record the amount of total filtration, if possible.
3. Using the light localizer, collimate to just cover the area of the ionization chamber.
4. Adjust the tube potential to 60 kVp.
5. Select a technique of mAs that will provide a reading that is nearly full scale on the ionization chamber.

6. Expose the ionization chamber sequentially three times, and record each measurement on the data sheet provided.
7. Insert 0.5 mm A1 filtration midway between the target and detector, and record three additional measurements.
8. Repeat this process with added aluminum filtration thicknesses of 1.0, 2.0, 3.0, 4.0, 6.0, and 8.0 mm. If an increase in mA, exposure time, or both is required at greater thicknesses of aluminum filtration, record these changes.
9. Repeat steps 4 through 8 at 90 kVp and again at 120 kVp.
10. Calculate the average intensity (mR) for each level of filtration at each kVp. Express the x-ray intensity in mR/mAs as follows:

X-ray intensity (mR/mAs) =

$$\frac{\text{Average intensity (mR)}}{\text{Tube current (mA)} \times \text{Exposure time(s)}}$$

RESULTS

Plot the x-ray intensity versus mm A1 added filtration for each kVp on the linear and semilog graph paper provided. Estimate the HVL for each curve.

TABLE E10-1	
	HVL, mm A1
60	
90	
120	

EXERCISES

1. Complete Table E10-1.
2. On the linear graph paper provided, plot HVL versus kVp. From the extrapolation of this curve, what would be the estimated HVL at 40 kVp? At 140 kVp?
3. Given the data obtained at 90 kVp, if an additional 1 mm A1 were added to the existing total filtration, what would the HVL be?
4. The homogeneity coefficient is defined as the ratio of the first HVL to the second HVL. From the data collected at 60 and 120 kVp, estimate the homogeneity coefficient for each condition.

DATA SHEET FOR EXPERIMENT 10: HALF-VALUE LAYER

CONSTANT FACTORS

- 100 cm source-to-ionization distance
- Total filtration: _____ mm Al

kVp	Added filtration, mm A1	Tube current, mA	Exposure time, ms	Exposure, mR			Average exposure, mR	mR/mAs
				First	Second	Third		
60	0.0							
60	0.5							
60	1.0							
60	2.0							
60	3.0							
60	4.0							
60	6.0							
60	8.0							
90	0.0							
90	0.5							
90	1.0							
90	2.0							
90	3.0							
90	4.0							
90	6.0							
90	8.0							
120	0.0							
120	0.5							
120	1.0							
120	2.0							
120	3.0							
120	4.0							
120	6.0							
120	8.0							

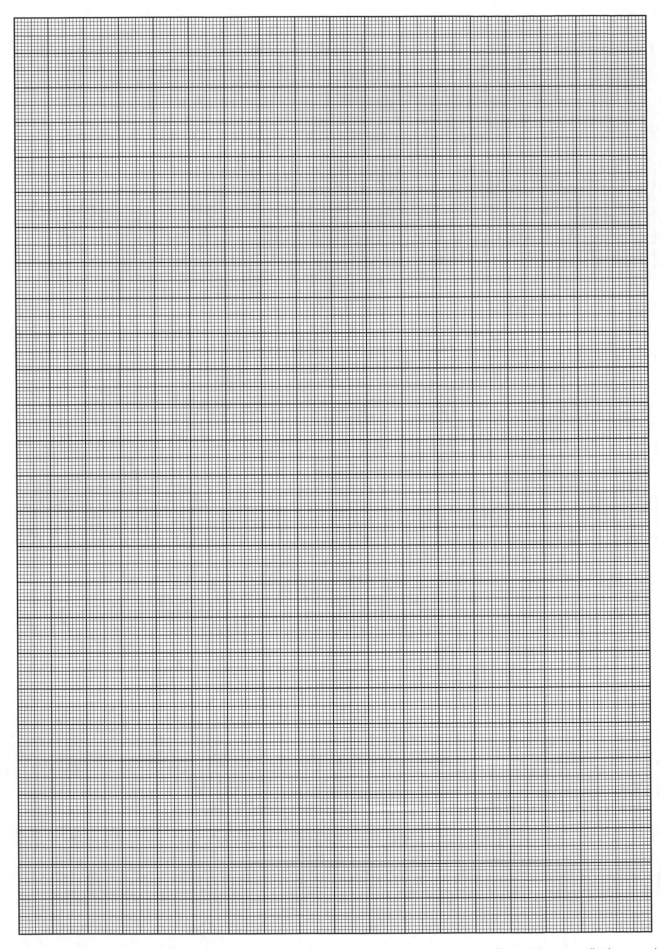

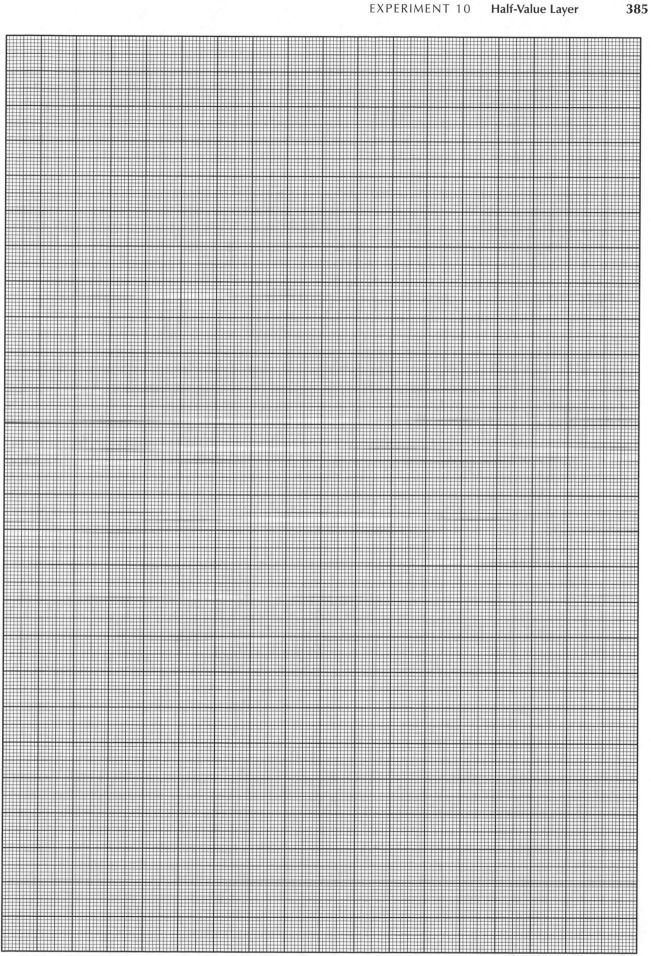

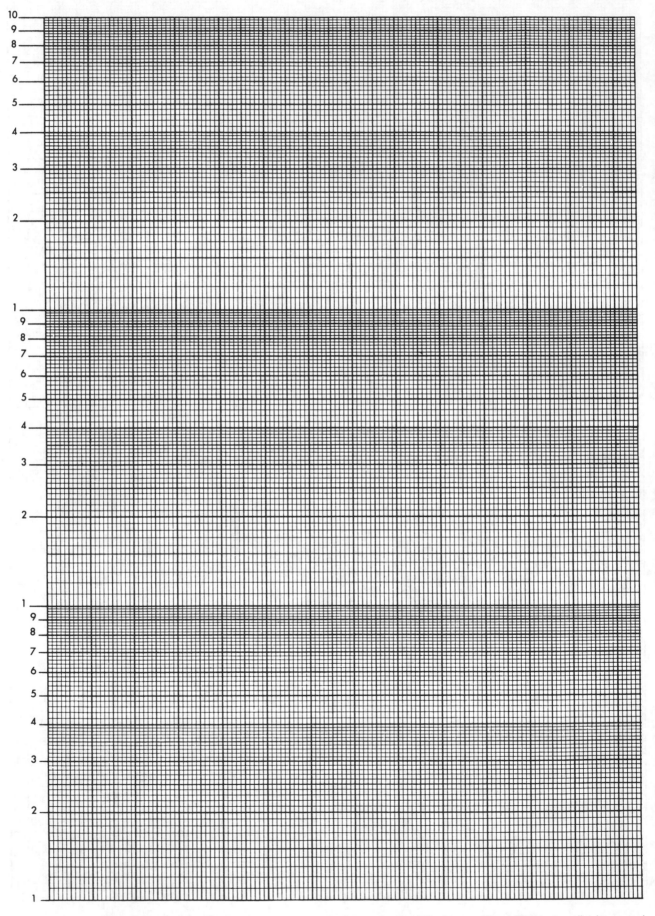

Effect of Field Size on Image Contrast

Name _____

Date _____

OBJECT

To demonstrate the effects of field size limitation (collimation) on optical density (OD) and image contrast.

DISCUSSION

When the size of the x-ray field is reduced, a smaller volume of tissue is exposed to radiation. The volume of tissue exposed determines the amount of scatter radiation produced and thus affects the amount of fog density on the radiograph. By collimating the x-ray field to a smaller size, less fog density is produced on the radiograph; this results in higher image contrast.

The total image OD is contributed to both by primary x-rays that penetrate to the image receptor and by scattered x-rays that are produced within tissues. When reducing scatter radiation by collimation of the x-ray field, one also produces an image with lower OD (lighter); therefore, mAs may have to be increased.

MATERIALS REQUIRED

- Radiographic imaging system
- Pelvis phantom or other phantom large enough to generate substantial scatter radiation
- X-ray film processor
- 400-speed screen-film cassettes, one 14 in × 17 in (35 cm × 43 cm) and one 10 in × 12 in (24 cm × 30 cm) or smaller
- Sponges, sandbags, or positioning clamps
- Lead numbers
- Viewbox
- Densitometer

PROCEDURE

1. Warm up the processor if needed, and run a couple of "scrap" films through it to stabilize temperature and circulation.
2. Set 86 kVp, 100 mA, and 100 ms exposure time. This will remain constant throughout the experiment.
3. Position the x-ray tube at 100 cm SID.
4. Have sponges and sandbags or clamps at hand to hold the pelvis phantom in a lateral position. If using another test object, position it with the thickest dimension vertical.
5. Number each film with a lead marker on the cassette. Take two exposures on separate films using the techniques listed here or alternate techniques to accommodate your equipment.

   Exposure 1 Load and place the large cassette lengthwise. Place the pelvis phantom in lateral position. Open the field size to 14 in × 17 in, and center over the lumbar vertebrae. Expose the film.

   Exposure 2 Load and place the small cassette lengthwise. Place the pelvis phantom in lateral position. Collimate the field size to a 5 in × 5 in square, and center over the lumbar vertebrae. Expose the film using the same technique.

6. Process the films.
7. On Exposure 2, select and circle two uniform OD areas within the anatomy to take densitometer measurements as follows: Area A must show a dark gray soft tissue OD. Area B must show a light gray bony OD. Now circle the same two areas on Exposure 1. Using the densitometer, determine the OD in these two areas for each exposure, and record below.

RESULTS

TABLE E11-1

	Field size	OD of area A	OD of area B
Exposure 1			
Exposure 2			

EXERCISES

1. What happened to the OD in Area A when the field size was reduced? Can you visually see the difference in Area A between the two films?
2. Why does this effect occur when field size is reduced?
3. Compute the radiographic technique change that would be required to maintain OD when field size is reduced in this case as follows: Divide Area A OD for Exposure 2 into that for Exposure 1. This is the factor by which mAs must be changed to maintain constant OD:

$$\frac{\text{Exposure 1, Area A}}{\text{Exposure 2, Area A}} = \underline{\hspace{3cm}} = \,?$$

4. Change the above answer into a percentage as follows: From this ratio, subtract 1.0, and then multiply the remaining decimal number by 100:

$$\underline{\hspace{1.5cm}} - 1.0 = \underline{\hspace{1.5cm}} \times 100 = \underline{\hspace{1.5cm}}\%$$

This is the percentage by which mAs must be changed to compensate. When collimating down to the smaller 5-in-square field, should mAs be increased or decreased by this percentage for OD to be maintained?
5. Compute the contrast for each exposure as follows. Subtract the OD of Area B from the OD of Area A, and record here:

Exposure 1 contrast (A − B): _____
Exposure 2 contrast (A − B): _____

6. Compare the computed contrast levels. What happened to the measured contrast for Exposure 2 when a much smaller field size was used?
7. Visually compare Exposure 2 with Exposure 1. When a much higher kVp is used, would the change in contrast be visible?
8. Briefly explain why this contrast change occurs with smaller field sizes. In Table E11-1, record for each exposure the field size used and the measured OD in Areas A and B.

Effect of Radiographic Grids on Optical Density and Image Contrast

Name _____

Date _____

OBJECT

To demonstrate the effect of radiographic grids on optical density (OD) and image contrast.

DISCUSSION

When thick body parts are radiographed, the quality of the image will be reduced by the scatter radiation produced. Radiographic grids should be used in such cases to improve image contrast.

The narrow slits of grid allow most of the primary x-rays to pass through while many of the scattered x-rays are absorbed. The effectiveness of a grid can be measured by comparing the image contrast produced with the grid versus that produced without the grid.

It is unfortunate that this reduction in scatter radiation, along with absorption of some of the primary beam, results in a loss of OD. To restore proper OD, mAs must be increased. This leads to an increase in patient dose, but this increase is necessary for adequate image quality. The higher the grid ratio, the more the mAs must be increased if OD is to be maintained.

MATERIALS REQUIRED

- Radiographic imaging system
- Pelvis phantom or other phantom large enough to generate substantial scatter radiation
- X-ray film processor
- Wafer grids (clamp-on or tape-on type) of different ratios as available; 10 in × 12 in size preferred
- 400-speed screen-film cassettes of the same size as the wafer grids
- Sponges, sandbags, or positioning clamps
- Lead or vinyl lead sheets
- Lead numbers
- Viewbox
- Densitometer

PROCEDURE

1. Warm up the processor if needed, and run a couple of "scrap" films through it to stabilize temperature and circulation.
2. Position the x-ray tube at 100 cm SID.
3. Position sponges, sandbags, or clamps to hold the pelvis phantom in a lateral position. If using another phantom, position it with the thickest dimension vertical.
4. Set 86 kVp. This will remain constant throughout the experiment.
5. Number each film with a lead marker on the cassette. Take exposures on separate films using the techniques listed here, or record any alternate techniques used.

Exposure 1 No grid: Collimate to a 14 in × 17 in lengthwise field, regardless of the film size used.
Technique: 200 mA, 10 mAs
Note: Process and check this film. It should be of medium OD, but it will appear quite gray with low contrast. If it is very light or very dark, adjust the mAs and repeat. Record this alternate technique:
Alternate Technique: _____

ADDITIONAL EXPOSURES WITH GRID

- Perform with the grid centered on the top of the film.
- Precisely center the light field to the grid, then arrange the phantom in lateral position on top of the grid. Do not change collimation.

Technique: Find the grid ratio labeled or embossed on one side of the grid. Refer to Table E12-1, and multiply the mAs used in the first exposure by the factor listed.

389

Grid ratio	Multiply nongrid mAs by:
TABLE E12-1	
5:1 or 6:1	2
8:1	3
10:1 or 12:1	4
15:1 or 16:1	5

(*Note:* The new mAs must be only an approximate value. Do not change the mA station unless there is no other way to approximate the needed mAs.) Record each ratio and the mAs used.

	GRID RATIO	mAs
Exposure 2	_____	_____
Exposure 3	_____	_____
Exposure 4	_____	_____

6. Process the films.
7. On the first exposure, select and circle two uniform OD areas within the anatomy for densitometer measurements. Area A must show a dark gray soft tissue density but must not be black. Area B must show a medium gray bony density. Now circle the same two uniform OD areas on all other exposures. Using the densitometer, determine the OD in these two areas for each exposure, and record in Table E12-2.

RESULTS

In Table E12-2, record for each exposure the grid ratio used and the measured OD in Areas A and B.

TABLE E12-2	Grid ratio	OD of area A	OD of area B
Exposure 1			
Exposure 2			
Exposure 3			
Exposure 4			

EXERCISES

1. Consider only the ODs for Area A. Compute the relative OD change for Exposures 2, 3, and 4 by dividing the OD of Area A for Exposure 1 into each of them, and record here:

   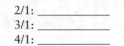

   2/1: _____
   3/1: _____
   4/1: _____

2. An OD change of 1.0 would indicate that the ODs produced by the different techniques are exactly the same. Consider the value above for Exposure 2. Is your computed average change within 20% of the original, that is, does it fall between 0.8 and 1.2? Did the value for the other grids also fall within this range? If not, list below the factors you would use in place of those from the table.
3. Visually compare Exposures 2, 3, and 4 with Exposure 1. Did the technique factors from the table reasonably maintain OD when the change was made from nongrid to grid exposures?
4. If these technique adjustments were not made, how would these radiographs have appeared? Why?
5. Compute the image contrast for each exposure as follows: Subtract the OD of Area B from the OD of Area A, and record here:

	GRID RATIO	CONTRAST (A − B)
Exposure 1	_____	_____
Exposure 2	_____	_____
Exposure 3	_____	_____
Exposure 4	_____	_____

6. Compare the computed contrast levels for Exposures 2, 3, and 4 with the contrast achieved when a grid is used. How do grids accomplish this change in contrast?

Effect of Grid Cutoff

Name _____

Date _____

OBJECT

To demonstrate grid cutoff.

DISCUSSION

Grid cutoff, a massive loss of optical density (OD), can be caused by laterally angling the grid to the central ray so that they are not perpendicular to each other, by placing the grid at an improper distance from the x-ray tube (outside of the grid radius), or by placing the grid upside down. The pattern of grid cutoff often can be used to determine which of these errors caused it.

MATERIALS REQUIRED

- Radiographic imaging system
- Pelvis phantom or other phantom large enough to generate substantial scatter radiation
- X-ray film processor
- Grids (clamp-on or tape-on type) of different ratios as available; 10 in × 12 in size preferred (Bucky may be used if you can determine the ratio of the grid within it)
- 400-speed screen-film cassettes of the same size as the wafer grids
- Sponges, sandbags, or positioning clamps
- Lead or vinyl lead sheets
- Lead numbers
- Viewbox
- Densitometer

PROCEDURE

1. Warm up the processor if needed, and run a couple of "scrap" films through it to stabilize temperature and circulation.
2. Position the x-ray tube at 100 cm SID.
3. Set 50 mA and 50 ms; this will remain constant throughout the experiment, except on the last exposure.
4. Use the highest-ratio 10 in × 12 in grid available to you; place it over each film and expose it directly to the x-ray beam.
5. Open the light field in the 10 in × 12 in grid, and leave it at this position throughout the experiment.
6. Number each film with a lead marker on the cassette. Take exposures on separate films, following the directions below. Different angles and kVp levels are required at different grid ratios for the experiment. Instructions are listed for an 8:1 grid and for a 12:1 grid. Use the instructions for the grid closest to the grid that you have.

TABLE E13-1

		If using 8:1 grid	If using 12:1 grid
Exposure 1	Angle beam parallel to grid strips, and center	30-degree angle, 70 kVp	20-degree angle, 80 kVp
Exposure 2	Angle beam perpendicular to grid strips, and center	30-degree angle, 70 kVp	25-degree angle, 80 kVp
Exposure 3	Off-center a perpendicular beam across grid strips by 3 in	65 kVp	75 kVp
Exposure 4	Turn grid over and expose upside down using a perpendicular, centered beam	62 kVp	70 kVp
Exposure 5	Use a perpendicular, centered beam, but change SID to 180 cm by placing the film and the grid on the floor. *Note:* Change exposure time to 0.1 ($^1/_{10}$) s	62 kVp	70 kVp

RESULTS

Visually observe the radiographs on a viewbox.

EXERCISES

1. Which of the preceding situations did not result in grid cutoff? Why?
2. Which of the preceding situations resulted in grid cutoff more severe toward one side of the film than the other?
3. Which of the preceding situations resulted in grid cutoff that is equal toward both sides of the film?
4. Which of the preceding situations caused the most severe grid cutoff overall?
5. If a higher ratio grid were used for this experiment, what change would you expect in all of the results? Why?

Effect of Intensifying Screens on Optical Density and Image Contrast

Name _____

Date _____

OBJECT

To demonstrate how intensifying screens work and their effect on optical density (OD) and image contrast.

DISCUSSION

Radiographic intensifying screens convert x-rays into light, which in turn, exposes the image receptor. The principal result is a reduction in patient dose. Such screens convert the energy and intensity of the x-ray beam into visible light, which then interacts with the image receptor more readily than x-rays do. An increase in kVp or an increase in mAs will cause the screen to glow brighter; this results in a darker image.

Radiographic intensifying screens can be made "faster" in several ways. Their absorption efficiency for x-rays can be increased with the use of thicker or rare Earth phosphors. Their emission efficiency for light emission can be increased by improvements in phosphor composition. Their x-ray–to–light emission conversion efficiency can be enhanced with the use of more effective phosphors, such as rare Earth elements. To maintain OD, techniques must be reduced by specified amounts when faster screens are used.

Generally, intensifying screens increase image contrast. This is not always measurable, but it is particularly pronounced when screen exposures are compared with nonscreen, direct exposures.

RECOMMENDED DEMONSTRATION

Open the different types of available screens, and lay them side by side on the tabletop. Open the light field to include portions of as many screens as possible. Turn off all lights in the examination room. Observe the different colors of light emitted by each screen when exposed through the following techniques:

1. 50 mA, 3 s, 50 kVp
2. 50 mA, 3 s, 90 kVp
3. 100 mA, 3 s, 50 kVp

At the same time, compare the brightness of light emitted by each screen. Discuss the reasons for the different brightness levels with different types of screens and with different radiographic techniques.

MATERIALS REQUIRED

- Radiographic imaging system
- Hand phantom or similar thin phantom
- Knee phantom or phantom of similar thickness
- X-ray film processor
- Direct exposure holder
- 100-speed screen-film cassettes, preferably the same size as the direct exposure holder
- 400-speed screen-film cassettes, preferably the same size as the direct exposure holder
- Small, dry bone such as a phalanx
- Rectangular sponge about 6 inches thick
- Lead numbers
- Viewbox
- Densitometer

PROCEDURE

1. Warm up the processor if needed, and run a couple of "scrap" films through it to stabilize temperature and circulation.
2. Position the x-ray tube at 100 cm SID.
3. Number each film with a lead marker on the cassette. Take exposures on separate films using the techniques listed here, or record alternate techniques that you may have to use.

Exposure 1
- Load and place the high-speed or rare Earth screen cassette on the tabletop.
- Place the knee phantom on the cassette, using sponges as needed to balance it. Collimate to the film size.

Technique: 200 mA, 5 mAs, 65 kVp

Note: Process and check this film. It should be of medium OD. If it is very light or very dark, adjust the mAs and start over. Write your alternate technique here:

Alternate Technique: _____

Exposure 2 Load and place the slow-speed ("extremity" or "fine") or par-speed screen cassette on the tabletop. Place the knee phantom on the cassette in precisely the same position as you did for Exposure 1. Do not change collimation from Exposure 1.

Technique: Refer to Table E14-1, which gives technique factors for intensifying screens, and determine the mAs to be used as follows: Divide the factor listed for the new screen to be used by the factor listed for the screen used in Exposure

1. Multiply the original mAs by your answer. (For example, if you used a rare Earth medium 200-speed screen on Exposure 1 and are using a slow [50-speed] screen now, divide 2 by ½, which equals 4. Use four times as much mAs as in Exposure 1. Record the technique you use here:

   Technique used: _____
   Total mAs used: _____

2. *Exposure 3* Again, use the slow-speed ("extremity" or "fine") or par-speed screen cassette on the tabletop. Collimate to the film size, and center. Then place thick rectangular sponges on the film to create an object-to-image distance receptor (OID) of about 6 inches. Place the hand phantom on the sponges with the resolution test pattern alongside it.

   Technique: 50 mA, 1.25 mAs, 54 kVp

   Note: Process and check this film. It should be of medium overall OD. If it is very light or very dark, adjust the mAs and start over. Write your alternate technique here:

   Alternate Technique: _____

3. *Exposure 4* Load a direct exposure holder with the same type of film used in the cassettes, and place it on the tabletop. Center the light field first (do not change collimation from Exposure 3). Place the 6 inches of sponge on the film with the hand phantom and resolution template alongside it, as was done in Exposure 3.

   Technique: 250 to 300 mAs, 54 kVp (This technique approximates the application of the factor for a direct exposure holder with screen film as listed in Table E14-1.)

4. Process the films.

5. On Exposure 1, select and circle two smooth OD areas within the anatomy to take densitometer measurements as follows: Area A must show a dark gray soft tissue OD, and Area B

must show a light gray bony OD. Now circle the same two smooth OD areas on Exposure 2. Repeat this procedure with Exposures 3 and 4. Using the densitometer, determine the OD in these two areas for each exposure, and record the information in Table E14-2.

TABLE E14-1 Technique factors for intensifying screen

Type of screen	Technique factor, mAs
Direct exposure holder with 80 screen film	80
Direct exposure holder with 30 direct exposure file	30
50 speed	2
100 speed	1
400 speed	0.25

RESULTS

In Table E14-2, record each type of screen used, the total mAs used, and the measured OD in Areas A and B.

TABLE E14-2

	Type of screen	mAs	OD of area A	OD of area B
Exposure 1				
Exposure 2				
Exposure 3				
Exposure 4				

EXERCISES

1. On a viewbox, visually compare the overall ODs for Exposures 1 and 2. Refer to Table E14-2. By what ratio was the mAs increased when the change was made from the higher-speed screen to the slower screen?

2. Did this technique change reasonably maintain OD when screens were changed? If not, what factor would you use in place of the one from Table E14-2?

3. If this change in screens were made without technique adjustment, what would happen to the resultant OD?

4. Compute the image contrast for each exposure as follows: Subtract the Area B OD from the Area A OD, and record here:
   Exposure 1 contrast (A − B):

   _____

   Exposure 2 contrast (A − B):

   _____

   Exposure 3 contrast (A − B):

   _____

   Exposure 4 contrast (A − B):

5. Compare the computed image contrast level for Exposure 2 versus the contrast for Exposure 1. Is there any difference? If so, which of these two screen speeds produces the greatest image contrast?

6. Now, compare the computed contrast level for Exposure 3 versus the contrast for Exposure 4. Which of these two methods of exposure produces the highest image contrast?

Effect of Intensifying Screens on Image Blur

Name _____

Date _____

OBJECT

To demonstrate how radiographic intensifying screens work and their effect on image blur.

DISCUSSION

Radiographic intensifying screens convert x-rays into light, which in turn, exposes the image receptor. The principal result is a reduction in patient dose. Such screens convert the energy and the intensity of the x-ray beam into visible light that interacts with radiographic film much more easily than x-rays. An increase in kVp or an increase in mAs will cause the screen to glow brighter; this results in a darker image.

The use of radiographic intensifying screens increases image blur as compared with direct exposure techniques. As light passes from the screen to the film, it spreads, increasing the blur of the image. This property is called *screen blur*.

MATERIALS REQUIRED

- Radiographic imaging system
- Hand phantom or similar thin phantom
- Knee phantom or phantom of similar thickness
- X-ray film processor
- Direct exposure holder
- 100-speed screen-film cassette, preferably the same size as the direct exposure holder
- 400-speed screen-film cassette, preferably the same size as the direct exposure holder
- Resolution test pattern (lp/mm)
- Rectangular sponge about 6 inches thick
- Lead numbers
- Viewbox
- Densitometer

PROCEDURE

1. Warm up the processor if needed, and run a couple of "scrap" films through it to stabilize temperature and circulation.
2. Position the x-ray tube at 100 cm SID.
3. Number each film with a lead marker on the cassette. Take exposures on separate films using the techniques listed here, or record any alternate techniques used.

Exposure 1
- Load and place the high-speed or rare Earth screen cassette. Place the resolution test pattern on the cassette, using sponges as needed to balance it.
- Collimate to the film size.

   Technique: 200 mA, 5 mAs, 65 kVp
   Note: Process and check this film. It should be of medium overall OD. If it is very light or very dark, adjust the mAs and start over. Write your alternate technique here:
   Alternate Technique: _____

Exposure 2 Load and place the slow-speed ("extremity" or "fine") or par-speed screen cassette on the tabletop. Place the resolution test pattern on the cassette. Note change collimation from Exposure 1.

   Technique: Refer to Table E14-2 to determine the mAs to be used as described for that experiment.

Technique Used: _____
Total mAs Used: _____

Exposure 3 Again, use the slow-speed ("extremity" or "fine") or par-speed screen cassette on the tabletop. Collimate to the film size, and center. Then place a thick rectangular sponge on the film to create an OID of about 6 inches. Place the resolution test pattern on the sponge.

Technique: 50 mA, 25 ms, 1.25 mAs, 54 kVp

Note: Process and check this film. It should be of gray OD. If it is very light or very dark, adjust the mAs and start over. Write your alternate technique here:

Alternate Technique: _____

Exposure 4 Load the direct exposure holder with the same type of film used in the cassettes and place it on the tabletop. Center the light field first (do not change collimation from Exposure 3). Place the 6-inch sponge on the film with the resolution test pattern on it as before.

    Technique: 250 to 300 mAs, 54 kVp

4. Process the films.

RESULTS

On the images of the resolution test pattern, scan downward across the black and white line pairs, from thickest to thinnest, and determine where they are blurred to the point that you cannot distinguish separate lines with clear edges. Note which line pair number this is. Refer to the resolution test pattern itself or to the table provided by your instructor to read off how many line pairs per millimeter correspond to this line pair number.

In Table E15-1, record each type of screen and the resolution in line pairs per millimeter.

TABLE E15-1

	Type of screen	Resolution, lp/mm
Exposure 1		
Exposure 2		
Exposure 2		
Exposure 4		

EXERCISES

1. On a viewbox, visually compare only Exposures 3 and 4. With which type of image receptor are more lines resolved? With which receptor do these lines appear to have sharper edges?
2. Refer to Table E15-1. Which receptor resolved the greatest number of line pairs per millimeter—the screen or the direct exposure holder? Does this agree with your visual observations in Exercise 1?
3. Why does this effect occur when the change is made from screen to direct exposures?
4. Refer to Table E15-1. Which of the two screen speeds, the higher or the lower speed, resolved the greatest number of line pairs per millimeter?

Processor Quality Control

Name _____

Date _____

OBJECT

To demonstrate a quality control program for automatic film processors.

DISCUSSION

When a film is too light or too dark, the most frequent cause is improper radiographic technique. However, the radiographic imaging system or the automatic processor is occasionally at fault. With establishment of a processor quality control program, problems with processors can be documented and sometimes corrected even before patient films are processed.

A process quality control program is begun by reserving a box of film to be used exclusively for processor monitoring. The standard or control film is exposed with a sensitometer. The sensitometer is a device that has an accurately reproducible light intensity combined with optical filters to produce a step-wedge image.

Each day, before patient film processing begins, an exposure of a test film is made with the sensitometer. With a busy processor, this test may be repeated several times each day. The test film then is compared with the standard film. No change should be observed because the same lot of film, an identical exposure of film, and the same processing are being used. A variation between the standard film and the test film represents a change in performance of the automatic film processor.

Because daily monitoring of a processor is not practical for a student laboratory exercise, perform suggested monitoring weekly at the beginning of each laboratory period. You will maintain a record of each week's results and graph the data weekly during the course of the experiment. These data will be used to evaluate the stability of performance of a single processor. During the final laboratory period, you will evaluate the uniformity of all processors within your department.

MATERIALS REQUIRED

- Empty film box that can be resealed without light leaks
- Sensitometer that produces steps discernible to the eye (i.e., approximately 15% exposure increase from one step to the next)
- Film illuminator
- 25 sheets of 8 in × 10 in (20 cm × 25 cm) film from the same manufacturer's lot
- Linear graph paper

PROCEDURE

FIRST WEEK

1. Set aside 25 sheets of film from the same manufacturer's lot (exclusively for this experiment) in an empty box that can be restored to its light-tight condition.
2. Allow the sensitometer to warm up for 5 minutes to ensure the stability of the light source.
3. Expose a film with the sensitometer.
4. Process the film in the automatic processor under investigation. Be careful to note the orientation of the transfer of film from the sensitometer into the processor, so the procedure can be identical each week.
5. Record all data indicated on the data sheet.
6. Save the film, and label it as standard or control.

EACH SUCCESSIVE WEEK

1. Repeat steps 2 to 5 of the instructions from the first week.
2. Label the film as "Test Film Week No. _____," and date it.
3. Using the same area of the illuminator each week, visually match the images of the step wedges of the test film with the standard film. Each step represents a change of 15% in exposure. A variance of two steps or greater indicates that the processor requires attention.

4. Record the OD difference, the developer temperature, and the water temperature on the data sheet, and plot data on the graph sheet provided.

FINAL WEEK

1. Expose the test film and record the data as usual.
2. During this laboratory period, compare the response of this processor with those of four other processors in your department. This can be done by using the sensitometer to expose films from the reserved package and processing them in the other processors in the same manner as all previous test films.

3. Identify the processor on each test film.
4. Compare the step-wedge images of these four processors with the test film from the processor that was monitored weekly, and record results on the data sheet.

EXERCISES

1. Discuss the stability of the processor that was monitored.
2. If the density difference varies by more than two steps, what can the radiologic technologist check before requesting a service call?
3. How do the processors within your department compare in uniformity?

DATA SHEET FOR EXPERIMENT 16: PROCESSOR QUALITY CONTROL

Processor identification: _____

Week no.	Optical density difference	Developer temperature, °F or °C	Water temperature, °F or °C
1			
2			
3			
4			
5			
6			
7			
8			
9			
10			
11			
12			
13			
14			
15			
16			
17			
18			

TABLE E16-2 **Processor 3**	1*	2	3	4	5
Optical density difference					

*Processor that has been monitored weekly.

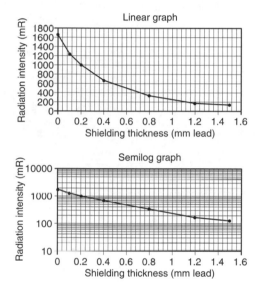

Effect of Focal-Spot Size on Image Blur

Name _____

Date _____

OBJECT

To demonstrate the effect that changing the focal-spot size has on image blur.

DISCUSSION

The size of the focal spot is the principal variable in radiography that affects image blur without affecting other image quality factors. It thus becomes the most important factor for controlling the spatial resolution of the imaging system. The smaller the focal spot used, the less will be the focal-spot blur on the image.

Generally, small focal spots should be used for any anatomy that is small enough to be radiographed tabletop (without a Bucky), to maximize diagnostic image quality. Small focal spots also are used for cerebral angiography (small vessels), mammography (microcalcifications), and other examinations of small, high-contrast structures.

MATERIALS REQUIRED

- Radiographic imaging system
- Small, dry bone such as a phalanx, or other small object
- Resolution test pattern (lp/mm)
- X-ray film processor
- 400-speed screen-film cassettes, 10 in × 12 in (24 cm × 30 cm)
- Lead or lead vinyl sheets
- Rectangular sponge approximately 4 inches thick
- Spherical object or head of a dry femur bone
- Lead numbers
- Viewbox
- Densitometer
- Magnifying glass

PROCEDURE

1. Warm up the processor, if needed, and run a couple of "scrap" films through it to stabilize temperature and circulation.
2. Set 50 kVp. This will remain constant throughout the experiment.
3. Set the SID to 100 cm. This will also remain constant throughout the experiment.
4. Load and place the 10 in × 12 in cassette on the table. Two exposures will be taken on one film.
5. Collimate the light field to a 4 in × 8 in area crosswise at one end of the film. Use the lead sheets to mask the other half of the film.
6. Place the 4-inch-thick flat sponge onto the film to create a large object-to-image receptor distance (OID); this must be kept constant on both exposures.
7. Place the resolution test pattern crosswise on one end of the sponge and the bone alongside it. Pay close attention to the position in which the bone is laid, because you must lay it precisely the same way on the second exposure. Both test objects must be within the light field.
8. Number each exposure with a lead marker on the cassette. Take two exposures using the following techniques or any necessary alternate techniques.
   Exposure 1: 50 mA, small focal spot, 35 ms
   Exposure 2: 200 mA, large focal spot, 8 ms
9. Process the film.

RESULTS

On images of the resolution test pattern, scan the black and white line pairs from thickest to thinnest, and determine where they are blurred first, so you cannot distinguish separate lines with clear edges. Use the magnifying glass, and note at which line pair number this first occurs. Refer to the resolution test pattern itself or to the table provided by your instructor to read off how many line pairs per millimeter correspond to this line pair number.

The unit "line pairs per millimeter" is a direct measurement of spatial resolution. The greater the number of line pairs per millimeter resolved, the less is the blur of the image. In Table E17-1, record each resolution in line pairs per millimeter.

When you have completed this, obtain a millimeter ruler and measure the length of the bone images of Exposures 1 and 2. Then, taking care to hold the bone as it was placed on the cassette and lining the ruler up precisely to the same points as you did on the radiographs, measure the length of the actual dry bone. Record these measurements also in Table E17-1.

TABLE E17-1

	Focal spot	Resolution, lp/mm	Bone image size
Exposure 1			
Exposure 2			

Actual bone size: _____

EXERCISES

1. Visually examine the marrow portion of the bone images for fine trabecular detail. With which focal-spot size is more detail resolved? With which focal spot does this detail appear to have sharper edges?
2. Refer to Table E17-1. Which focal spot resolved the greater number of line pairs per millimeter? Does this agree with your visual observations in Exercise 1?
3. What general rule of thumb can you make for focal-spot size to consistently produce radiographs with maximum resolution?
4. From Table E17-1, compute the magnification factors for the two exposures using the formula below, and record them:

$$\text{Magnification} = \frac{\text{Measured image length}}{\text{Actual bone length}}$$

Exposure 1 magnification: _____
Exposure 2 magnification: _____

5. Did one focal spot cause more magnification than the other? Does focal spot affect the size of the image?

Effect of Object-to-Image Receptor Distance on Image Blur and Magnification

Name _____

Date _____

OBJECT

To demonstrate the effects of changing object-to-image receptor distance (OID) on image blur and magnification, and to describe the influence of changing source-to-image receptor distance (SID).

DISCUSSION

OID affects image blur and magnification in the image. Ideally, the anatomic part that is being examined should be placed in direct contact with the image receptor so that the OID is minimized, but a substantial OID is often unavoidable. This increases focal-spot blur and loss of image detail. It also results in image magnification. The only way to compensate for both of these problems is by increasing the SID as well.

MATERIALS REQUIRED

- Radiographic imaging system
- Small, dry bone such as a phalanx, or other small object
- Resolution test pattern (lp/mm)
- X-ray film processor
- 400-speed screen-film cassettes, 14 in × 17 in (35 cm × 43 cm)
- Lead or vinyl lead sheets
- Rectangular sponge approximately 4 inches thick
- Additional rectangular sponge approximately 2 inches thick (must be one-half the thickness of the other sponge)
- Spherical object or head of a dry femur bone
- Lead numbers
- Viewbox
- Densitometer

PROCEDURE

1. Warm up the processor if needed, and run a couple of "scrap" films through it to stabilize temperature and circulation.
2. Set 50 kVp. This will remain constant throughout the experiment.
3. Load and place the 14 in × 17 in cassette on the table. Three exposures will be taken on one film.
4. Collimate the light field to a 5 in × 8 in area crosswise at one end of the film. Use the lead sheets to mask the adjacent film area. Both test objects must be within the light field.
5. Number each exposure with a lead marker on the cassette. Take three exposures using the following techniques or necessary alternate techniques.

Exposure 1 Place the 2-inch sponge on one end of the film. Place the resolution test pattern crosswise and the bone alongside it, resting on the sponge. Pay close attention to the position in which the bone is laid because you must lay it precisely the same way for Exposure 2.

Set the SID precisely to 50 cm from the tabletop. Be sure to visually check the light field, and open it up to include the test objects.

Technique: 50 mA, 8 ms

Exposure 2 Place the 4-inch sponge in the middle of the film. Place the resolution test pattern crosswise on the sponge and the bone alongside it, exactly as you did for Exposure 1. Keep the same SID. Check the light field to be sure that the test objects are within it.

Technique: 50 mA, 8 ms

Exposure 3 Place the 4-inch sponge at the remaining end of the film. Place the resolution test pattern crosswise on the sponge and the bone alongside it, exactly as you did for Exposure 1. Keep the same SID. Collimate the light field down to the remaining cassette area.

Technique: 50 mA, 35 ms

6. Process the film.

RESULTS

On the images of the resolution test pattern, scan the black and white line pairs from thickest to thinnest, and determine where they are blurred first, so you cannot distinguish separate lines with clear edges. Note at which line pair number this first occurs. Refer to the resolution test pattern itself or to the table provided by your instructor to read off how many line pairs per millimeter correspond to this line pair number. In Table E18-1, record each OID, the SID, and the resolution in line pairs per millimeter.

With a millimeter ruler, measure the length of the bone images for each exposure. Then, taking care to hold the bone as it was placed on the cassette and lining the ruler up precisely to the same points as you did on the radiographs, measure the length of the actual dry bone. Record these measurements also in Table E18-1.

TABLE E18-1				
	OID	SID	Resolution, lp/mm	Bone image size
Exposure 1				
Exposure 2				
Exposure 3				
Exposure 4				

EXERCISES

1. Visually examine the marrow portion of the bone images for fine trabecular detail. With which OID/SID combination is the detail most blurred?
2. Refer to Table E18-1 and compare Exposures 1 and 2. At which OID was the greater number of line pairs per millimeter resolved?
3. What general rule of thumb can you make for OID to consistently produce radiographs with maximum resolution?
4. Now compare the results from Table E18-1 with regard to the lp/mm resolved for Exposures 3 and 1. For Exposure 3, both OID and SID were doubled. Is the resolution different? Why or why not?
5. From Table E18-1, compute the magnification factor for the three exposures using the following formula:

$$\text{Magnification} = \frac{\text{Measured image length}}{\text{Actual bone length}}$$

Exposure 1 magnification: _____
Exposure 2 magnification: _____
Exposure 3 magnification: _____

6. Compare the magnification for Exposures 1 and 2. At which OID was magnification the greatest?
7. What general rule can you make for OID, to consistently produce radiographs with minimum magnification?
8. Now compare the magnification for Exposures 2 and 3. For Exposure 3, the OID and the SID were doubled. Is the magnification different? Why or why not?
9. On the basis of your answers to Exercises 4 and 8, with regard to control of magnification and resolution, what is the relationship between OID and SID?

Effect of Object Alignment on Image Distortion

Name _____

Date _____

OBJECT

To demonstrate the distorting effects of misalignment of the x-ray beam, the object, and the image receptor.

DISCUSSION

Misalignment problems include off-centering of the central ray from the anatomic part, angling of the image receptor or anatomic part so that one is not parallel to the other, and angling of the central ray so that it is not perpendicular to the anatomic part or the film.

Generally, these conditions cause distortion of object shape on the image of the anatomic part that is being radiographed. When the anatomic part and the image receptor cannot be placed parallel to each other, shape distortion is minimized by angling the central ray to one-half the angle formed between the part and the image receptor.

There are two types of shape distortion: elongation of the image and foreshortening of the image. Distortion is always undesirable and should be minimized.

MATERIALS REQUIRED

- Radiographic imaging system
- X-ray film processor
- 400-speed screen-film cassettes, 14 in × 17 in (35 cm × 43 cm)
- Lead or vinyl lead sheets
- Rectangular sponge approximately 2 inches thick
- 45-degree-angle sponge
- Coin
- Spherical object or head of a dry femur bone
- Lead numbers
- Viewbox

PROCEDURE

1. Warm up the processor if needed, and run a couple of "scrap" films through it to stabilize temperature and circulation.
2. Set 50 kVp. This will remain constant throughout the experiment.
3. Load and place the 14 in × 17 in cassette on the table. Six exposures will be taken on one film; it will be divided it into two rows of three exposures each.
4. Collimate the light field to a 5-inch-square area in one corner of the film. Use the lead sheets to mask the adjacent film areas.
5. Place the 2-inch-thick flat sponge on the film to create a larger object-to-image receptor distance (OID). All views must be taken at the same OID.
6. Number each exposure with a lead marker on the cassette. Take six exposures using the following techniques.
7. Set 50 mA and 50 kVp.

   Exposure 1 Place the spherical object or head of a femur on the sponge in the corner of the film. Pay close attention to how you place this object because it must be placed exactly the same way on Exposure 2. Center a 100-cm SID perpendicular beam to the sphere.

   Exposure 2 Place the spherical object on the sponge in the same position as you did for Exposure 1. Angle the x-ray beam 35 degrees, and maintain SID by reducing the tabletop-to-tube distance to 84 cm to the center of the sphere.

   Exposure 3 Place the coin on the sponge lying parallel to the film. Center a 100-cm SID perpendicular beam to the coin.

407

Exposure 4 Tape the coin to a 45-degree-angle sponge at a spot that maintains exactly the same OID as the flat sponge in Exposure 3. Angle the x-ray beam 45 degrees so that the central ray is perpendicular to the coin, and maintain SID by adjusting the tabletop-to-tube distance to the center of the coin.

Exposure 5 Keep the coin taped to the same spot on the 45-degree-angle sponge as it was in Exposure 4. Center a vertical beam perpendicular to the film. The SID should be 100 cm.

Exposure 6 Keep the coin taped to the same spot on the 45-degree-angle sponge as it was in Exposure 4. Angle the x-ray beam isometrically to 22.5 degrees (one half of the angle formed between the coin and the film). Maintain SID by adjusting the tabletop-to-tube distance to the center to the coin.

RESULTS

Visually observe the images on a viewbox. If distortion effects are not obvious, use a ruler to measure objects and images along the axis at which the beam or the coin was angled.

EXERCISES

1. Visually compare Exposures 1 and 2. Does angling the x-ray beam distort the true shape of a spherical object?
2. Note the width of the spherical image at the axis crosswise to the direction the beam was angled. Compare Exposure 2 with Exposure 1. You can superimpose the images with a bright light for visual comparison or use a ruler and measure the width. For magnification to occur, both the length and the width of the image should be increased from Exposure 1. Did angulation of the beam cause magnification of the image when distances were maintained?
3. Compare the coin image on Exposure 4 with that on Exposure 3. Is distortion caused when the object is angled in relation to the film and the beam is kept perpendicular to the object? If so, what specific type of distortion occurs?
4. Compare the coin image on Exposure 5 with that on Exposure 3. Is distortion caused when the object is angled in relation to the film and the beam is kept perpendicular to the film? If so, what specific type of distortion occurs?
5. Compare the coin image on Exposure 6 with that on Exposure 3. Is distortion caused when the object is angled in relation to the film and the beam is angled isometrically between the object and the film?

Anode Heel Effect

Name _____

Date _____

OBJECT

To demonstrate the variation of x-ray intensity in a plane perpendicular to the central axis of the useful beam.

DISCUSSION

The radiation intensity across the useful x-ray beam is higher on the cathode side than on the anode side. Along a line perpendicular to the anode–cathode axis, the radiation intensity is constant. The x-rays produced from a depth in the tube target must traverse a greater thickness of target material on the anode side than on the cathode side. Because of this self-absorption of x-rays in the "heel" of the anode, the resultant distribution of x-ray intensity is known as the heel effect.

MATERIALS REQUIRED

- Radiographic imaging system
- Ionization chamber
- 50 cm × 50 cm grid marked in 5-cm intervals
- Linear graph paper

PROCEDURE

1. Tape the 50 cm × 50 cm grid to the tabletop so the central axis of the x-ray beam intersects the center of the grid.
2. Position the x-ray tube target 80 cm above the tabletop.
3. The x-ray imaging system may be used as it is normally filtered. Record the amount of total filtration, if known. Adjust the tube potential to 70 kVp, and select an appropriate mAs that will produce a response of the ionization chamber that is at least half-scale. The kVp, mA, and exposure time will remain constant throughout the experiment.
4. Position the ionization chamber on the central ray and, using the data sheet provided, record the response. Three measurements are necessary at each position.
5. Reposition the ionization chamber at 5-cm intervals along the four major radii from the central axis (two along the anode–cathode axis and two perpendicular to that axis).
6. Calculate the average intensity (mR) at each location.
7. Calculate the percentage of the central ray intensity at each location as follows:

Intensity as % of central ray Intensity =

$$\frac{\text{Intensity at grid location (mR)}}{\text{Intensity at central ray (mR)}} \times 100$$

RESULTS

On the linear graph paper provided, plot the percentage of the central ray intensity versus the position of the x-ray beam along the anode–cathode axis and versus the position of the x-ray beam along the axis perpendicular to the anode–cathode axis.

EXERCISES

1. If a 10 in × 12 in film were centered on a grid with the 12 inch (30 cm) dimension along the anode–cathode axis, what percentage of the central ray exposure would exist along the four sides of the film?

2. Discuss the effect, if any, that a change from the small focal-spot station to the large focal-spot station would have on the magnitude of the heel effect.

3. Discuss the effect, if any, that a change in the target angle would have on the magnitude of the heel effect.

4. In each of the following examinations, how should the anode–cathode axis of the x-ray tube be oriented with respect to the patient, or does it matter?
   a. Extremity _____
   b. Chest _____
   c. Skull _____
   d. Pelvis _____
   e. Mammogram _____

DATA SHEET FOR EXPERIMENT 20: ANODE HEEL EFFECT

CONSTANT FACTORS
- 70 kVp mA _____
- Exposure time (ms): _____
- 75 cm source-to-detector distance
- Filtration: _____ mm Al

Grid position	Exposure, mR			Average exposure, mR	Percent of central ray
	First	Second	Third		
Central ray					
1					
2					
3					
4					
5					
6					
7					
8					
9					
10					
11					
12					
13					
14					
15					
16					
17					
18					
19					
20					
21					
22					

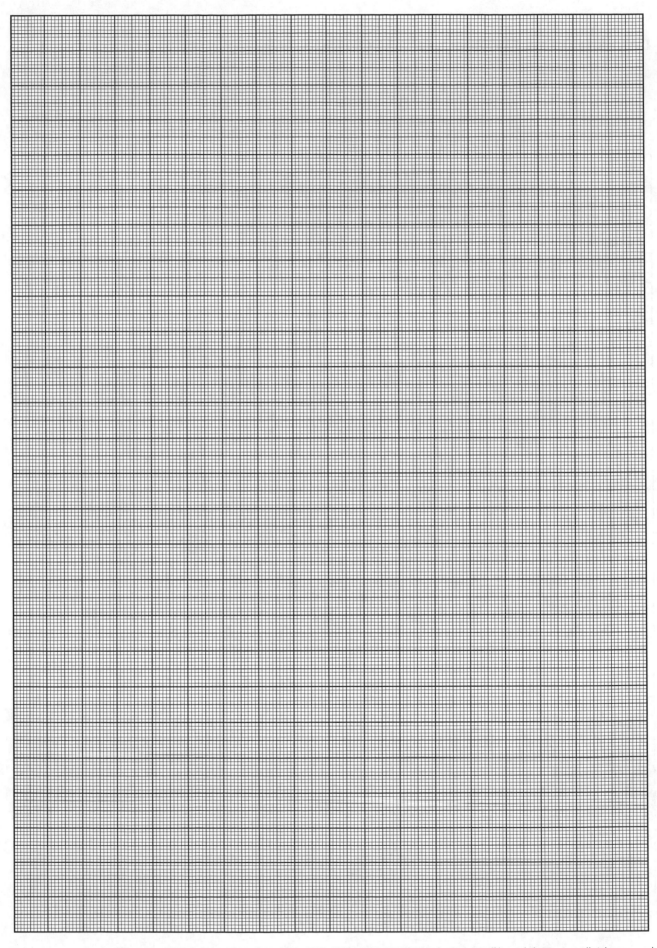

Effective Focal-Spot Size

Name _____

Date _____

OBJECT

To measure the effective focal-spot size (EFS) under differing conditions of x-ray tube current.

DISCUSSION

Currently, three methods are used for measuring effective focal-spot size while the tube is energized. The **pinhole camera** is simplest in concept but somewhat difficult to use. When x-rays from the focal spot are incident on an aperture or pinhole, which is much smaller than the focal spot and is positioned midway between the source and the image receptor, the resultant image will have the same size and shape as the effective focal spot. If the pinhole is located at any other position between target and film, magnification or minification will occur. Positioning of the pinhole is critical; it must lie on the central ray of the x-ray beam midway between the source and the image receptor and in a plane parallel with the image receptor, yet it must be perpendicular to the central axis.

Then:

$$EFS = AFS \times \sin \theta$$

where *EFS* is the effective focal-spot size, *AFS* is the actual focal-spot size, and θ is the target angle.

The use of a **star test pattern** is much easier, but the theoretical basis for its use is more complicated. The star test pattern must be centered on the central ray of the x-ray beam and perpendicular to it. With this device, however, precise positioning is less necessary. The EFS is calculated from measurements made from the star test pattern image as follows:

$$EFS = \frac{N}{57.3} \times \frac{D}{m - 1}$$

where *EFS* is the effective focal-spot size in millimeters, *N* is the star pattern angle in degrees (usually 1 or 2 degrees and indicated on the pattern), *D* is the

blur diameter measured in millimeters from the image, and *m* equals

Image size (magnification factor)

Object size

The blur diameter should be measured across the image along the anode–cathode axis and its perpendicular axis. Results may demonstrate that the EFS is not square.

The third method employs a **slit camera**. The slit camera is used in much the same way as the pinhole camera; when used correctly, it is the most accurate of the three. The slit camera is used by manufacturers in their laboratories and by medical physicists in the clinic.

MATERIALS REQUIRED

- Dual-focus radiographic imaging system
- Pinhole camera with approximate 0.03-mm opening
- 360-degree star test pattern
- Pinhole camera
- Tape measure
- Magnifying glass
- 0.1-mm increment rule
- Magnified reticule

PROCEDURE

PINHOLE CAMERA

1. Select 50 kVp and an mA station for which both large and small focal-spot sizes are available. Usually, the 100 mA station is suitable. Begin with the small focal-spot station.
2. Position the pinhole camera midway between the target and the image receptor and cone down the useful beam to about 5 cm × 5 cm on the film, centered on the pinhole. The source-to-image receptor distance (SID) should be about 75 cm.

3. Adjust the pinhole alignment until an acceptable image is obtained. At least 1000 mAs may be required; therefore, multiple exposures may be necessary.
4. Change to the large focal-spot station and repeat Step 3.
5. Using the large focal spot, increase the mA to the highest possible value while maintaining a constant mAs, and repeat Step 3.

STAR TEST PATTERN

1. Replace the pinhole camera with the star test pattern. It is acceptable to tape the test pattern to the light-localizing collimator.
2. Repeat Steps 3, 4, and 5 of the pinhole camera procedure. A much lower mAs will be required. Try 50 mAs as a starter.

SLIT CAMERA

1. Position the slit camera on the central axis and midway between the focal spot and image receptor. The slit should be parallel to the anode–cathode axis. Image the slit at low kVp and high mAs: try 50 kVp, 1000 mAs. Rotate the slit camera 90 degrees and repeat the exposure.
2. Measure the width of each slit with a magnified reticule.

RESULTS

With the magnifying glass and scale ruled to the nearest 0.1 mm, measure the length and width of each of the three focal-spot images obtained with the pinhole camera. Measure the perpendicular blur diameters from the three star test pattern exposures. Use the attached data sheet as a guide, and calculate the EFS. Complete Tables E21-1 and E21-2, which show results.

EXERCISES

1. When mA is increased, the EFS often increases in size. This effect is called *blooming*. Using these test device data, calculate the percentage increase in EFS with an increase in mA.

TABLE E21-1 Focal spot size (mm × mm)

	Small spot, low mA	Large spot, low mA	Large spot, high mA
Pinhole camera			
Star test pattern			

TABLE E21-2 Focal spot size (mm × mm)

	Slit camera	Anode–cathode axis	Perpindicular axis
Slit camera			
Star test pattern			

2. Describe the shape and optical density (OD) distribution of each of the images obtained with the pinhole camera.
3. If the actual focal spot of a 13-degree target angle tube measures 4.8 mm × 1.0 mm, what will be the EFS?
4. If the EFS is 0.6 mm × 0.6 mm and the target angle is 10.5 degrees, what is the actual focal-spot size (AFS)?

DATA SHEET FOR EXPERIMENT 21: EFFECTIVE FOCAL-SPOT SIZE

Pinhole Camera

d = _____ cm, the distance on the pinhole plate separating the large localizing holes, which is usually 1.27 cm.

d^1 = _____ cm, the distance on the image separating the localizing holes.

Small focal spot (low mA)
Focal-spot image length = _____ mm
Focal-spot image width = _____ mm

Large focal spot (low mA)
Focal-spot image length = _____ mm
Focal-spot image width = _____ mm

Large focal spot (high mA)
Focal-spot image length = _____ mm
Focal-spot image width = _____ mm

Effective focal point size (mm) =
Image size
($d/d^1 - d$)

Star Test Pattern

N = _____ degrees, the star test pattern angle.

Object size = _____, the diameter of the star test pattern.

Image size = _____, the diameter of the image of the star test pattern.

m = _____.

Small focal spot (low mA)
Blur diameter = _____ mm × _____ mm

Large focal spot (low mA)
Blur diameter = _____ mm × _____ mm

Large focal spot (high mA)
Blur diameter = _____ mm × _____ mm

Effective focal spot size (mm) =
$$\frac{N}{57.3} = \frac{Blur\ diameter}{m - 1}$$

Slit Camera

Effective focal spot, large (mm) = _____
Effective focal spot, small (mm) = _____

Repeat Analysis

Name _____

Date _____

OBJECT

To demonstrate how a repeat analysis is conducted.

DISCUSSION

Repeat analysis can be conducted for an individual radiographer or for an entire radiology department. Studies have shown that, when an imaging department initiates a quality control program that includes repeat analysis, sensitometric processor monitoring, and the use of technique charts, the exposures repeated because of improper optical density (OD) can be cut by one third to one half. This saves money for the department, reduces unnecessary patient dose, and should be taken seriously by every radiologic technologist.

By analyzing and categorizing repeated exposures, the department can identify specific areas of need for attention and continuing education. The individual radiologic technologist can recognize areas for improvement, as well as personal strong points. The more detailed the analysis is, the more useful it will be.

MATERIALS REQUIRED

- A box, drawer, or file in which to store throwaway films for each individual or group under study

PROCEDURE

1. For a period of 2 to 4 weeks, as directed by your instructor, place all of your throwaway films in a separate box, drawer, or file with your name on it so no one will inadvertently misplace it.

2. During this time, you also must keep accurate records of the total number of radiographs you made. For accuracy, it is best to use the following Record A, which you must mark after every procedure, summing the number of views taken (not films used). However, if you do not have time to do this, a fair estimate can be made to the best of your memory by using Record B, which must be filled out at the end of each working day. The totals then will be estimated at the end of the study period by multiplying the number of views taken for that procedure. Choose Record A or Record B and fill in the required information.

3. At the end of the study period, insert the data in the following section and complete the exercises.

RECORD A FOR REPEAT ANALYSIS

After each procedure is performed, fill in the number of views (*not* films) taken in the appropriate category below.

Note: "Torso" includes chest films, abdomen films, and intravenous pyelograms (IVPs).

"Extremity" includes pelvic and shoulder girdle films. "Fluoroscopic" includes upper gastrointestinal films, barium enemas, and air-contrast barium enemas.

RECORD B FOR REPEAT ANALYSIS

At the end of each working day, fill in the number of procedures of each type that are performed that day. At the end of the study period, fill in the routine number of views taken for each type of procedure. Multiply the number of views by the number of each procedure done to obtain a total.

TABLE E22-1 **Type of procedure**					
Torso	Head	Spine	Extremity	Fluoroscopic	Other

Total for period: _____
Grand total: _____
Number of views for period (add all columns): _____

RESULTS

Refer to Record A or Record B and record here the total number of views taken:

_____

Record the number of views taken in each of the following:

    Torso: _____
    Head: _____
    Spine: _____
    Extremities (and girdles): _____
    Fluoroscopic procedures: _____
    Other: _____

Record the total number of repeat exposures made:

_____

Now carefully examine each film in the throwaway file, and determine the primary cause for its being repeated. Sort films into the following groups. When this has been done, count and record the number of films in each group.

REASON FOR REPEAT	NUMBER OF REPEATS
Optical density too dark:	_____
Optical density too light:	_____
Not flashed or not properly marked:	_____
Artifacts on patient, film, or table:	_____
Motion:	_____
Blank film or processing artifacts:	_____
Positioning, alignment, and collimation:	_____

TABLE E22-2 Type of procedure

Torso	Head	Spine	Extremity	Fluoroscopic	Other

Total for period: _____
Grand total: _____
Number of views for period (add all columns): _____

From the positioning category only, sort and total the following:

    Torso: _____
    Head: _____
    Spine: _____
    Extremities (and girdles): _____
    Fluoroscopic procedures: _____
    Other: _____

period by the total number of views taken. Multiply the result by 100.

$$\text{Repeat rate} = \frac{\text{Total repeats}}{\text{Total view}} \times 100$$

Repeat rate: _____%

EXERCISES

1. Refer to the "Results" section and determine the overall repeat rate as follows. Divide the total number of repeats taken for the entire

2. Compute the percent of all repeats caused by each of the following problems, as follows: Divide the number of repeats taken for this reason by the total number of repeats taken for the entire period. Multiply this result by 100. Record here for each category:

Optical density too dark: _____%

Optical density too light: _____%

Not flashed or not properly marked: _____%

Artifacts on patient, film, or table: _____%

Motion: _____%

Blank film or processing artifacts: _____%

Positioning, alignment, and collimation: ____%

3. What type of problem caused the greatest number of repeat exposures? What type of problem caused the second greatest number of repeats?

4. What type of problem caused the lowest number of repeats?

5. Refer to the "Results" section and compute the repeat rate for each of the following types of procedures as follows: Divide the number of repeats taken for each procedure by the total number of views taken for each procedure. Multiply this result by 100. Record here:

Torso: _____

Head: _____

Spine: _____

Extremities (and girdles): _____

Fluoroscopic procedures: _____

Other: _____

6. Which general type of procedure has the highest repeat rate? What could be done to improve this?

Procedure	Routine number of views	Day of month or of study period																														Total procedures	Total views taken
		1	2	3	4	5	6	7	8	9	10	11	12	13	14	15	16	17	18	19	20	21	22	23	24	25	26	27	28	29	30	31		
Torso																																			
Chest																																			
Abdomen																																			
IVP																																			
Head																																			
Skull																																			
Sinus/facies																																			
Mandible																																			
Orbits																																			
Other																																			
Spines																																			
Cervical																																			
Thoracic																																			
Lumbar																																			
Sacrum/C																																			
Extremities																																			
Hand/finger																																			
Wrist																																			
Forearm																																			
Elbow																																			
Humerus																																			
Shoulder																																			

Procedure	Routine number of views	Day of month or of study period																															Total procedures	Total views taken
		1	2	3	4	5	6	7	8	9	10	11	12	13	14	15	16	17	18	19	20	21	22	23	24	25	26	27	28	29	30	31		
Clavicle/scapula																																			
Foot/toe																																			
Ankle																																			
Leg																																			
Knee																																			
Femur																																			
Hip																																			
Pelvis																																			
Fluoroscopic																																			
Upper GI																																			
Air contrast																																			
barium enema																																			
Barium enema																																			
Other																																			

Grand total no. of views for period: _____

Tomography

Name _____

Date _____

OBJECT

To demonstrate the effect of the tomographic angle on the tomographic image.

DISCUSSION

Obtaining an acceptable radiograph is frequently difficult because of the superimposition of anatomic structures. For example, examination of the bronchi is difficult with a conventional radiograph because of adjacent sternal and vertebral bony structures. A tomographic motion will blur the image of the overlying sternum and underlying spine while maintaining detail of structures in the plane of focus (the plane that contains the pivot or fulcrum).

During tomography, the x-ray tube and the image receptor are separated by a fixed distance and move in synchrony about the pivot or focal point. A variety of motions are available, including linear, circular, and elliptical. Linear tomography prevails as the one that is most often used.

A range of tomographic angles is permitted for linear tomography. Complex motions produce increased blurring of objects outside the plane of focus compared with simple motions. This has the effect of increasing the contrast of objects in the plane of focus.

Similarly, an increase in tomographic angle will increase the blurring of objects outside the plane of focus. Additionally, an increase in tomographic angle will reduce the thickness of the in-focus layer.

MATERIALS REQUIRED

- Tomographic test object
- Linear tomographic imaging system
- Film marking pencil
- Lead diaphragm with pinhole
- 400-speed cassette, 10 in × 12 in (25 cm × 30 cm)
- Viewbox

PROCEDURE

PART I: PINHOLE TRACING

Place a lead diaphragm containing a pinhole on the examination table, and position it 17 cm above the plane of focus. Shield a large area around the pinhole with lead masks or a lead apron. With the collimators fully open, make a separate exposure on 10 in × 12 in (25 cm × 30 cm) film, using each of the possible movements of the tomograph (try 65 kVp, 120 mAs). The pinhole tracings that you obtain can be used to evaluate the following tomographic characteristics:

1. **Geometric form of the motion.** Any gross deviations from the intended motion will be observed.
2. **Mechanical stability.** Unwanted motion in the x-ray tube housing or the image receptor assembly will result in a wavy tracing or "wobble."
3. **Completeness of exposure.** Open sections in the image tracing indicate incomplete exposure, whereas overlapped sections indicate unnecessary double exposure.
4. **Uniformity of intensity.** Undesirable changes in radiation intensity during exposure will appear on the tracing as variations in optical density (OD).

Observations of each of these characteristics are to be made on the data sheet.

PART II: THICKNESS OF CUT

Section thickness can be measured and compared with that stated by the manufacturer.

Center the tomographic test object on the table, set the focal plane at the level of the scale 4.0 cm above the table, and make an exposure (try 120 mAs at 50 kVp). The test object should be positioned perpendicular to the direction of the tube movement for linear motion. Examine the image of the inclined wires next to the scale. One wire measures in millimeter increments, whereas the other measures in centimeter increments.

Place the film on a viewbox and use a film marking pencil to mark lightly where each end of the wire comes into focus. Lay a piece of paper next to the wire image and mark the in-focus length of wire. Use the paper as a guide and lay it next to the image of the scale. Read the thickness of cut using the appropriate scale, and record these values on the data sheet.

Compute the percent error as follows:

$$\% \text{ Error} = \frac{\text{Difference between indicated and measured thickness}}{\text{Indicated thickness}}$$

Observe the quality of the image of the bone lesion.

PART III: EFFECT OF TOMOGRAPHIC ANGLE

Center the tomographic phantom on the table and adjust the focal plane to the level of the scale. Make an exposure of the tomographic phantom (try 120 mAs at 50 kVp) using tomographic angles of 10, 20, and 30 degrees in the linear mode. Remember to place the tomographic phantom perpendicular to the tube movement. Compare the blur images of the circle and star patterns. Patterns nearest the scale are in the plane of focus, and their image should be sharp. Patterns farthest from the scale are 5 mm above the plane of focus, and their image should demonstrate the effect of the blurring of objects out of the plane of focus.

Using the technique in Part II, measure the thickness of cut. Observe the quality of the image of the bone lesion. Record your observations and values on the data sheet.

RESULTS

Complete the data sheet that follows.

EXERCISES

1. Briefly discuss the clinical application of each motion you studied and the reason it was selected for that examination.

DATA SHEET FOR EXPERIMENT 23: TOMOGRAPHY
PART I PINHOLE TRACING

TABLE E23-1

Type of motion	Integrity of motion	Mechanical stability	Completeness of exposure	Intensity uniformity
Linear				
Circular				
Elliptical				
Trispiral				
Hypocycloidal				

PART II THICKNESS OF CUT
Tomographic angle: _____

TABLE E23-2

Type of motion	Indicated section thickness	Measured section thickness	% Error	Quality of image of bone lesion
Linear				
Circular				
Elliptical				

PART III EFFECT OF TOMOGRAPHIC ANGLE
Type of motion: _____

TABLE E23-3

Tomographic angle	Angle thickness	Width of blur	Quality of image of bone lesion
10 degrees			
20 degrees			
30 degrees			

Radiographic Quality Control Survey

Name _____

Date _____

OBJECT

To evaluate the performance of a radiographic imaging system in terms of image quality and radiation safety.

DISCUSSION

In the United States, two organizations are directly concerned with the safe design and operation of medical x-ray apparatus: the National Council on Radiation Protection and Measurement (NCRP) and the Center for Devices and Radiological Health (CDRH), an arm of the U.S. Food and Drug Administration (FDA). The NCRP is an advisory group that has no authority to enforce compliance with its recommendations. The CDRH has the authority to set standards and enforce them. In addition to the CDRH, most state government radiation control departments subscribe to NCRP recommendations.

The tests included in this experiment are adopted from CDRH and NCRP documents and are designed as relatively simple evaluations that the radiologic technologist can perform to maintain good image quality and to control the radiation exposure of patients and radiologic personnel.

MATERIALS REQUIRED

- Radiographic imaging system with variable-aperture light-localizing collimator
- Tape measure
- Paper clips
- Exposure timer
- Portable ionization chamber survey meter
- Aluminum filters
- Aluminum step-wedge penetrometer
- 400-speed cassette

PROCEDURE

The format of this experiment is slightly different from that of previous experiments. A statement will be made regarding proper operation of a specific component of the radiographic imaging system; it will be followed by instructions on how to determine whether the given operation is consistent with acceptable radiation control characteristics.

1. **Coincidence of the x-ray beam and light field**
   The error of coincidence must not exceed 2% of the source-to-image receptor distance (SID) on any side of the field.

   Place a cassette at 100-cm SID, outline the light field with paper clips, and make an exposure. Measure the deviation in both directions, and determine whether the degree of coincidence is acceptable.

2. **Accuracy of the distance indicator**
   The SID indicator should be correct to within 2% of the indicated distance.

   Locate the position of the target of the x-ray tube. It is marked on many tube housings. If it is not, the target position may be estimated by the procedure demonstrated in Experiment 1: Inverse Square Law.

   With a tape measure, determine the actual distance from the target to the image receptor when the indicator shows 100 cm. Repeat this measurement at maximum and minimum travel of the tube.

3. **Exposure switch location**
   The exposure switch should be so located that it cannot be conveniently operated outside a shielded area.

   Examine the exposure switch to see whether the cord is too long or the console-mounted button is in such a position that it allows the radiologic technologist to make an exposure while part of her or his body is outside the shielded area. If the cord is too long, it should be shortened or permanently affixed to the console. If the console is too close to the edge of the protective barrier, warning tape should be placed on the floor.

4. Exposure timer accuracy

Exposure timers should be accurate to within 10% of the time indicated when the exposure set is 100 ms or longer. At shorter exposure times, a 20% variance is allowed.

The timer on any radiographic imaging system can be checked with a number of commercially available direct-reading instruments. Place the instrument at any convenient SID and expose it to a range of exposure times. Compare the measured exposure time with the set exposure time.

5. Indication of "beam-on"

The control panel should include a device (usually a light or milliammeter) that gives a positive indication of the production of x-rays whenever the x-ray tube is energized.

Check for a positive indication of beam-on by deflection of the needle of the mA meter during an exposure. Most imaging systems provide a separate lamp and an audible signal as well.

6. Exposure linearity

The radiation exposure obtained when operated at adjacent mA stations at constant exposure time should not vary more than 10% when expressed as mR/mAs.

If a direct-reading ionization chamber is used, the results are directly obtainable; exposure time should remain constant while mA is increased. Try 80 kVp at 100 mA as follows:

100 mA = 10 mAs
200 mA = 20 mAs
400 mA = 40 mAs
800 mA = 60 mAs

7. Reproducibility

The radiation intensity obtained during sequential exposures at a fixed technique should exhibit a coefficient of variation (C) of not more than 0.05, where the following is true:

$$c = \frac{\sqrt{\Sigma(X_i \ X)2}}{n-1}{X} \le 0.05$$

This requirement essentially states that variation in radiation intensity at a constant technique shall not exceed 5%. To test this, 10 successive exposures

are made, and the radiation intensity for each is recorded. From these measurements, the coefficient of variation is calculated.

8. X-ray quality

The following total filtration is required:

TABLE E24-1		
Operating kVp	Minimum total filtration (inherent plus added)	Minimum acceptable HVL
Below 50 kVp	0.5 mm Al	0.6 mm Al at 50 kVp
50 to 70 kVp	1.5 mm Al	1.3 mm Al at 60 kVp
Above 70 kVp	2.5 mm Al	2.2 mm Al at 70 kVp

If the added filtration is not directly measurable, determine the half-value layer at 70 kVp as demonstrated in Experiment 10: Half-Value Layer. If the unit is ever operated above 70 kVp, 2.5 mm Al or an HVL of 2.2 mm Al must exist.

RESULTS

1. Coincidence of the x-ray beam and light field

SID _____

2% SID _____

Misalignment Width: _____ + _____ = _____

≤ 2% SID?   Yes   No

Length: _____ + _____ = _____

≤ 2% SID?   Yes   No

Is this acceptable?   Yes   No

2. Accuracy of the distance indicator

Selected SID = _____

2% selected SID = _____

Measured SID = _____

Difference = _____

≤ 2% selected SID?   Yes   No

3. Exposure switch location

Is the exposure switch adequately located?

Yes   No

4. Exposure switch location

TABLE E24-2

Set time, ms	Measured time, ms	Acceptable?
10		
50		
100		
500		

5. Indication of "beam-on"
Visible: Yes No
Audible: Yes No

6. Exposure linearity
70 kVp

TABLE E24-3

No.	mA	Time, ms	mAs	Exposure, mR 1st	2nd	3rd	Average exposure, mR	mR/mAs
1								
2								
3								

Is $(mR/mAs_1 - mR/mAs_1) < 0.1 (mR/mAs_1 + mR/mAs_2)$?

Yes   No

_____ − _____ < 0.1 (_____ + _____)

Is $(mR/mAs_2 - mR/mAs_3) < 0.1 (mR/mAs_2 + mR/mAs_3)$?

Yes   No

_____ − _____ < 0.1 (_____ + _____)

Is this acceptable?

Yes   No

7. Reproducibility

TABLE E24-4

Exposure number, n	X_i, mR	$X_i - X$	$(X_i - X)^2$
1			
2			
3			
4			
5			
6			
7			
8			
9			
10			

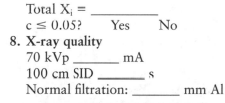

Total X_i = _____
$c \leq 0.05$?   Yes   No

8. X-ray quality
70 kVp _____ mA
100 cm SID _____ s
Normal filtration: _____ mm Al

TABLE E24-5

Added filtration, mm Al	Exposure, mR 1st	2nd	3rd	Average exposure	mR/mAs
0					
0.5					
1.0					
2.0					
3.0					
4.0					
5.0					

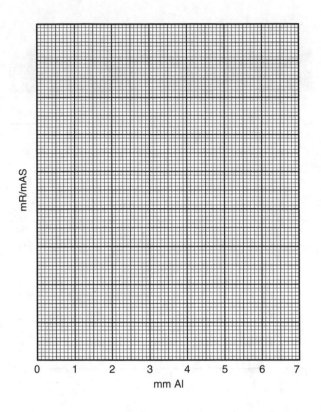

Plot the resultant mR/mAs as a function of mm Al on the graph above, and estimate the half- value layer.

HVL = _____ mm Al

HVL ≥ 2.2 mm Al?   Yes   No

EXERCISES

1. A 23 cm × 40 cm (10 in × 16 in) light field is set at an SID of 100 cm (40 in). The x-ray beam has exactly the same dimensions, but it misses superimposition by 1 cm on all sides. Is this acceptable? What is the limit of acceptability in this instance?

2. The SID indicator shows 91 cm, but actual measurement shows 89 cm. Is this acceptable? What is the range of acceptability for this situation?

3. A mobile unit (single-phase, half-wave rectified) is operated with the exposure timer at $\frac{1}{30}$ second. How many dashes from the image of the spinning top would be expected?

4. The following exposure data are obtained from a conventional radiographic unit operated at 70 kVp:
   50 mA, 500 ms, 210 mR
   100 mA, 500 ms, 390 mR
   200 mA, 500 ms, 704 mR
   Are these acceptable?

Fluoroscopic Quality Control Survey

Name _____

Date _____

OBJECT

To evaluate the performance of a fluoroscope in terms of image quality and radiation safety.

DISCUSSION

Similar to the previous experiment, this experiment consists of a series of measurements and observations, each designed to test compliance with a specific radiation control recommendation of the NCRP or the CDRH. The procedure section contains statements of requirements followed by directions for measuring compliance with those requirements.

MATERIALS REQUIRED

- Fluoroscopic imaging system
- Aluminum block patient phantom
- Lead attenuation block
- Ionization chamber
- Portable ionization chamber survey meter
- Tape measure
- Aluminum filters

PROCEDURE

Caution must be exercised during this experiment to ensure that the image intensifier is not damaged because of exposure to an unattenuated primary beam. Always position the aluminum block phantom, the lead attenuator, or both in the useful beam during exposure.

1. **Protective curtain and Bucky slot cover**
   Shielding devices of at least 0.25 mm Pb equivalent must be available to intercept scatter radiation that would otherwise reach the radiologic technologist and the radiologist standing to the side of the table.

This is a visual inspection. See that a protective curtain of adequate design is affixed to the intensifier tower and that it drapes all the way to the tabletop, regardless of SID. When the Bucky is moved to the end of the table, a cover for the space between the tabletop and the side panel (the Bucky slot cover) should automatically move into place.

2. **Exposure switch and timer**
   A dead-man type of switch is required for energizing the fluoroscopic x-ray tube. A 5-minute preset timer also is required, and an audible alarm should sound at the end of 5 minutes. This sound should continue until the timer has been reset.

   Check all exposure switches to be sure that continuous pressure by the operator is required during the entire exposure. Set approximately 15 s on the timer, and observe whether the audible alarm functions properly when the time expires.

3. **X-ray tube target position**
   The source-to-tabletop distance should be at least 38 cm.

   Place a flat, regularly shaped metal object on the tabletop and take a spot film of it. Measure the tabletop-to-image receptor distance, and calculate the distance of the x-ray tube target to the tabletop as follows:

   $$SOD = (SID)\ O/I$$

   where *SOD* is the source-to-tabletop distance, *SID* is the source-to-image receptor distance, *O* is object size, and *I* is image size.

4. **Beam quality**
   Total filtration, including the tabletop, should be at least 2.5 mm Al equivalent.

   Position the ionization chamber approximately 20 cm above the tabletop, and sequentially insert graduated thicknesses of aluminum filtration between the ionization chamber and the tabletop. When the fluoroscope is operated at 80 kVp, if the estimated half-value layer (HVL) is 2.4 mm Al or greater, total filtration is sufficient.

If it is possible to operate only in the automatic exposure mode, the total thickness of aluminum filtration must remain constant. Begin with the total thickness of aluminum filtration positioned in the x-ray beam above the ionization chamber. Each aluminum filter positioned between the ionization chamber and the tabletop should come from the stack above.

5. Beam quantity

When operated at 80 kVp, the tabletop exposure rate should not exceed 3.2 R/mAmin, and under no conditions of operation should the output intensity exceed 10 R/min.

Adjust the fluoroscopic tube potential and, with the ionization chamber on the tabletop, record the tube mA and output intensity in R/m. It is helpful if the mA is first adjusted to an integer value (1, 2, or 3). Next, adjust the kVp and mA to their maximum values and record the R/m.

6. Primary protective barrier

The entire cross section of the useful beam should be intercepted by a primary protective barrier at all SIDs.

When the image-intensifier tower is in the parked position, it should not be possible to energize the undertable x-ray tube. On equipment that fails this test, a simple microswitch interlocked with the x-ray exposure switch will satisfy the requirement.

With the tower at maximum SID and in a position to intercept the wide-open beam, the exposure rate above the tower must not exceed 2 mR/hr for every R/m at the tabletop. This is measured with the portable survey meter.

7. Primary beam limitation

When the adjustable collimators are fully open, the primary beam should be restricted to the diameter of the input phosphor.

Open the collimators wide and elevate the tower so that the input phosphor is 38 cm from the tabletop.

With the x-ray tube energized, an unexposed border should be visible on four sides of the image field. As the elevation of the tower is changed, the collimators should automatically compensate to continue the unexposed borders on the viewing system.

RESULTS

1. Protective curtain and Bucky slot cover
Is an adequate protective tower curtain present?
        Yes   No
Is there a tightly fitting Bucky slot cover?
        Yes   No

2. Exposure switch and timer
Is a dead-man type of exposure switch in use?
        Yes   No
Is there a properly functioning 5-minute reset timer?
        Yes   No
Is the signal audible?
        Yes   No
Is the signal visual?
        Yes   No
Does the timer terminate the exposure?
        Yes   No
For how long? _____

3. X-ray tube target position
Object size (O): _____
Image size (I): _____
Tabletop-to-image receptor distance (TTID): _____

$$STTD = \frac{TTID\ O/I}{1\ O/I}$$

Source-to-tabletop distance (STTD): _____
<38 cm?   Yes   No

4. Beam quality
80 kVp
Normal filtration: _____ mA

TABLE E25-1	
Added filtration, mm A1	**Exposure rate, R/min**
0	
0.5	
1.0	
2.0	
3.0	
4.0	
5.0	

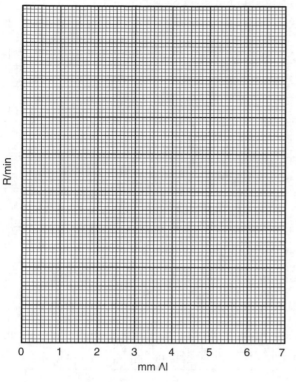

Plot the resultant R/min as a function of mm Al on the above graph, and estimate the half-value layer.

HVL = _____ mm Al

HVL ≥ 2.4 mm Al?   Yes   No

5. Beam quantity

Tube current: _____ mA

Tabletop exposure rate: _____ R/min

Output intensity: _____ R/mAmin × 3.2 R/mA

Maximum output intensity: _____ R/m

Obtained at _____ kVp and _____ mA < 10 R/min?

          Yes   No

TABLE E25-2							
Added filtration, mm Al	0	0.5	1	2	3	4	5
aR/min	5.3	4.5	3.9	3.1	2.5	1.9	1.5

6. Primary protective barrier

Is the intensifier tower assembly properly connected and interlocked with the x-ray tube?

          Yes   No

Table output intensity: _____ R/min

Exposure rate above and around the intensifier tower: _____ mR/hr

_____ (mR/r)/_____ (R/min) = _____

mR/hr ≤ 2 mR/hr ?   Yes   No
R/min R/min

7. Primary beam limitation

Do the primary beam collimators function properly?

          Yes   No

EXERCISES

1. Calculate the quantity of R/mAmin for each of the following conditions of operation:
   a. 70 kVp, 1.5 mA, 3.2 R for 2 min
   b. 95 kVp, 4.2 mA, 4.1 R for 30 s
   c. 115 kVp, 2.7 mA, 6.8 R for 5 min
2. A silver dollar measures 38 mm in diameter. Its image on a spot film measures 91 mm, and the object and image planes are separated by 30 cm. What is the x-ray tube target-to-tabletop distance? Is it sufficient?
3. The following beam quality data were obtained at 80 kVp and 5 mA, and the detector was positioned 20 cm above the tabletop. The x-ray target-to-tabletop distance was 40 cm.

   Is the total filtration adequate? Is the tabletop exposure rate acceptable? Use the graph paper provided to assist in obtaining the solution.

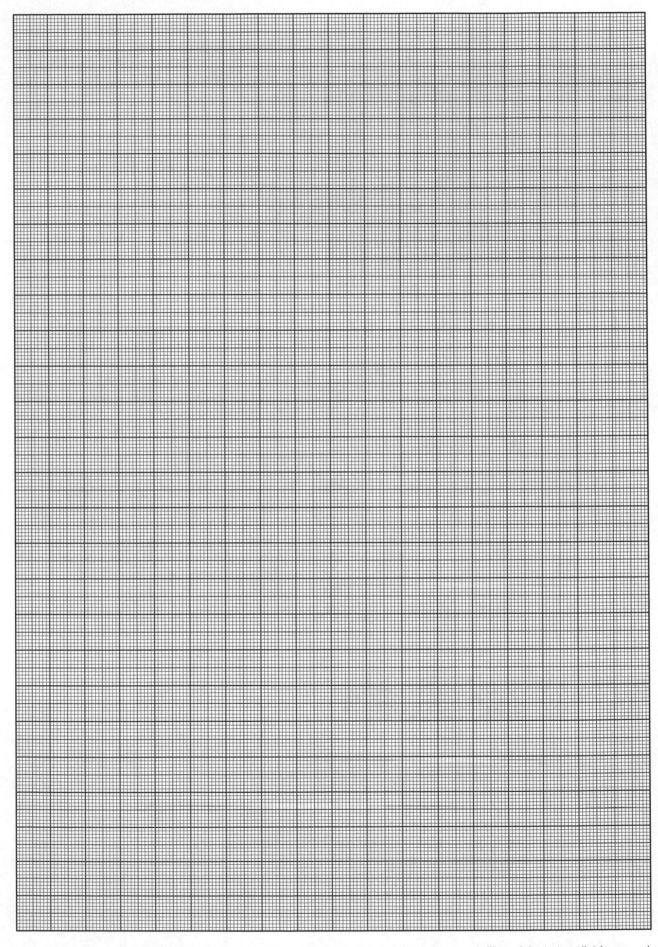

WORKSHEET
ANSWER KEY

WORKSHEET 1-1

1. e	6. d	11. d	15. b
2. b	7. a	12. b	16. c
3. c	8. c	13. d	17. b
4. b	9. e	14. b	18. b
5. b	10. e		

WORKSHEET 1-2

1. c	7. a	13. c
2. a	8. a	14. d
3. a	9. a	15. e
4. c	10. e	16. a
5. e	11. c	
6. a	12. c	

WORKSHEET 1-3

1. e	6. c	10. d	14. b
2. d	7. d	11. a	15. d
3. d	8. a	12. e	16. d
4. e	9. e	13. e	17. d
5. e			

WORKSHEET 2-1

1. 737	29. 53.5
2. 319,090	30. $^{-7}/_{24}$
3. 66,705	31. 1:4
4. 37,652	32. 6 mR
5. 21,310.802	33. 224 mAs
6. 352,080	34. 375mAs
7. 2.69094	35. 200 mAs
8. 10	36. 35 mAs
9. 1358.9	37. 7
10. 114.5913	38. b
11. ¾	39. b
12. $^{11}/_{16}$	40. 2.74192×10^3
13. ¾	41. 9.174843×10^6
14. $^{3}/_{16}$	42. 7.713×10^3
15. $^{-33}/_{20}$	43. 5.58×10^2
16. $^{57}/_{32}$	44. 8.9482×10^2
17. $^{5}/_{8}$	45. 3.7617×10^4
18. $^{2365}/_{128}$	46. 1.6×10^{-3}
19. 1½	47. 1.26×10^7
20. 2	48. 2.49×10^{-1}
21. 189.0	49. 10^{20}
22. 5.21	50. 10^9
23. 94.25	51. 10^{-16}
24. 5.58	52. 3×10^8
25. 2.35	53. 20:1
26. 9.7	54. 2.18×10^{-22} g
27. −126	55. 100,000:1
28. 15/8	

WORKSHEET 2-2

Note: Where two answers are given, the first is the rounded answer using number pairs as described in the "Math Tutor Section," and the second is the computed answer for comparison.

PART I: DECIMAL/FRACTION CONVERSIONS

1. 0.2	11. 0.15	20. ⅖
2. 0.05	12. 0.13 (0.133)	21. $^{1}/_{60}$
3. 0.13 (0.125)	13. 0.7	22. $^{1}/_{40}$
4. 0.017 (0.0167)	14. 0.6	23. $^{1}/_{7}$
5. 0.07 (0.067)	15. 0.35	24. ¾
6. 0.025	16. $^{1}/_{20}$	25. $^{1}/_{12}$
7. 0.008 (0.0083)	17. ⅓	26. $^{1}/_{15}$
8. 0.67 (0.666)	18. $^{1}/_{80}$	27. ⅘
9. 0.033	19. $^{1}/_{50}$	
10. 0.4		

PART II: DECIMAL TIMES

28. 7 mAs	42. 3 mAs	55. 80 mAs
29. 1.3 mAs	43. 24 mAs	56. 140 mAs
30. 3.3 mAs	44. 15 mAs	57. 0.8 mAs
31. 25 mAs	45. 150 mAs	58. 35 mAs
32. 0.9 mAs	46. 60 mAs	59. 20 mAs
33. 8 mAs	47. 48 mAs	60. 200 mAs
34. 14 mAs	48. 100 (99) mAs	61. 2 mAs
35. 5 mAs	49. 10 (9.9) mAs	62. 2.5 mAs
36. 7 mAs	50. 4.5 mAs	63. 300 mAs
37. 70 mAs	51. 0.6 mAs	64. 12 mAs
38. 24 mAs	52. 32 mAs	65. 90 mAs
39. 40 mAs	53. 12 mAs	66. 1.8 mAs
40. 120 mAs	54. 14 mAs	67. 75 mAs
41. 1 mAs		

PART III: FRACTIONAL TIMES

68. 13 (12.5) mAs	88. 7 (6.7) mAs
69. 0.8 (0.83) mAs	89. 42 (41.5) mAs
70. 7 (6.7) mAs	90. 33 (33.3) mAs
71. 2.5 mAs	91. 25 mAs
72. 17 (16.7) mAs	92. 15 mAs
73. 2.5 mAs	93. 20 mAs
74. 0.4 mAs	94. 5 mAs
75. 0.6 mAs	95. 24 mAs
76. 2.5 mAs	96. 120 mAs
77. 17 (16.7) mAs	97. 13 (13.3) mAs
78. 13 (13.3 mAs)	98. 35 mAs
79. 5 mAs	99. 160 mAs
80. 7 (6.7) mAs	100. 60 mAs
81. 33 (33.4 mAs)	101. 240 mAs
82. 60 mAs	102. 40 mAs
83. 5 mAs	103. 90 mAs
84. 20 mAs	104. 240 mAs
85. 2.5 mAs	105. 60 mAs
86. 20 mAs	106. 75 mAs
87. 5 mAs	107. 90 mAs

WORKSHEET 2-3

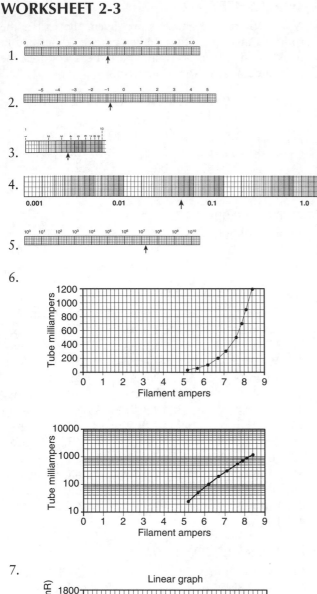

1.

2.

3.

4.

5.

6.

7.

8.

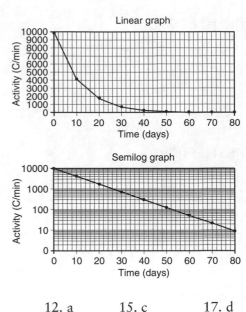

9. b	12. a	15. c	17. d
10. b	13. b	16. d	18. b
11. b	14. a		

WORKSHEET 2-4

1. c	10. a	18. a
2. d	11. c	19. d
3. d	12. c	20. 0.000001L, 10^{-6}L
4. c	13. e	21. 0.1 m, 10^{-1}m
5. d	14. b	22. 10kg, 10^1 kg
6. e	15. d	23. 1.2 A, $1.2 \times 10°$A
7. c	16. c	24. 0.007R, 7×10^{-3}R
8. a	17. d	25. 10
9. e		

WORKSHEET 2-5

1. b 2. e 3. e 4. d 5. d 6. c 7. e 8. b 9. e 10. c
11. c 12. e 13. d 14. a 15. e 16. a or c

WORKSHEET 2-6

1. d 2. d 3. c 4. c 5. b 6. d 7. a 8. d 9. e 10. b
11. e 12. a 13. a 14. e 15. e 16. c 17. d 18. b
19. a

WORKSHEET 2-7

1. a	5. d	9. c	13. d or e	17. c
2. a	6. a	10. a	14. e	18. c
3. c	7. e	11. a	15. c	19. d
4. a	8. d	12. c	16. c	

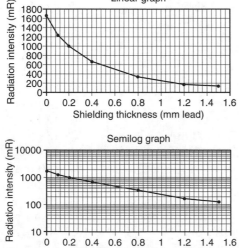

WORKSHEET 2-8

1. c, f	8. d	16. d
2. a, b, e,	9. d	15. e
3. a, c	10. d	17. b
4. a, c	11. c	18. a
5. a, b	12. d	19. c
6. c	13. d	20. e
7. a	14. d	21. d

WORKSHEET 3-1

1. a	6. e	11. e	16. d
2. e	7. c	12. b	17. a
3. c	8. b	13. d	18. b
4. b	9. d	14. d	19. b
5. b	10. a	15. b	20. b

WORKSHEET 3-2

1. b	5. b	9. c	13. c	16. d
2. b	6. c & d	10. a	14. c	17. e
3. d	7. e	11. b	15. b	18. b
4. d	8. b	12. b		

WORKSHEET 3-3

1. g	7. d	13. d	18. e	23. c
2. h	8. h	14. c	19. e	24. a
3. a	9. j	15. d	20. d	25. e
4. i	10. e	16. e	21. a	26. c
5. c	11. b	17. d	22. a	27. a
6. f	12. d			

WORKSHEET 3-4

1. d	5. b	9. e	13. c
2. d	6. e	10. d	14. c
3. b	7. e	11. b	15. d
4. c	8. a	12. a	

WORKSHEET 3-5

1. e	5. b	9. e	13. a	16. a
2. b	6. d	10. e	14. a	17. d
3. b	7. e	11. a	15. a	18. d
4. d	8. a	12. a		

WORKSHEET 4-1

1. c	5. b	9. e	13. e	17. e
2. e	6. b	10. d	14. e	18. d
3. d	7. b	11. b	15. b	19. a
4. d	8. c	12. e	16. d	20. b

WORKSHEET 4-2

1. e	5. c	9. a	13. a	16. e
2. d	6. d	10. c	14. d	17. c
3. c	7. a	11. d	15. b	18. e
4. b	8. b	12. e		

WORKSHEET 4-3

1. a	6. c	11. b	15. a	19. e
2. e	7. c	12. c	16. b	
3. d	8. c	13. b	17. b	
4. c	9. e	14. b	18. d	
5. d	10. e			

WORKSHEET 4-4

1. b	5. c	9. d	12. e	15. a
2. c	6. e	10. b	13. c	16. d
3. c	7. d	11. e	14. e	17. e
4. c	8. c			

WORKSHEET 4-5

1. d	6. d	11. c	16. e
2. e	7. e	12. e	17. d
3. e	8. c	13. e	18. a
4. c	9. c	14. d	19. b
5. a	10. e	15. d	

WORKSHEET 4-6

1. c	4. b	7. d	10. a	13. b	16. e
2. c	5. d	8. c	11. b	14. b	17. a
3. a	6. e	9. c	12. d	15. e	18. d

WORKSHEET 5-1

1. d	5. e	9. e	13. e	17. b
2. e	6. c	10. c	14. b	18. a & d
3. e	7. a	11. d	15. d	19. e
4. a	8. b	12. d	16. e	20. d

WORKSHEET 5-2

1. e	6. e	11. d	16. c	21. a
2. d	7. e	12. a	17. d	22. e
3. d	8. e	13. a	18. b	23. d
4. c	9. b	14. d	19. e	24. c
5. a	10. d	15. b	20. a	25. b

WORKSHEET 5-3

1. c	5. d	9. a	13. e
2. b	6. a	10. c	14. b
3. c	7. c	11. e	15. c
4. d	8. a	12. d	16. a

WORKSHEET 5-4

1. d	6. c	11. d	16. a	20. c
2. b	7. d	12. b	17. d	21. a
3. a	8. a	13. c	18. d	
4. d	9. e	14. c	19. c	
5. b	10. c	15. d		

WORKSHEET 5-5

1. d	5. a	9. e	13. a	17. b
2. c	6. a	10. c	14. c	18. b
3. c	7. c	11. d	15. e	19. b
4. d	8. b	12. c	16. b	20. d

WORKSHEET 5-6

1. b	5. e	9. d	13. d	17. a
2. a	6. a	10. c	14. b	
3. b	7. a	11. b	15. e & b	
4. b	8. a	12. b	16. c	

WORKSHEET 5-7

1. e	5. d	9. d	13. e	17. a
2. a	6. d	10. e	14. e	18. a
3. c	7. b	11. a	15. c	19. b
4. c	8. c	12. c	16. e	

WORKSHEET 5-8

1. c	6. a	10. b	14. d	18. a
2. b	7. c	11. c	15. e	19. c
3. c	8. e	12. c	16. c	20. b
4. a	9. b	13. a	17. e	21. e
5. b				

WORKSHEET 6-1

1. e	5. b	9. a	13. d	16. c
2. e	6. d	10. b	14. a	17. e
3. c	7. b	11. c	15. a	18. c
4. c	8. a	12. b		

WORKSHEET 6-2

1. d	5. b	9. c	13. e	17. c
2. b	6. c	10. a	14. c	18. d
3. e	7. d	11. d	15. b	19. d
4. b	8. a	12. d	16. d	20. a

WORKSHEET 6-3

1. c	4. c	7. b	10. a	13. d
2. c	5. b	8. b	11. e	14. e
3. b	6. d	9. e	12. e	15. d

WORKSHEET 6-4

1. a	5. a	9. a	13. b	16. a
2. a	6. d	10. c	14. e	17. c
3. a	7. e	11. d	15. e	18. b
4. d	8. d	12. a		

ACROSS

1. Diodes

2. Ionize

3. Size

4. Square

5. Time

6. Half-value

7. Timing

8. Step

9. Quantity

10. Autotransformer

11. Reverse

12. Falling

13. Supply

14. Therm

DOWN

1. Sinus

2. Single

3. Image

4. Half

5. Electromagnetic

6. Quality

7. Inverter

8. Low

9. Negatively

10. Temperature

11. Current

12. Turn

13. Filament

14. Ripple

15. Serial

WORKSHEET 7-1

1. c	6. d	11. a	16. c
2. e	7. d	12. c	17. e
3. d	8. d	13. c	18. 200 mA
4. b	9. b	14. e	19. 4.6 A
5. b	10. c	15. a	

WORKSHEET 7-2

1. a	6. b	10. c	14. a	18. a
2. e	7. d	11. d	15. a	19. b
3. d	8. a	12. a	16. b	20. d
4. d	9. a	13. c	17. e	21. a
5. d				

WORKSHEET 7-3

1. a	13. a	25. 1.5 minutes
2. a	14. a	26. c
3. b	15. b	27. a
4. b	16. a	28. e
5. b	17. a	29. a
6. b	18. b	30. d
7. a	19. b	31. d
8. b	20. a	32. a
9. b	21. 7500 HU	33. d
10. b	22. 300,000 HU	34. e
11. b	23. 8 minutes	35. a
12. a	24. 6.5 minutes	

WORKSHEET 8-1

1. d	5. e	9. a	13. b
2. c	6. d	10. a & d	14. c
3. e	7. c	11. e	15. d
4. b	8. c	12. b & c	

WORKSHEET 8-2

1. c	5. b	9. e	13. c	17. a
2. e	6. d	10. e	14. e	
3. a	7. d	11. d	15. e	
4. b	8. a	12. a	16. c	

WORKSHEET 8-3

1. d	5. a	9. c	13. a
2. a	6. e	10. c	14. b
3. e	7. d	11. c	15. e
4. d	8. b	12. c	16. c

WORKSHEET 8-4

1. e	5. a & e	9. a	13. e
2. e	6. b	10. e	14. e
3. b	7. a	11. b	
4. c	8. d	12. c	

WORKSHEET 8-5

1. d	4. d	7. c	10. c
2. b	5. c	8. b	11. b
3. d	6. b	9. e	

WORKSHEET 9-1

1. d	5. e	9. c	13. a
2. c	6. e	10. d	14. a
3. a	7. e	11. c	15. c
4. a	8. b	12. d	

WORKSHEET 9-2

1. b	8. d	15. e	22. c	28. b
2. c	9. c	16. c	23. d	29. e
3. b	10. c	17. d	24. a	30. c
4. b	11. c	18. a	25. c	31. a
5. d	12. a	19. b	26. e	32. c
6. c	13. d	20. b	27. a	33. e
7. e	14. b	21. e		

WORKSHEET 9-3

1. c	6. b	11. d	16. d
2. c	7. d	12. b	17. a
3. c	8. c	13. a	18. d
4. d	9. a	14. e	19. b
5. c	10. a	15. c	

WORKSHEET 10-1

1. a	5. a	9. c	12. b	15. e
2. a	6. d	10. c	13. b	16. a
3. c	7. e	11. a	14. a	17. b
4. b	8. d			

WORKSHEET 10-2

1. c	5. c	9. d	13. e
2. a	6. a	10. c	14. b
3. a	7. a	11. a	15. a
4. d	8. a	12. b	16. e

WORKSHEET 10-3

1. a	8. e	14. c	20. c	26. b
2. e	9. a	15. c	21. e	27. e
3. c	10. c	16. d	22. d	28. e
4. b	11. e	17. b	23. e	29. d
5. b	12. e	18. b	24. c	30. d & e
6. c	13. b	19. b	25. a	31. b
7. c & d				

WORKSHEET 11-1

1. d	5. a & b	9. a	13. e	17. e
2. e	6. d	10. a	14. e	18. d
3. b	7. a	11. b	15. a	19. d
4. d	8. a	12. a	16. d	

WORKSHEET 11-2

1. e	5. e	9. d	13. c	17. d
2. e	6. a	10. a	14. d	18. e
3. b	7. e	11. d	15. e	19. b
4. b	8. a & c	12. c	16. d	

WORKSHEET 11-3

1. d	6. b	10. e	14. b	18. b
2. d	7. a	11. e	15. b	19. d
3. e	8. c	12. d	16. b	20. a
4. e	9. a	13. b	17. a	21. c
5. b				

WORKSHEET 12-1

1. a	6. b	10. e	14. a	18. a
2. c	7. b	11. d	15. a	19. e
3. a	8. b	12. e	16. e	20. c
4. d	9. c	13. e	17. c	21. b
5. d				

WORKSHEET 12-2

1. e	5. a	9. c	13. a	16. e
2. a	6. a	10. a	14. e	17. b
3. e	7. a	11. c	15. c	18. e
4. d	8. a	12. d		

WORKSHEET 12-3

1. e	5. b	9. a	13. c	17. c
2. b	6. a	10. c	14. b	18. c
3. c	7. b	11. c	15. c	19. b
4. a	8. b	12. c	16. c	20. a

WORKSHEET 13-1

1. e	6. c	10. d	14. c
2. d	7. b	11. e	15. e
3. e	8. d	12. e	16. e
4. c	9. a	13. e	17. d
5. b			

WORKSHEET 13-2

1. a	5. d	9. c	13. c	17. e	21. c
2. b	6. a	10. d	14. e	18. d	22. c
3. c	7. e	11. c	15. e	19. b	23. a
4. d	8. e	12. b	16. b	20. e	

ACROSS	DOWN
1. kVp	1. K-shell
2. Quantum mottle	2. Intensifying
3. Outer	3. Bent
4. Ground state	4. Yttrium tantalate
5. Felt	5. mA
6. Interact	6. Greater
7. High atomic	7. Thermal
8. Light	8. Absorption
9. Single	9. To light
10. Tungstate	10. Increased
11. Decreases	11. Spatial
12. Line	
13. Heat	
14. Spec	

WORKSHEET 14-1

1. c	5. d	9. e	13. e	16. b
2. b	6. b	10. b	14. b	17. c
3. a	7. d	11. e	15. d	
4. b	8. a	12. d		

WORKSHEET 14-2

1. d	5. d	9. c	13. c	16. b
2. c	6. b	10. b	14. a	17. c
3. e	7. e	11. d	15. e	
4. e	8. b & e	12. c		

WORKSHEET 14-3

1. b	5. a	9. b	12. d	15. d
2. b	6. b	10. c & d	13. b	16. c
3. d	7. d	11. e	14. e	17. b
4. c	8. d			

WORKSHEET 14-4

1. d	5. b	9. d	12. d	15. e
2. c	6. c	10. a	13. d	16. e
3. a	7. d	11. b & d	14. a	17. a
4. d	8. b			

WORKSHEET 14-5

1. a	4. e	7. e	10. a	12. b
2. b	5. c	8. a	11. e	13. c & d
3. e	6. b	9. e		

WORKSHEET 15-1

1. d	4. b	7. b	10. a
2. e	5. a	8. a	11. b
3. b	6. c	9. c	12. a

WORKSHEET 15-2

1. c	5. d	9. a	13. a	17. b
2. e	6. e	10. d	14. b	18. d
3. b	7. a	11. e	15. d	19. e
4. d	8. b	12. b	16. d	

WORKSHEET 15-3

1. a	4. d	7. a	10. d
2. d	5. d	8. b	11. d
3. d	6. e	9. a	12. d

WORKSHEET 15-4

1. b	5. e	9. b	13. a
2. c	6. d	10. e	14. c
3. b	7. b	11. a	15. d
4. c	8. a	12. a or c	16. c

WORKSHEET 15-5

1. c	6. b	11. c	16. b
2. d	7. b	12. a	17. a
3. d	8. d	13. e	18. e
4. b	9. e	14. b	19. b
5. c	10. a	15. e	20. e

WORKSHEET 16-1

1. d	5. c	9. d	13. e	17. a
2. d	6. b	10. b	14. c	
3. d	7. c	11. e	15. d	
4. b	8. c	12. b	16. b	

WORKSHEET 16-2

1. c	6. c	11. b	15. c
2. a	7. d	12. b	16. a
3. a	8. b	13. a	17. a
4. a	9. a	14. e	18. b
5. c	10. b & e		

WORKSHEET 16-3

1. a	5. c	9. b	12. e	15. b
2. b	6. b	10. b	13. c	16. b
3. e	7. e	11. e	14. e	17. c
4. e	8. d			

WORKSHEET 16-4

1. a	5. c	9. a	13. e	17. c
2. e	6. e	10. e	14. c	18. d
3. b	7. b	11. d	15. e	19. e
4. d	8. a & c	12. e	16. e	

WORKSHEET 16-5

1. d	5. b	9. b	13. d	17. c
2. e	6. b & d	10. b	14. b	18. a
3. a	7. c	11. b	15. e	19. d
4. a	8. a	12. c	16. e	

WORKSHEET 16-6

1. a	4. b	7. a	10. d	13. b	16. c
2. d	5. b	8. d	11. b	14. e	17. a
3. c	6. c	9. a	12. b	15. c	18. b

WORKSHEET 16-7

1. b	5. c	8. e	11. e	14. d
2. a	6. b	9. e	12. b	15. e
3. e	7. b	10. d	13. d	16. e
4. e				

WORKSHEET 16-8

1. d	5. a	9. a, b	12. e	15. e
2. a, b	6. d	10. c, d, e	13. e	16. a
3. b	7. d	11. e	14. a	17. e
4. e	8. b			

WORKSHEET 17-1

1. d	4. c	7. e	10. a	13. e
2. d	5. d	8. a	11. b	14. e
3. d	6. a	9. c	12. d	15. c

ACROSS	DOWN
1. Chemical	1. Warped
2. Geometric	2. Optical density
3. Pi lines	3. Smoothness
4. Radiation	4. Wet pressure
5. Curtain	5. Dichroic
6. Double exposures	6. Static
7. Cutoff	
8. Fingernail	
9. Unsharp	
10. Sludge	

WORKSHEET 18-1

1. b	5. c	9. d	13. a	16. d	19. c
2. a	6. e	10. c	14. b	17. d	
3. d	7. b	11. d	15. e	18. b	
4. a	8. c	12. b			

ACROSS	DOWN
1. Stereoradiography	1. Position
2. Blurring	2. Vascular
3. Superimposition	3. Grids
4. Thinner	4. Fixed
5. Hypocycloidal	5. Virtual
6. Small	6. Stereoscopy
7. Linear	7. Uniform
8. Nephrotomography	8. Tomography
9. Dominant	

WORKSHEET 19-1

1. c	5. e	9. e	12. b	15. b
2. e	6. e	10. b	13. e	16. d
3. c	7. b	11. e	14. d	17. b
4. c	8. c			

WORKSHEET 19-2

1. c	4. a	7. a	10. e
2. d	5. e	8. d	11. a
3. c	6. c	9. d	12. c

WORKSHEET 20-1

1. a	9. b	17. e	24. a	31. c
2. d	10. d	18. a	25. d	32. c
3. c	11. d	19. b	26. a	33. b
4. c	12. e	20. b	27. a	34. b
5. e	13. c	21. d	28. d	35. b
6. b	14. b	22. a	29. c	36. a
7. d	15. d	23. d	30. c	37. b
8. a	16. c			

WORKSHEET 21-1

1. a	5. d	9. a	13. d	17. e
2. d	6. b & d	10. a	14. c	18. e
3. b	7. e	11. d	15. d	19. d
4. b	8. a	12. c	16. a	

WORKSHEET 21-2

1. b	5. c	9. b	13. e	17. c
2. a	6. e	10. a	14. a	18. e
3. a	7. b	11. c	15. d	19. c
4. d	8. a	12. b	16. c	

WORKSHEET 21-3

1. d	5. d	9. a	13. e	17. d
2. d	6. d	10. b	14. a	18. b
3. d	7. a	11. d	15. a	19. c
4. b	8. c	12. d	16. e	20. e

ACROSS
1. Plumbicon
2. Phototopic
3. Chamberlain
4. Thermionic
5. Scotopic
6. Edison
7. Contrast
8. Active

DOWN
1. Bandpass
2. Visual
3. Photocathode
4. Brightness
5. Vignetting
6. Minification
7. Cesium

WORKSHEET 22-1

1. b	8. d	15. d	21. d	27. d
2. d	9. c	16. d	22. e	28. a
3. e	10. b	17. d	23. b	29. b
4. c	11. c	18. d	24. c	30. a
5. c	12. c	19. b	25. b	31. c
6. e	13. e	20. b	26. c	32. e
7. c	14. e			

WORKSHEET 23-1

1. a	5. b	9. a	13. b	17. d
2. a	6. d	10. c	14. d	18. d
3. a	7. a	11. a	15. b	19. c
4. e	8. b	12. e	16. c	20. e

WORKSHEET 23-2

1. d	5. c	9. d	13. e	16. c
2. c	6. b	10. b	14. c	17. a
3. c	7. c	11. b	15. c	18. c
4. d	8. c	12. d		

WORKSHEET 23-3

1. b	7. b	13. c	18. d	23. b	28. a
2. b	8. a	14. a	19. d	24. d	
3. b	9. c	15. e	20. b	25. a	
4. d	10. d	16. d	21. a	26. e	
5. a	11. e	17. e	22. e	27. e	
6. e	12. b				

WORKSHEET 24-1

1. c	5. b	9. b	13. d	17. c
2. a	6. c	10. e	14. e	18. c
3. e	7. d	11. e	15. a	19. b
4. e	8. e	12. c	16. c	

WORKSHEET 24-2

1. c	6. c	11. c	15. d	19. a
2. b	7. e	12. d	16. b	20. e
3. e	8. c	13. b	17. b	21. c
4. b	9. e	14. c	18. b	22. e
5. b	10. e			

ACROSS
1. Scram
2. Hollerith
3. Integrated circuit
4. Atansoff
5. VDT
6. Chip
7. Software
8. Pascal
9. Batch
10. Mauchly
11. Central processing
12. Electronic

DOWN
1. Shockley
2. Random access
3. Microprocessor
4. Control unit
5. Input
6. Semiconductor
7. Output
8. Optical disc
9. Babbage
10. Hardware
11. Hard disk

WORKSHEET 25-1

1. a 2. d 3. a 4. e 5. e 6. b 7. a 8. b 9. a 10. c
11. d 12. b 13. c 14. b 15. c

WORKSHEET 25-2

1. b 2. b 3. c 4. b 5. c 6. a 7. a 8. a 9. c 10. c
11. a 12. e 13. a 14. b 15. d

WORKSHEET 26-1

1. d	5. d	9. d	13. c	17. a
2. b	6. e	10. d	14. c	18. e
3. d	7. e	11. c	15. d	19. e
4. d	8. e	12. e	16. b	20. a

WORKSHEET 27-1

1. a	9. a	17. c	24. c	31. d
2. d	10. c	18. c	25. c	32. a
3. b	11. e	19. d	26. b	33. b
4. a	12. b	20. e	27. a	34. e
5. d	13. c	21. c	28. e	35. e
6. d	14. a	22. d	29. a	36. b
7. c	15. b	23. a	30. b	37. e
8. c	16. b			

WORKSHEET 28-1

1. c 2. b 3. c 4. d 5. d 6. b 7. d 8. a 9. a 10. b
11. b 12. d 13. a 14. c 15. e 16. e 17. b 18. a
19. a

WORKSHEET 28-2
1. e 2. c 3. a 4. c 5. b 6. a 7. e 8. a 9. a 10. b
11. b 12. a 13. d 14. e 15. e

WORKSHEET 29-1
1. b 2. e 3. b 4. c 5. d 6. e 7. a 8. e 9. e 10. e
11. b 12. d 13. e 14. d 15. a 16. b 17. b

WORKSHEET 30-1
1. a 2. b 3. d 4. d 5. c 6. d 7. d 8. d 9. e 10. e
11. d

WORKSHEET 31-1
1. c 2. a 3. c 4. d 5. c 6. a 7. a 8. a 9. b 10. d

WORKSHEET 32-1
1. d	5. b	9. c	13. a
2. c	6. e	10. a	14. a
3. a	7. a	11. b	15. c
4. e	8. c	12. d	

WORKSHEET 32-2
1. b	7. a	13. b	19. e	25. a
2. b	8. a	14. a	20. b	26. a
3. a	9. c	15. e	21. e	27. b
4. a	10. c	16. b	22. c	28. b
5. e	11. e	17. a	23. d	29. e
6. e	12. c	18. d	24. b	30. b

WORKSHEET 33-1
1. b	5. d	9. d	13. c	17. e
2. d	6. d	10. d	14. b	18. a
3. a	7. c	11. d	15. d	19. c
4. c	8. a	12. c	16. c	

WORKSHEET 33-2
1. b	5. a	9. a	13. b	16. e
2. a	6. b	10. d	14. e	17. e
3. b	7. b	11. a	15. c	18. a
4. a	8. a	12. c		

WORKSHEET 34-1
1. d 2. b 3. b 4. d 5. c 6. c 7. a 8. c 9. c 10. d
11. b 12. b 13. a 14. e 15. d

WORKSHEET 34-2
1. d	5. e	9. a	12. a	15. c	18. a	21. b
2. d	6. a	10. d	13. d	16. a	19. d	22. d
3. a	7. a	11. e	14. d	17. e	20. a	23. a
4. c	8. e					

WORKSHEET 35-1
1. c	5. d	9. c	13. a	17. a
2. b	6. b	10. b	14. a	18. a
3. c	7. e	11. d	15. c	19. b
4. d	8. e	12. d	16. b	

WORKSHEET 35-2
1. c	5. a	9. a	13. c	17. a
2. b	6. a	10. c	14. d	18. d
3. d	7. a	11. d	15. a	19. d
4. d	8. e	12. b	16. a	20. e

ACROSS	**DOWN**
1. Thrombocytes	1. Erythema
2. Gastrointestinal	2. Acute
3. Prodromal	3. Basal
4. Lymphopenia	4. Desquamation
5. Dermis	5. Granulocytopenia
6. Erythrocytes	6. Gametogenesis
7. Epilation	7. Cytogenetics
8. Granulocytosis	8. Manifest
9. Atrophy	9. Epidermis
10. Oogonia	10. Leukocytes
11. Granulocytes	11. Thrombocytes
12. Leukopenia	13. Grenz
14. Oocytes	
15. Latent	

WORKSHEET 36-1
1. e	5. b	9. c	13. b	16. b
2. d	6. a	10. e	14. b	17. c
3. b	7. d	11. c	15. b	18. b
4. b	8. d	12. a		

WORKSHEET 36-2
1. b	5. b	9. e	12. e	15. b
2. c	6. b	10. b	13. c	16. c
3. d	7. b	11. b	14. d	17. c
4. a	8. c			

WORKSHEET 37-1
1. d   6. c   11. c   15. b
2. b   7. a   12. a   16. d
3. a   8. d   13. e   17. c
4. c   9. c   14. b
5. d   10. c

WORKSHEET 38-1
1. b   5. b   9. c   13. d   16. d   19. b
2. d   6. a   10. b   14. d   17. b
3. e   7. d   11. d   15. c   18. b
4. d   8. a   12. c

WORKSHEET 38-2
1. e   5. d   9. a   13. c   16. a
2. b   6. c   10. a   14. b   17. a
3. c   7. e   11. a   15. a   18. a
4. d   8. b   12. b

WORKSHEET 39-1
1. d 2. d 3. b 4. a & c 5. b 6. d 7. a
8. b 9. b 10. b 11. e 12. a 13. b 14. e
15. c 16. e

WORKSHEET 39-2
1. c   5. a   8. a   11. e   14. d
2. c   6. a   9. d   12. b   15. e
3. e   7. a   10. b   13. a   16. c
4. d

WORKSHEET 40-1
1. a 2. d 3. e 4. e 5. b 6. c 7. d 8. a 9. e 10. e
11. e 12. d 13. e 14. c 15. e 16. c 17. a 18. c
19. a

ACROSS	DOWN
1. Millirem	1. Millirad
2. Milliroentgen	2. Control
3. Quarter	3. Gender
4. Effective dose	4. Fluoroscopy
5. Exposure	5. Patient dose
6. Genetically	6. Dose
7. rem	7. Weighted

MATH TUTOR
ANSWER KEY

PART ONE:
BASIC MAS AND TIME CONVERSIONS
WORKING WITH DECIMAL TIMERS

Exercise 1: Calculating Total mAs Values
1. 5 mAs
2. 6.4 mAs
3. 1.9 mAs
4. 12.5 mAs
5. 80 mAs
6. 4 mAs
7. 10 mAs
8. 12.8 mAs
9. 3 mAs
10. 0.3 mAs
11. 25 mAs
12. 60 mAs
13. 80 mAs
14. 1.6 mAs
15. 0.6 mAs
16. 7 mAs
17. 9 mAs
18. 21 mAs
19. 210 mAs
20. 30 mAs
21. 150 mAs
22. 480 mAs
23. 3.6 mAs
24. 4.8 mAs
25. 30 mAs
26. 90 mAs
27. 12 mAs
28. 4.5 mAs
29. 75 mAs
30. 7.5 mAs
31. 45 mAs
32. 1.8 mAs
33. 1.2 mAs
34. 4 mAs
35. 16 mAs
36. 32 mAs
37. 64 mAs
38. 6.4 mAs
39. 132 mAs
40. 320 mAs
41. 280 mAs
42. 2.8 mAs
43. 40 mAs
44. 15 mAs
45. 100 mAs
46. 350 mAs
47. 3.5 mAs
48. 62.5 mAs

WORKING WITH FRACTIONAL TIMERS

Exercise 2: The 100 mA Station
1. 50 mAs
2. 5 mAs
3. 2 mAs
4. 20 mAs
5. Approx. 12 mAs
6. Approx. 1.2 mAs
7. Approx. 8 mAs
8. Approx. 0.8 mAs
9. Approx. 15 mAs
10. Approx. 7 mAs
11. 2.5 mAs
12. Approx. 33 mAs
13. Approx. 3.3 mAs
14. Approx. 16 or 17 mAs
15. Approx. 1.6 or 1.7 mAs
16. Approx. 66 or 67 mAs

Exercise 3: The 200 mA and 50 mA Stations
1. Approx. 24 or 25 mAs
2. 2.5 mAs
3. 40 mAs
4. 4 mAs
5. Approx. 6 mAs
6. Approx. 2.4 or 2.5 mAs
7. Approx. 16 or 17 mAs
8. Approx. 1.6 or 1.7 mAs
9. Approx. 4 mAs
10. Approx. 0.4 mAs
11. Approx. 7 to 8 mAs
12. Approx. 14 mAs
13. 5 mAs
14. Approx. 16 or 17 mAs
15. Approx. 1.6 or 1.7 mAs
16. Approx. 66 or 67 mAs
17. Approx. 6.6 or 6.7 mAs
18. Approx. 32 to 34 mAs
19. Approx. 3.2 to 3.4 mAs
20. Approx. 132 to 134 mAs
21. Approx. 8 to 9 mAs
22. Approx. 0.8 to 0.9 mAs
23. Approx. 0.6 to 0.7 mAs
24. Approx. 30 mAs

Exercise 4: The 300 mA Station
1. 60 mAs
2. 50 mAs
3. 6 mAs
4. 5 mAs
5. 15 mAs
6. 150 mAs
7. 20 mAs

8. 25 mAs
9. 2.5 mAs
10. 12 mAs
11. 75 mAs
12. 7.5 mAs
13. Approx. 36 mAs
14. Approx. 3.6 mAs
15. Approx. 45 mAs
16. 10 mAs

Exercise 5: The 400, 500, and 600 mA Stations

1. 20 mAs (4 sets of 5)
2. 25 mAs (5 sets of 5)
3. 30 mAs (6 sets of 5)
4. 80 mAs (4 sets of 20)
5. 120 mAs (6 sets of 20)
6. 8 mAs (4 sets of 2)
7. 12 mAs (6 sets of 2)
8. 125 mAs (5 sets of 25)
9. 150 mAs (6 sets of 25)
10. 12.5 mAs (5 sets of 2.5)
11. 15 mAs (6 sets of 2.5)
12. 20 mAs (⅓ of 60, or 6 sets of 3.3)
13. Approx. 13 mAs (4 sets of 3.3)
14. Approx. 6.4 mAs (4 sets of 1.6)
15. Approx. 60 mAs (4 sets of 15)
16. Approx. 48 to 50 mAs (4 sets of 12 or 12.5)
17. Approx. 4.8 to 5 mAs (4 sets of 1.25)
18. Approx. 60 mAs (5 sets of 12)
19. Approx. 48 to 50 mAs (6 sets of 8)
20. Approx. 5 mAs (6 sets of .8)
21. Approx. 40 mAs (5 sets of 8)
22. Approx. 3.2 to 3.3 mAs (4 sets of 0.8)
23. Approx. 28 mAs (4 sets of 7)
24. Approx. 35 mAs (5 sets of 7)
25. Approx. 16 mAs (4 sets of 4)
26. Approx. 20 mAs (5 sets of 4)
27. Approx. 24 mAs (6 sets of 4)
28. Approx. 120 to 132 mAs (4 sets of 33)

Exercise 6: Complex Fractions

1. 40 mAs
2. Approx. 14 mAs (2 sets of 7)
3. Approx. 21 mAs
4. 15 mAs (3 sets of 5)
5. 35 mAs
6. 150 mAs
7. 80 mAs (2 sets of 40)
8. 120 mAs
9. 160 mAs
10. 60 mAs
11. 140 mAs
12. Approx. 28 to 30 mAs (2 7 2)
13. Approx. 42 mAs (2 7 3)
14. 30 mAs (3 sets of 10)

15. 70 mAs
16. 160 mAs (2 sets of 80)
17. 240 mAs
18. 320 mAs
19. 120 mAs (3 × 40)
20. 280 mAs
21. 200 mAs
22. 120 mAs (2 × 60)
23. 180 mAs
24. 240 mAs
25. 90 mAs
26. 210 mAs (7 × 30)
27. 40 mAs (2 × 20)
28. 60 mAs
29. 45 mAs (3 × 15)
30. 60 mAs
31. 140 mAs
32. 200 mAs
33. 150 mAs
34. 350 mAs (7 × 50)
35. 75 mAs (3 × 25)
36. 240 mAs (2 × 120)
37. 360 mAs
38. 180 mAs (3 × 60)
39. 90 mAs (3 × 30)
40. 120 mAs*

(*Note that on question 40 you may simply take double the answer you would get at the 300 mA station. If you have memorized that 15 s and 20 s go together at the 300 mA station, then a 15th at 600 would be double 20 or 40. Then take 3 sets of 40. Many problems at the 600 mA station can be solved this way—by just doubling the answer you would get at 300 mA. Also, many mAs values can be figured at the 400 mA station in a similar manner by doubling numbers you are familiar with using at the 200 mA station.)

TIMERS: CONVERTING FRACTIONS INTO DECIMALS AND VICE VERSA

Exercise 7: Converting Fractions Into Decimals

1. 0.75
2. 0.667
3. 0.25
4. 0.2
5. 0.167
6. 0.142
7. 0.125
8. 0.083
9. 0.0667
10. 0.05
11. 0.04
12. 0.033
13. 0.025
14. 0.02

15. 0.0167
16. 0.0125
17. 0.01
18. 0.0083
19. 0.7
20. 0.133
21. 0.15
22. 0.4
23. 0.6
24. 0.8
25. 0.33
26. 0.2
27. 0.35
28. 0.0067
29. 0.375
30. 0.3125
 4. $\frac{1}{15}$
 5. $\frac{1}{6}$
 6. $\frac{1}{12}$
 7. $\frac{1}{30}$
 8. $\frac{1}{60}$
 9. $\frac{1}{80}$
10. $\frac{1}{120}$
11. $\frac{2}{5}$ (2 sets of 20)
12. $\frac{1}{30}$
13. $\frac{1}{20}$
14. $\frac{1}{40}$
15. $\frac{1}{8}$
16. $\frac{1}{5}$
17. $\frac{3}{5}$ (3 sets of 40)
18. $\frac{1}{40}$
19. $\frac{1}{40}$
20. $\frac{2}{15}$ (2 sets of 7)
21. $\frac{1}{6}$
22. $\frac{1}{50}$
23. $\frac{1}{15}$
24. $\frac{1}{120}$
25. $\frac{3}{20}$ (3 sets of 15)
26. $\frac{3}{5}$ (3 sets of 60)
27. $\frac{4}{5}$ (4 sets of 60)
28. $\frac{1}{4}$ (cut in half twice)
29. $\frac{1}{5}$
30. $\frac{3}{5}$ (3 sets of 80)

Exercise 8: Converting Decimals Into Fractions

 1. $\frac{1}{20}$
 2. $\frac{1}{30}$ (common denominator is 333)
 3. $\frac{1}{5}$
 4. $\frac{3}{4}$
 5. $\frac{1}{40}$
 6. $\frac{2}{3}$
 7. $\frac{1}{7}$ (common denominator is 143)

 8. $\frac{1}{500}$
 9. $\frac{4}{5}$
10. $\frac{1}{6}$ (common denominator is 167)
11. $\frac{1}{8}$
12. $\frac{3}{5}$
13. $\frac{1}{16}$
14. $\frac{1}{12}$ (common denominator is 833)

FINDING mA AND TIME COMBINATIONS FOR A DESIRED mAs

Exercise 9: Warm-up Calculations

 1. 2 sets of 40
 2. 3 sets of 15
 3. 2 sets of 33
 4. 3 sets of 25
 5. 3 sets of 60
 6. 3 sets of 40 *or* 2 sets of 60
 7. 2 sets of 80 *or* 4 sets of 40
 8. 3 sets of 80 *or* 4 sets of 60
 9. 3 sets of 30
10. 4 sets of 80

Exercise 11: Calculations Using Decimals

 1. 0.04
 2. 0.025
 3. 0.67
 4. 0.07
 5. 0.16
 6. 0.08
 7. 0.033
 8. 0.017
 9. 0.4
10. 0.05
11. 0.025
12. 0.125
13. 0.2
14. 0.6
15. 0.025
16. 0.0125
17. 0.7
18. 0.17
19. 0.02
20. 0.07
21. 0.6
22. 0.25
23. 0.2
24. 0.6

Exercise 10: Calculations Using Fractions

 1. $\frac{1}{50}$
 2. $\frac{1}{40}$
 3. $\frac{2}{3}$ (2 sets of 33)

PART TWO:
MATHEMATICS OF RADIOGRAPHIC
TECHNIQUES

Exercise 13: Adjusting for Distance Changes, the Inverse Square Law, the Square Law: Rules of Thumb for Distance Changes

1. Approx. 75
2. Approx. 30
3. Approx. 30
4. Approx. 36
5. 15
6. 10
7. 15
8. 25
9. 68 to 70
10. Four times
11. Two times
12. ¼
13. ½
14. 62.5
15. 3.47
16. 0.77
17. 0.28
18. 70
19. 12 in
20. 30 in
21. 40 in
22. 60 in
23. 1.17
24. 4.34
25. 8.1
26. 0.31
27. 0.69
28. 1.93
29. 0.56

TECHNIQUE ADJUSTMENTS

Exercise 12: Applying the 15% Rule for kVp, Applying the Rule in Steps, Applying the Rule in Portions

1. 6
2. 4.5
3. 4
4. 2.5
5. 3
6. 10.5
7. 6
8. 9
9. 16.5
10. 3
11. Approx. 5
12. 6
13. Approx. 4
14. Approx. 7
15. 9
16. 102 kVp
17. 46 kVp
18. 64 to 65 kVp
19. 74 kVp